IMMUNOLOGY

Readings from
**SCIENTIFIC
AMERICAN**

IMMUNOLOGY

*With Introductions and
Additional Material by*
F. M. Burnet
University of Melbourne

W. H. Freeman and Company
San Francisco

Cover illustration: Antibodies distinguish among different antigens by recognizing differences in their shapes, as is illustrated by the relationship of this hapten antigen to a surrounding antibody-active site. According to the idea of selective immunity, an antigen selects cells that are already making antibodies that happen to fit. It then stimulates those cells to make large quantities of antibodies. Illustration is from "The Structure and Function of Antibodies," by Gerald M. Edelman, pages 39–48.

Most of the SCIENTIFIC AMERICAN articles in IMMUNOLOGY are available as separate Offprints. For a complete list of more than 950 articles now available as Offprints, write to W. H. Freeman and Company, 660 Market Street, San Francisco, California 94104.

Library of Congress Cataloging in Publication Data

Main entry under title:

Immunology: readings from Scientific American.

    1. Immunology—Addresses, essays, lectures.
I. Burnet, Frank Macfarlane, Sir, 1899–   II. Scientific American. [DNLM: 1. Immunology—Collected works. QW505 I33]
QR181.5.I46   616.07′9′08   75–19356
ISBN 0–7167–0525–7
ISBN 0–7167–0524–9 pbk.

Printed in the United States of America

9 8 7 6 5 4 3 2 1

PREFACE

Immunology in its modern sense is very much a creation of the last twenty years, and to produce an anthology of articles on immunology from *Scientific American* means that one can aim at providing a fairly comprehensive picture of present day immunology as well as something of a history of how that knowledge was obtained.

It may sound presumptuous to date modern immunology from 1955 or thereabouts when every reader will be well aware that most of the great practical achievements of immunization came well before that date. Occasionally I have found 1955 useful as the milestone that marked the completion of the effective conquest of infectious disease, primarily because the Salk vaccine against polio came into general use that year. Effective immunization against smallpox, diphtheria, whooping cough, yellow fever, and tetanus had been in regular use for many years. Less comprehensive means of immunization against cholera, plague, typhoid fever, and influenza had also been used, and, if immunization was unavailable or unsatisfactory, antibiotics were available for chemoprophylaxis or therapy.

The advances since 1955 have been specially concerned with bringing immunology into step with the rest of biology, notably in reinterpreting it in contemporary terms, just as the disciplines of biochemistry and genetics gave birth to molecular biology in the 1950s. When virtually nothing was known of the biological synthesis of proteins, no useful hypothesis on the nature and formation of antibody at the molecular level was even thinkable. At every stage of scientific development there are current hypotheses about most or all of the phenomena being investigated. Necessarily they will always be expressed in contemporary terms. Looking through a monograph I wrote with Frank J. Fenner in 1948–1949 on the production of antibodies, I can sense how the stage was being set for the great leap forward. It was obvious that Linus Pauling's formulation, in 1940, of antibody production was inadequate, yet there was nothing to replace it. Plasma cells had been recognized as the dominant producers of "gamma globulin" and lymphocytes had been recognized as probable producers of antibodies. The different qualities of tuberculin reactions and other types of sensitization were well recognized but the concept of cell-mediated immunity had not yet crystallized. P. B. Medawar had laid the foundations of an immunological interpretation of the phenomena of transplantation, and Fenner's and my ideas that immunological tolerance was not something inborn but that it developed during embryonic life could be expressed fairly explicitly. However, it was not until the expression of information coded in DNA as protein structure was understood that any consideration of immunology at a molecular level became possible. I am quite certain that there can never be a detailed interpretation of the immune system in molecular terms, but during the last twenty years we have at least achieved the central requirement for any biological understanding: a knowledge in fairly precise detail of the chemical structure of the agents we are primarily interested in—in this instance, antibodies.

The articles from *Scientific American* that remain relevant to modern immunology are therefore virtually limited to those that have appeared since 1955. None earlier than this date has been selected, and the great majority have appeared since 1961. It seemed reasonable to divide the articles into two major categories: the first concerned essentially with the physiology of all aspects of the immune system, and the second with medical implications and applications of immunology.

I have written brief introductions to most of the sections of the book; other sections and the epilogue are original essays written for those places where I felt a proper understanding of the scope of the field of immunology warranted further discussion. These, and two essays within other sections, all appear in this book for the first time.

November 1975   *F. M. Burnet*

CONTENTS

PART TWO   **Immunity in Relation to Medicine**

Note on cross-references: References to articles included in this book are noted by the title of the article and the page on which it begins; references to articles that are available as Offprints, but are not included here, are noted by the article's title and Offprint number; references to articles published by *Scientific American,* but which are not available as Offprints, are noted by the title of the article and the month and year of its publication.

IMMUNOLOGY

Immunity of the Normal Organism

I

ANTIBODIES
AND RECEPTORS

I ANTIBODIES AND RECEPTORS

INTRODUCTION

Ever since people began to think about the immunity to reinfection that follows diseases with easily recognizable symptoms, such as smallpox, measles, chicken pox, and mumps, the specificity of the immunity has interested philosophically-minded physicians. Slowly during the nineteenth century experimental approaches developed. Pasteur extended Edward Jenner's concept of vaccination to attenuated cultures of bacteria, and attention turned to the antibacterial qualities of freshly drawn blood. Immunology came into being in the last decade of the nineteenth century with Emil von Behring's production of antitoxins and the crystallization of the concepts of "antibody" and "complement" by Jules Bordet, Paul Ehrlich, and soon many others. It became evident that when a bacterium or its toxin entered the body, some tissue or population of cells reacted to its presence by producing a substance, a soluble protein, which carried a pattern allowing it to attach specifically to the surface of the bacterium or to a toxin molecule. Thus a lock-and-key relationship of complementary pattern was spoken of at an early stage as a basis for specific union and for the initiation of various types of defense against the invaders. The medical importance of antibody was obvious; so was its fascination and convenience as an object for laboratory study. So antibody—its nature, its origin, its medical and biological significance—became and has remained the central theme of immunology.

Many aspects of the defense of the body against infection are only indirectly related to antibody action. Invertebrate animals had effective defense against casual bacteria long before any antibody-based system evolved. Yet with only minor qualification one can say that no invertebrate ever developed anything comparable to the mammalian lymphocyte-antibody immune system, most of the qualities of which can be recognized in all vertebrates down to the most primitive cyclostomes: lamprey and hagfish. [*See the illustration on page 5.*] To the pioneer immunologists and to their successors, the central theme of specific antibody was the key to understanding defense against infection and the nature of post-infectious immunity. We know now that there is much more to immunology than was dreamed of fifty years ago, but the specificity and diversity of antibody has retained its central fascination and must take priority in this volume.

IMMUNOGLOBULINS AND ANTIBODIES

Most immunologists would probably agree that the concept of clonal selection is the characteristic feature of contemporary immunological theory, and it seems reasonable to select as the first *Scientific American* reading in

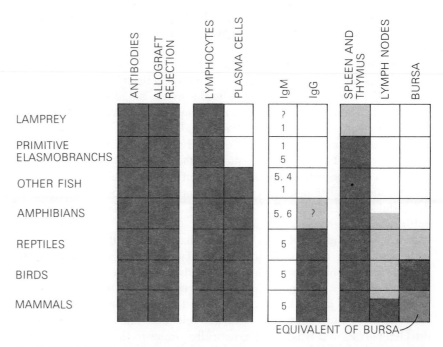

EQUIVALENT OF BURSA

AN OVERALL VIEW of the development of vertebrate immunity can be seen in this chart, the columns of which are separated into four categories. From the left, these are: immune functions, morphological cell types associated with immunity, immunoglobulins, and presence or absence of immunologically significant organs. All vertebrates from the lamprey onward possess circulating cells having the qualities of lymphocytes and the capacity to produce antibodies and to reject grafts from other individuals of the same species. Immunoglobulin G (IgG) appears relatively late but is preceded by monomeric IgM of similar molecular size. In the IgM column the number of subunits found to exist in the macromolecule in various species is shown for the various animal groups. Note that birds are the only vertebrates that have an unequivocal bursa of Fabricius, though in a sense any animal with plasma cells can be said to have an equivalent. The light gray areas show findings that are weak or doubtful. Where two shadings are shown in a square, differences are present within an order. The diagram has been prepared from data in J. J. Marchalonis, *Immunity in Evolution*, Harvard University Press, 1975.

this volume my own article of 1961. This was the first account in *Scientific American* of an immunological topic in which clonal selection was discussed. On rereading the article today, my chief impression is that, though the general concept is expressed in terms that are still reasonably valid, the intervening years have introduced many refinements and shown how, as is the way of science, each advance toward clarification has introduced a new set of uncertainties. With hindsight, the sentence in the article which pleases me the most is that the clonal selection approach "must stimulate attempts to define the potentialities of single cells and to analyze the population dynamics of the immunological cells of the body." This is in fact a fair description of the recent course of basic immunological research.

No area of active research can persist unchanged for even a year, and any good text on immunology will aspire to be not more than a year behind the growing edge of significant discoveries. However, much that is worth appreciating can be derived from a collection of articles written by people who were sure that they had something new and exciting to tell an audience wider than their co-workers in the same field. To understand how a tentative hypothesis became an established concept and how an erroneous idea unexpectedly led to a useful one—things like this can often give a more meaningful grasp of current interpretations of immunology and underline the certainty that, whatever the accepted views are or have been, they will certainly change with the years.

With that in mind, some points in my 1961 article may be singled out for comment on the way things subsequently developed or now look like they will develop in the future.

1. Probably the greatest theoretical difficulty presented by the selection theories was how to picture the generation of genetically based diversity of antibody pattern. The only suggestion in the article is that somatic mutation in stem cells of the lymphocyte series is responsibile, followed at a later stage of development by phenotypic restriction and stabilization of antibody patterns. Further enlightenment would obviously have to wait until something was known about the chemical nature of the specificity of different antibodies. As will become progressively evident in subsequent articles in this volume, the elucidation of the structure of antibodies has been magnificently successful—but there are still three mutually incompatible theories of how antibodies are genetically determined.

2. The second aspect of clonal selection that is vital to the whole concept is the significance of natural tolerance—the fact that the constituents of the body do not provoke a production of antibody or any type of self-damaging immune responses. We know now that in certain states of human disease, and as a result of rather drastic and unnatural manipulation in experimental animals, there can be exceptions to the rule that immune responses are directed only against what is not genetically proper to the body. The beginning of an understanding of the way in which "self" could, as it were, be differentiated from "not-self" came largely from the study of such accidental occurrences as the fusion of placental circulations in cases of multiple birth. From immunological study of such situations one could deduce that the recognition of self was something that had to be developed during embryonic life; it was not a primary genetic quality. In that conclusion there was a seed of hope for the eventual achievement of organ replacement by surgery. The germination and eventual success of that idea can be followed in the articles on transplantation in Section VII of this volume.

3. A third topic given important subsequent development is the graft-versus-host reaction, illustrated by the cellular "pocks" that develop on the chorioallantoic membrane of the chick embryo when adult chicken leucocytes are deposited on its surface. Each pock represents a point at which an adult lymphocyte recognizes the presence of a foreign antigen (i.e., host cells) with which it can react and be induced to proliferate: the graft recognizes the foreign quality of the host instead of the more usual relationship; hence the term "graft versus host." Already in 1961 there seemed to be too many pocks being produced in such experiments. The proportion of lymphocytes in chicken blood that reacted with a single foreign antigen was too high for the results to accord with a clonal selection theory. As work continued, the disparity became more and more evident, and in Morten Simonsen's hands it remains a potent, and I believe successful, argument against a fully unified clonal selection theory.

4. The chicken, both before and after hatching, is an important test object for immunology, and as part of our work on the nature of the "immune" pocks on the chorioallantois, Noel L. Warner and I became interested in the observation by Bruce Glick a few years previously that chickens whose bursa of Fabricius had been removed immediately after hatching failed subsequently to produce antibody. The fact that, in experiments by Warner and Aleksander Szenberg, chickens whose bursal function had never developed produced normal foci on the chorioallantoic membrane even though they were quite incapable of producing antibodies was, I believe, the seminal discovery from which the concept of T (for thymus) and B (for bursa) cells, and all that has grown from it, developed.

THE ELUCIDATION OF ANTIBODY STRUCTURE
AND ITS IMPLICATIONS FOR THE GENERATION
OF ANTIBODY DIVERSITY

In the contributions of Rodney R. Porter and Gerald M. Edelman, who together shared a Nobel prize in 1972 for the work they report, all the essen-
tials of the story of antibody structure will be found. The only addition that
seems to be needed is to bring up to date the still unsolved problem of how
the immense variety of antibodies is produced. By 1970 Edelman was able to
be confident that the chemical differences responsible for the specificity of
antibodies were embodied in the amino acid sequences of their variable regions. If the antibody structure is thought of at the very simplest as having
a "Y" or "T" shape, the variable regions are at the upper outer arms. All subsequent work has confirmed Edelman's conclusions, but there have been
some elaborations.

It is now accepted that in the final three-dimensional configuration of the
antibody molecule the variable regions of the light and heavy chains take up
an accurately aligned relationship that defines a shallow groove, which is the
specific combining site to which the antigenic determinant becomes attached.
The significant atomic groupings in the two variable segments concerned are
in what are now known as the *hypervariable* regions of these domains. By
using a convention due to T. T. Wu and E. A. Kabat of Columbia University
Medical School, it is possible to illustrate the range of replacement amino
acids that has been found to be present at each numbered position in the
variable region of those kappa myeloma light chains that have been studied
[*see the illustration below*]. The higher the bar, the more heterogeneous the

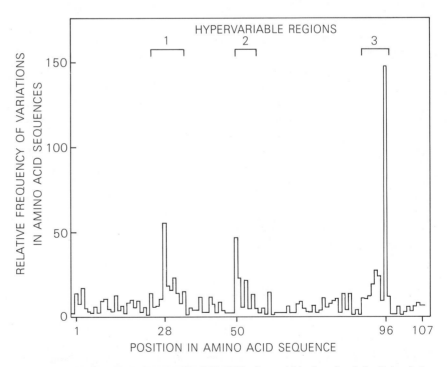

IN THE ANTIBODY MOLECULE IN HUMANS, the variable domain of the light chains
shows several hypervariable regions. The diagram gives a measure of the relative heterogeneity
of the amino acid residues occupying the places from 1 to 107 of the V domain. Note that each
of the three hypervariable regions shows one position with much greater heterogeneity than
any other. The diagram is adapted, with slight modifications, from T. T. Wu and E. A. Kabat,
Journal of Experimental Medicine, **132:211–250 (1970).**

amino acids that have been found at that point. Clearly three limited regions are well demarcated from the rest, and a wide range of consistent evidence now points to those hypervariable regions as being responsible for the differences of antibody specificity. Learning what the genetic origin of the hypervariable regions is thus becomes the essential problem.

As yet none of the three possible explanations briefly outlined in Edelman's article has been ruled out. One can still argue that all the differences between antibodies are of germ-line origin, that for each antibody type there is a structural gene just as there is for all the standard proteins synthesized in the body. Likewise, one may assume that though there must be a complex set of structural genes concerned, most of the detailed differences must arise at the somatic level as the stem lines of lymphocytes develop. Those changes can be called somatic mutations, but the phrase is a rather vague one which nowadays requires qualification about what genetic process is being assumed to occur. Several have been suggested for this particular role, but they all have the quality of armchair hypotheses not easily accessible to experimental test.

The one that I prefer because of its potential susceptibility to experimental test is due to David Baltimore of Massachusetts Institute of Technology. In essence it assumes a quite special form of excision and repair of short sections of the structural genes corresponding to the variable regions. The key suggestion is that in place of a normal repair DNA polymerase, the enzyme concerned in refilling the gaps is a terminal transferase, which introduces at random any nucleotides that happen to be available. It is characteristic of all normal DNA polymerases that only the "right" nucleotides should be inserted; errors in the sequence result in point mutations. [*See the illustration on page 9.*] On Baltimore's hypothesis, evolution seems to have solved the problem of diversification by greatly increasing the error-proneness of nucleotide insertion. The terminal transferase was at first known to be present only in the thymus, but small amounts have also been found within bone marrow. There are suggestions that it may be characteristic of undifferentiated stem cells of the hematopoietic series.

Baltimore's theory is far from being fully established, but it has the experimentally accessible aspect of focusing on a distinctive enzyme to allow further study. As one very much interested in mutation and error-prone enzymes, I have an intuitive feeling that the special need for diversification of one unique set of gene products could best be met by relaxing the demand for fidelity in the repair and replication of DNA. My guess, however, is that there is a better chance of finding the crucial type of error-prone DNA polymerase in the avian bursa rather than in the thymus. What can be said with conviction is that a serious test of the Baltimore hypothesis in a collaboration of molecular geneticists with immunologists is more likely than any other project to provide the best explanation of the diversification.

THE POPULATION DYNAMICS OF THE CELLS OF THE IMMUNE SYSTEM

To understand the function of antibodies, much more is needed than to know their molecular structure and to have some idea of how the diversity of chemical structure is determined at the genetic level. An antibody and the various manifestations of cellular immunity must be brought to bear on the job at hand, at the proper time and place and with the right specificity. To understand how this happens we have to analyze an immensely complex system of almost completely mobile cells, heterogeneous populations that somehow achieve a miracle of coordinated function. In the articles by G. J. V. Nossal, Niels Kaj Jerne, and Max D. Cooper and Alexander R. Lawton III, one can follow some of the important stages by which our understanding has increased.

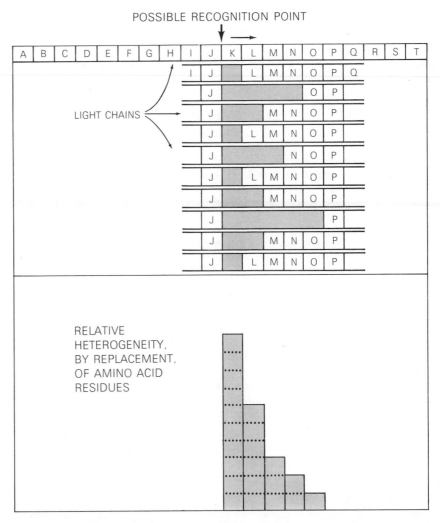

SEVERAL EXPLANATIONS CAN BE GIVEN for the data in the illustration on page 7.
David Baltimore's interpretation is that an incising enzyme (endonuclease) initiates a removal
of one or more nucleotides, starting at a constant point in the sequence and ceasing after one
or a small number have been removed. The gaps are then filled at random by another enzyme,
terminal deoxyribonucleotidyl transferase. In the absence of complicating factors the recognition point would show the highest incidence of replacement by "wrong" nucleotides and
hence the greatest heterogeneity of amino acid residues at the corresponding point. In this
illustration, to avoid unnecessary complication, one nucleotide is shown as equivalent to one
amino acid residue. The general form of the lower section of the figure is the same as would
be obtained if the consequences of the 3 : 1 ratio had been elaborated.

The first requirement for the verification of the clonal selection hypothesis
at the cellular level was to show experimentally that the almost foolhardy
dogma of "one cell, one antibody" (or "one clone, one antibody") did actually
correspond to the facts. Nossal himself showed that when animals were
injected with two distinct antigens—semipurified flagella from two sero-
logically distinct bacterial cultures—their antibody-producing cells liberated
one antibody or the other, never both. Another group of equally reliable
experimenters, using bacteriophages as antigens, found irrefutably that rabbits
given two distinct phages produced some cells liberating antibody that could
neutralize both types: I have a very clear memory still of how Nossal and I
spent a morning at Stanford University with Edwin S. Lennox and Melvin
Cohn, going over their data and trying to understand why the experiments
disagreed so categorically. As Nossal indicates in his article, neither team at
that time could provide a convincing reason, and to the best of my knowledge

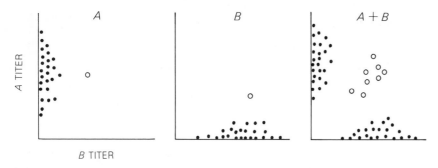

A PROBABLE INTERPRETATION of the Attardi-Lennox-Cohn experiment, which appeared to show production of two different antibodies by single cells from doubly immunized rabbits. Two bacteriophages, A and B, were used and the titer of the antibody produced by single cells against each phage was plotted as shown. Only the general character of the results is indicated; the "double-antibody producers" (open circles) from A + B rabbits are presumed to be derived from the very rare cells with a single pattern of antibody that can react with both antigens. Consequently the cells were disproportionately stimulated in the doubly immunized animals.

none has ever been published. It is, however, now fairly clear why Nossal's experiments gave the "right" answer and those with bacteriophages the "wrong" one. It was because the bacterial flagellin was essentially a pure antigen, with only one type of antigenic determinant for each bacterial type, while bacteriophages are highly complex structures. One must add to this something not realized at the time: that even with a pure antigen an individual animal may produce several hundred physicochemically distinguishable antibodies. What happened in the Attardi-Cohn-Lennox experiments was that an occasional antibody had some reactivity against both A and B bacteriophages. [*See the illustration above.*] Remember that an antigen does not in any sense direct the formation of any given pattern of antibody; it merely reacts with those patterns current in the body *that happen to fit.* In an animal injected only with A, a very rare antibody pattern that reacted with both A and B would be present in only a tiny proportion of the cells to be tested, and would almost certainly be overlooked. It would be equally inconspicuous in the responding cell population of a rabbit given B alone. On the other hand, when such a cell arises in the rabbit given A + B, the antibody pattern will be stimulated by antigen twice as often as any other pattern of cell and a descendant clone will consequently become conspicuous. The cells that seemed to be producing two distinct antibodies were producing a single type of antibody molecule, but it was a molecule capable of reacting with a significant determinant on both A and B antigens. Phenomena of this type are now well known even among antibodies against a simple hapten like dinitrophenyl.

There are two other results described in Nossal's article that arose from his special interest in handling single cells concerned with immune responses. One was the discovery that although a cell produced only one sort of antibody, i.e., having one set of variable regions, it could produce two different types of immunoglobulin, IgM and IgG. The further development of that discovery is brought fully up to date in Cooper and Lawton's article. The second result concerns the discovery of dendritic phagocytic cells in the germinal centers of lymph nodes. These cells have a special propensity to hold antigen—often in the form of antigen-antibody complexes—on the surface of slender cytoplasmic extensions that wind among the closely packed proliferating cells. If one reflects on the intensely dynamic quality of a lymph node, most of the cells of which are in active movement and are constantly making new contacts with other cells, these dendritic cells seem to have the best possibility of presenting antigen to the appropriate lymphocytes as these pass by.

Jerne's account of the immune system brings us almost to the growing edge of immunological theory. An eigen-system based on the well-established fact that the combining site of a newly prevalent antibody is itself an antigenic determinant foreign to the body is probably still too sophisticated a concept for most immunologists. For one thing, it does not lend itself at all to easy experimental analysis, and for another, the complex idiotope-antiidiotope interactions that are postulated in such a system must be further complicated by a whole range of other controls and inhibitors. One has only to look through Cooper and Lawton's article to realize how much more there is to the immune system than antigen, antibody, and antibody-producing cells, with which Jerne's theoretical picture is almost wholly concerned. Cooper and Lawton discuss the role of T cells, the factors that determine the predominant routes along which the different types of relevant cells move and the sites where they settle, the change in cells from producing IgM to IgG, IgA, and perhaps IgD, and the largely unstudied processes by which originally antigenic material is ultimately eliminated from the body. There is not the least doubt about the importance of Jerne's concept, but it is still not possible to assess it fully; it probably represents only the beginning of the next major turn in immunological theory.

1

The Mechanism of Immunity

by Sir Macfarlane Burnet
January 1961

How does an animal make an antibody that neutralizes a single foreign substance, or antigen? The evidence favors the theory that cells able to make the antibody are "selected" by the antigen and then multiply

Deliberate defense against infectious disease started in the late 18th century with Edward Jenner's discovery of the principle of immunity, so triumphantly demonstrated by the success of Jenner's vaccine against smallpox. Today the technique of immunization provides protection against all the significant diseases that have not been eliminated by public-health measures or that do not yield readily to chemotherapy. Much public-health work remains to be done, particularly in the underdeveloped areas of the tropics, but without important exception man can now control all the infectious diseases that seriously threaten human life.

Although the practical problems of immunization have been solved, immunology remains an important branch of medicine. The immunologist of today, however, is not so much interested in finding out how to immunize people more effectively against diphtheria or poliomyelitis as he is concerned with understanding what happens when people become immune. He asks more sophisticated questions than in the past. For example: Why can a surgeon successfully graft skin or other tissue from one part of the body to another but not from one individual to another, except in the case of grafts between identical twins? How is it that occasionally a pair of fraternal (nonidentical) twins share two blood groups and accept skin grafts from each other? How can an individual who had suffered a single attack of a virus disease 20, 30 or even 60 years ago continue to produce antibody against the virus? And why are there "autoimmune" diseases, such as rheumatoid arthritis, acquired hemolytic anemia and Hashimoto's disease of the thyroid, in which an abnormal immune reaction is directed against the body's own cells and tissues? Any modern formulation of immunolog-

ical theory must supply at least provisional answers to these and other equally complex questions.

But immunology is not simply a branch of medicine. It is a discipline in its own right, potentially able to make a rich contribution to the understanding of the central problems of biology, notably the nature of genetic information and the mechanism of protein synthesis. Both of these problems are intimately tied to any theory of immunity.

In its modern form orthodox immunological theory holds that the central feature of immunity is the production of antibody by a specialized group of tissue cells known as plasma cells. Antibody is a globular protein of blood plasma which can be identified by its physical behavior as a "gamma globulin." Each antibody has a highly specific affinity with the particular antigen which stimulates its production. An antigen may be part of a virus, bacterium or foreign tissue cell, or a fragment of some such structure, a protein or a polysaccharide (a large molecule made of many simple sugar units). Antibody protects the organism against a foreign substance by combining with it and thereby rendering it inactive.

Antigen and antibody are both large in the chemical sense, that is, the molecules of both consist of a great many atoms. Antibody globulin has a molecular weight of about 160,000 (10,000 times the weight of the oxygen atom). Typical antigens are of the same order of size. The sites of chemical activity which bring antibody and antigen together into combination, however, represent relatively small portions of these complex molecules. A single site may be thought of as equivalent to the region occupied by three to five of the several hundred amino-acid units in an average

protein (a protein being composed of combinations of any of 20-odd different amino acids), or an equally small number of the monosaccharide units in a polysaccharide. These small regions of active union are called antigenic determinants on the antigen and specific patches on the antibody. According to the classical theory, the two combine because the geometrical configuration of the specific patch is complementary to the pattern of the antigenic determinant. They fit each other just as a particular key matches its lock. In this scheme, which bears the strong imprint of such figures as Paul Ehrlich, Karl Landsteiner and Linus Pauling, the specific patch on the antibody acquires its pattern by being synthesized in contact with the antigenic determinant. The antigen itself is presumably taken into the cell and comes into action after the amino-acid units of the globulin molecule have been assembled by the cell's machinery of synthesis and are in process of being folded into globular form. At the folding stage the globulin is brought into contact with the antigen and is molded into the required complementary pattern.

This is the simplest form of what Joshua Lederberg of Stanford University has called the "instructive" theory of antibody formation: the antigenic determinant itself supplies the information from which each highly specific antibody is constructed. The instructive theory does not, however, account satisfactorily for several significant processes associated with immunity, such as the persistence of immunity and the origin of the autoimmune diseases. A fundamentally different view has accordingly been advanced by the proponents of the so-called selection theory.

This theory holds that antibody molecules are made in essentially the same way that other proteins are synthesized,

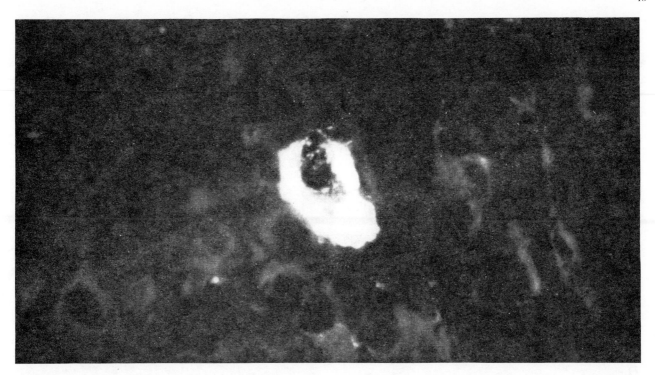

MATURE PLASMA CELL containing rheumatoid factor is made visible by reaction with a fluorescing compound. Neighboring cells have no rheumatoid factor, hence do not combine with fluorescing compound and are barely visible. Interpretation according to selection theory would be that fluorescing cell "inherited" a particular antibody pattern which is carried in its genetic material.

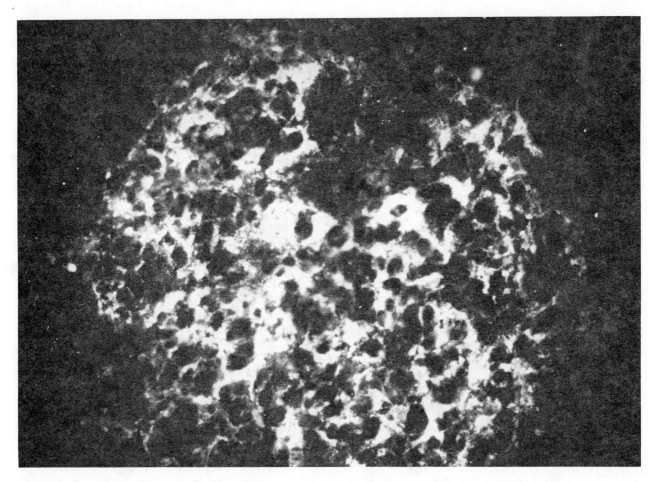

NODULAR AGGREGATION of cells in lymph node fluoresces because cells contain rheumatoid factor, a giant molecule with antibody-like characteristics found in blood of majority of patients with rheumatoid arthritis. It may indicate an autoimmune response. The photomicrographs were made by Robert C. Mellors, Hospital for Special Surgery, New York Hospital-Cornell Medical Center.

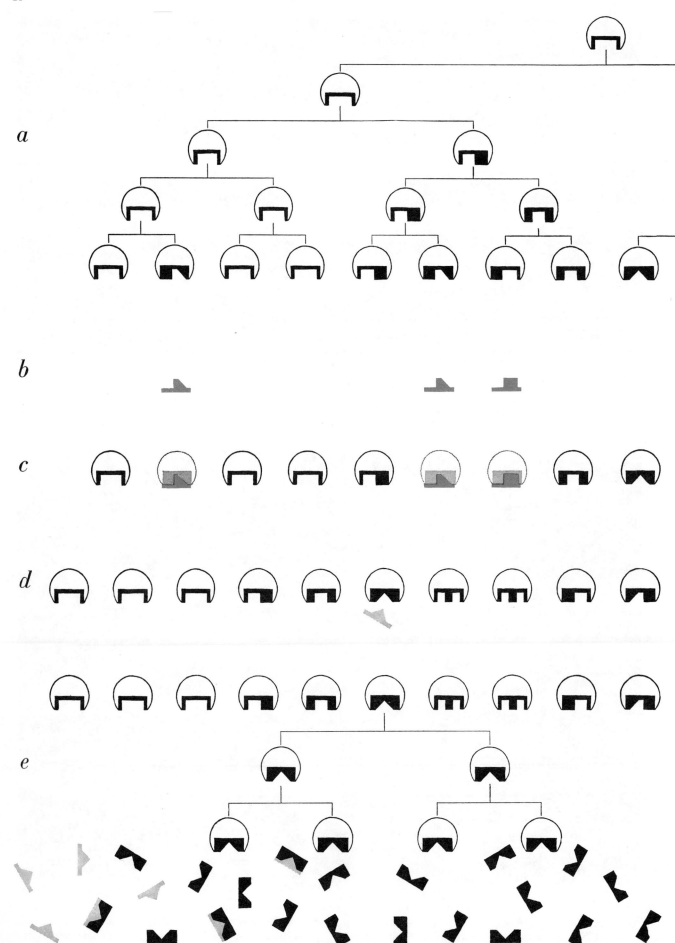

a

b

c

d

e

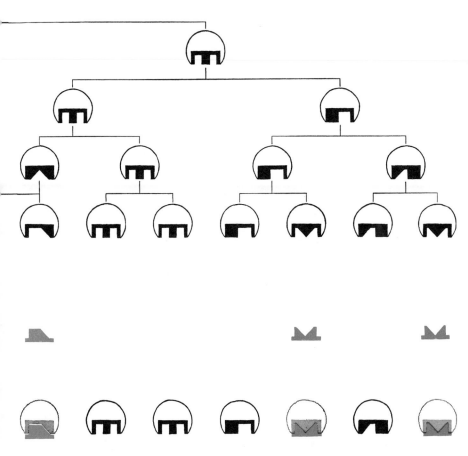

SELECTION THEORY OF IMMUNITY proposes that early in embryonic life immunological cells mutate frequently (*a*), producing all possible antibody patterns, represented here by only 11 different symbols. Some will match antigens native to the body (*b*). These antigens will kill immunological cells having the complementary pattern (*c*), leaving only the cells with antibody patterns which correspond to foreign antigens (*d*). When these cells have matured, a foreign antigen reaching one of them (*d*) stimulates it to proliferate rapidly (*e*). Its descendants produce antibody which combines with and inactivates foreign antigen.

view that a bacterium can produce a given enzyme only if the necessary information is incorporated in its genetic mechanism; the experimental change in the environment allows the emergence into activity of what was formerly only a latent capacity.

It is likely that views of antibody formation will change in the same direction, toward a wider acceptance of selection theories. Certainly this approach leads more directly to the central process in immunology, which I defined a long time ago as the differentiation between the self and the not-self. The body does not normally produce antibodies against its own tissues, although it is at least potentially capable of producing antibodies against any protein or any other substance of appropriate molecular character that is not present in the body. The implications of this fact are the most important reasons for favoring a selection theory of immunity.

Most proteins are antigenic to an organism that has not been concerned in producing them. At the present time only one protein is known well enough to permit a comparison of its chemical structure with its immunological activity. This is insulin, one of the smallest proteins; the full sequence of amino-acid units has been worked out for the insulins of several animal species. Of course insulin is not antigenic in the animal that produces it, and it also happens that it is a rather mild antigen. Most diabetics can receive beef or sheep insulin for years without any trouble. Some, however, become resistant to insulin because they are making antibodies against it. This difficulty can usually be circumvented by using pig insulin. The difference between beef insulin and pig insulin is known [*see illustration on pages 18 and 19*]. Of the 51 amino-acid units in the insulin molecule, 48 have the same arrangement in the insulins of different species; the sequence of units in one segment of three units varies. If an insulin is antigenic for a mammal, it is because this sequence differs from the corresponding sequence of the animal's own insulin.

In these days when genetics has come so close to biochemistry it is worth pointing out that an antigen, like a gene, is a purely relative concept. A gene is an entity devised to explain an observable hereditary difference between two interbreeding stocks or individuals. Long stretches of a chromosome must remain genetically silent if there are no regions of observable difference between available stocks. An antigen, or more strictly

that is, according to genetic instructions contained in the nucleus of the manufacturing cell. At no time does information enter the cell from outside. Instead, for each one of the thousands of possible foreign antigens, the body already contains a cell or group of cells genetically capable of synthesizing the appropriate antibody. Each of these cells or groups of cells "knows" how to make the specific antibody even if the complementary antigen never enters the body. The function of the antigen is simply to select and stimulate the proliferation of the appropriate group of cells, thus increasing production of the required antibody.

The idea of selection has been central to biology ever since the publication of the *Origin of Species*: The environment selects among organisms for the differential survival attributes or potentiali-

ties which are conferred upon them by genetic processes. The sun does not breed maggots in a dead dog unless the fertilized fly deposits the necessary genetic information in the carrion. No one now seriously argues that evolution produced the whale and the giraffe by the Lamarckian formula according to which function in the environment molds form —first physically and then inheritably— in the right direction. Recently, however, some investigators have held that bacteria show a wide capacity to produce "adaptive" enzymes on demand. It was indeed observed that bacterial cultures can start producing new enzymes when presented with unusual substances in their nutrient. But it soon became clear that adaptive-enzyme formation is a much subtler phenomenon. Current interpretation tends toward the

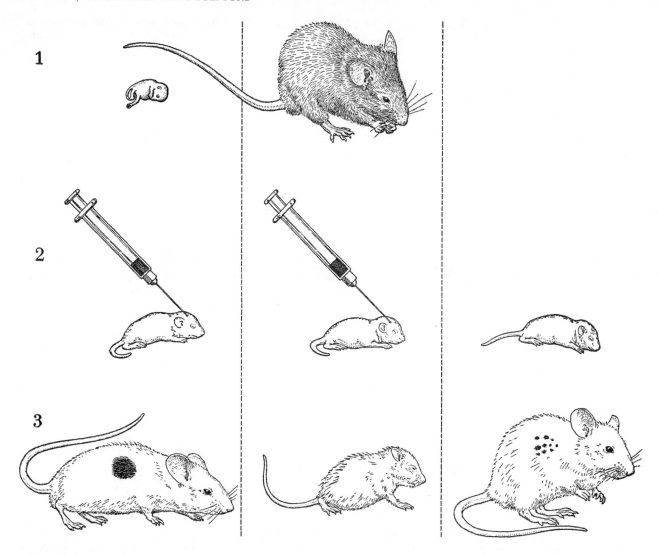

GRAFT AND HOST INTERACT in mice. At left spleen cells from embryo mouse of strain B (1) are injected into newborn mouse of strain A (2). Later skin graft from B takes on A (3), showing mutual tolerance of host and graft. In center spleen cells from adult mouse B are injected into second newborn A mouse, which develops runt disease (3) because injected cells set up immune response to it. Third newborn B mouse (*right*) receives no injection at birth to establish tolerance, later (3) rejects skin graft from strain A.

an antigenic determinant, is also an expression of difference. It contains certain patterns which differ from any pattern present in the animal in which it is tested for antigenicity. In one kind of animal one part of a foreign protein molecule may be antigenic; in another species an entirely different segment of the same molecule may stimulate the antibody reaction.

Even though insulin is a poor antigen, it still presents rather clearly the central question: How does the insulin-resistant diabetic "recognize" the tiny difference between beef insulin and his own insulin and so make antibody against the former? Basically this is a problem of information. How does the body acquire or generate the information needed to distinguish foreign chemical configurations from its own?

The most important clue is provided by experimental manipulations that trick an organism into accepting as its own a substance or a cell that genetically speaking has no right to be there. Probably the most impressive example comes from the rare experiments of nature by which genetically dissimilar human twins share a common placental circulation in their mother's uterus. This will ensure that each twin receives a variety of cells from the other, including cells that can settle down in the bone marrow and multiply to produce the red blood cells. Three pairs of such twins have been recognized in adult life. When their blood was typed prior to their acting as blood donors, they were found to have two blood groups: their own and that which was genetically appropriate to their twin. Such fraternal twins have a second striking difference from an ordinary pair of dissimilar twins. Fraternal

twins who have developed in the usual fashion from two separate placentas will not accept skin transplants from each other. An immune reaction kills the grafts. But fraternal twins with double blood groups (at least the only pair of twins so far tested) have been found to accept cross skin-grafting as happily as if they were genetically identical twins. This indicates that self-recognition in the antibody-producing system is not due simply to hereditary traits. Rather, self-recognition seems to develop as a secondary process sometime during embryonic life.

Much work has been done in recent years on the experimental demonstration of immunological tolerance, most often in mice and rats. Laboratories now possess many lines of mice so inbred and so similar genetically that each individual will accept grafts of skin or other tissue from any other member of its strain. Two very illuminating experiments can be carried out with two suitable strains: A and B. In both experiments an emulsion of living cells from a mouse of strain B is inoculated into a vein on the face of a newborn mouse of strain A. This requires steady hands and a good eye, but it is done routinely.

In the first experiment cells from the spleen and kidney of an embryo of mouse B are inoculated into a newborn mouse of strain A. The mouse develops normally. If a piece of B skin is grafted to the mouse when it is sufficiently grown, the graft "takes" and persists in a healthy condition. If the A mice are white and the B mice are black, the A mouse presents the unprecedented anomaly of a patch of healthy black hair.

In the second experiment another mouseling of strain A is inoculated with cells from the spleen of an adult B mouse, not an embryo. The result is disastrous. Depending upon the number of cells and the particular pair of mouse strains being used, the mouseling either dies within two or three weeks or develops slowly into an undersized, scruffy-looking individual suffering from what has been called runt disease [*see illustration on opposite page*].

A slightly oversimplified explanation is that in the first experiment host A becomes tolerant of the B cells implanted in its tissues just after birth. As a result A subsequently tolerates a graft of B skin. But it is important to note that the cells that are implanted have qualities just as definite as those of the host. If an equilibrium is to be reached, the implanted B cells must become tolerant of their foreign host as well as vice versa. The embryonic B cells do become tolerant. But in the second experiment the adult B cells set up their own immune reaction against their host and produce runt disease or death.

A detailed consideration of many phenomena of the same general quality permits the formulation of the key question in the self and not-self problem: What is the process by which the body learns during development to differentiate its own substance from that of others? As Niels K. Jerne of the World Health Organization has put it, where or what is the dictionary that the body must consult to decide whether such and such a word (chemical configuration) is foreign or belongs to its own language? Along with Lederberg and other investigators, he believes that the dictionary lists only foreign words and that it has in it a list of all the foreign words without ever having heard them!

Such a dictionary can be pictured in several possible ways, but basically it must contain a large, though not infinite, number of patterns (words) which among them can offer a complementary specific antibody patch to correspond with every possible antigenic determinant. The proposal is not as outrageously unlikely as it sounds, because the number of antigenic determinants is not impossibly large. Both the antigenic determinants and the specific patches are small configurations. The number of different three- and four-letter combinations for the 20-letter alphabet of amino-acid units in proteins is respectively 8,000 and 160,000; these are very few compared with the number of cells in

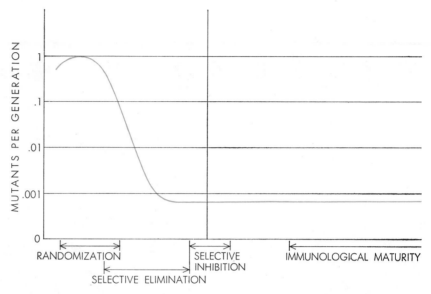

MUTATION RATE per cell-generation of genes carrying antibody patterns is high in early embryonic life (*vertical line down chart indicates birth*). Then mutation rate slows and most cells carrying "self"-antibody patterns are eliminated; later others are selectively inhibited. Immunological maturity occurs some time after birth. Mutations continue to appear throughout life, but at a much lower rate than in an individual's early embryonic life.

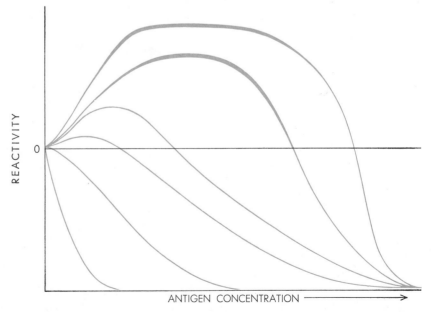

MATURITY CHANGES REACTION of immunological cells to increasing concentration of antigen. The most immature cells are represented by bottom curve; the most mature cells, by top curve. Zero line indicates no reaction to antigen. Above it, cells proliferate, and the thickened curves indicate development of plasma cells and production of antibody. Below the zero line immune cells are first inhibited and then, as the curves indicate, further concentration of antigen can drive them to dormancy and can even destroy the very immature cells.

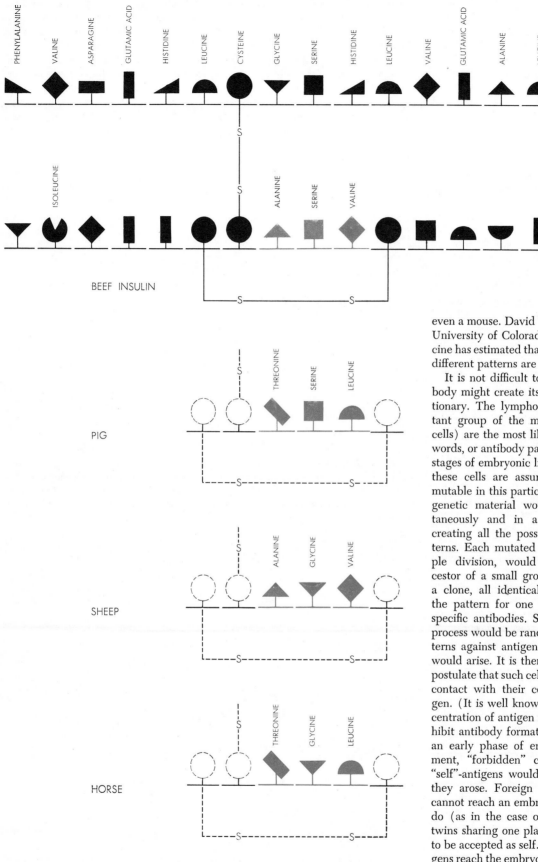

DIFFERENCES IN INSULIN MOLECULES produced by various mammals are slight. Sequence of amino-acid units in entire beef-insulin molecule appears at top. Only three units (*color*) differ from those found in pig, sheep and horse, as indicated below.

even a mouse. David W. Talmage of the University of Colorado School of Medicine has estimated that only some 10,000 different patterns are needed.

It is not difficult to imagine how the body might create its foreign-word dictionary. The lymphocytes (one important group of the mobile white blood cells) are the most likely carriers of the words, or antibody patterns. In the early stages of embryonic life the ancestors of these cells are assumed to be highly mutable in this particular quality. Their genetic material would change spontaneously and in a random fashion, creating all the possible antibody patterns. Each mutated cell, through simple division, would become the ancestor of a small group of cells, called a clone, all identical and all carrying the pattern for one or at most a few specific antibodies. Since the mutation process would be random, antibody patterns against antigens within the body would arise. It is therefore necessary to postulate that such cells are destroyed by contact with their corresponding antigen. (It is well known that a high concentration of antigen in an adult will inhibit antibody formation.) Thus during an early phase of embryonic development, "forbidden" clones that match "self"-antigens would be eliminated as they arose. Foreign antigens normally cannot reach an embryo, but when they do (as in the case of the nonidentical twins sharing one placenta), they come to be accepted as self. If no foreign antigens reach the embryo, it presumably retains all the foreign patterns.

Later in embryonic life the rate of mutations in immunological cells would decrease drastically to the mutation rate

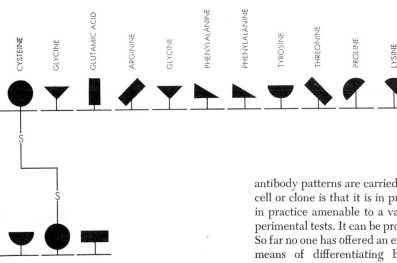

CYSTEINE   GLYCINE   GLUTAMIC ACID   ARGININE   GLYCINE   PHENYLALANINE   PHENYLALANINE   TYROSINE   THREONINE   PROLINE   LYSINE   ALANINE

found everywhere in the body throughout life. (It has been estimated that as many as a million body cells undergo mutation each day.) Forbidden clones would continue to arise, though infrequently, and would normally be killed off, or at least inhibited, while still immature. Mature immunological cells, instead of being destroyed by the appropriate antigen, would be stimulated by it to proliferate [*see illustration on pages 14 and 15*], producing among their offspring a great many of the plasma cells that probably manufacture the actual antibody molecules to combine with and deactivate foreign antigens.

The theory is called the clonal-selection theory because the action of the antigen is simply to select for proliferation that particular clone of cells which can react with it. In the original form of the hypothesis each clone was believed to carry only one pattern, but two patterns per clone now seems to accord better with evidence from observations.

Many immunologists are highly sympathetic to the general idea of a clonal-selection theory, but are skeptical of the necessity of limiting the capacity of a given cell or clone to one, two or at most three patterns. They would prefer a substantial number, perhaps 10 to 20 related patterns per clone. Some even press the idea to its logical conclusion and assume that every cell which is a potential antibody producer carries its own complete foreign-word dictionary and can therefore recognize any antigenic determinant and through its descendants produce antibody against it.

The main virtue of the clonal-selection theory in which not more than three

antibody patterns are carried by a single cell or clone is that it is in principle and in practice amenable to a variety of experimental tests. It can be proved wrong. So far no one has offered an experimental means of differentiating between an instructive theory and the theory that every immunological cell carries all possible antibody patterns. Furthermore, it is extremely difficult to picture how every one of these cells could contain all the information needed for the recognition of every foreign antigenic determinant.

In biology the only function of a generalization is to present clearly a statement in such a form that any interested worker can grasp the type of experimental or observational information that will be needed to disprove it or to compel its modification. No theory can ever be proved to be correct. The only major

virtue of the clonal-selection hypothesis is that it draws attention to the essential role of cells, rather than of antigens, in antibody production and immunity. Hence it must stimulate attempts to define the potentialities of single cells and to analyze the population dynamics of the immunological cells in the body.

Several experimental approaches are possible. One is the study of the ability of single cells to produce antibody and of the number of types of antibody that a single cell can produce. It is now established that in an animal immunized with more than one antigen most cells produce only one type of antibody, but that an occasional cell can undoubtedly produce two. Another type of experiment is based on finding a situation in which a small proportion of cells with some special antibody pattern can be sorted out from a large population of immunological cells. At our laboratory in Melbourne we have recently been engaged in producing immunological "pocks" on the chorioallantois of the chick embryo, the membrane in the egg which supplies the chick with oxygen [*see illustration below*]. We do this by inoculating the membrane with white blood cells from a mature chicken. The inoculation produces one focus, or pock, for roughly every 20,000 white cells. One focus, we believe, represents one cell; our provi-

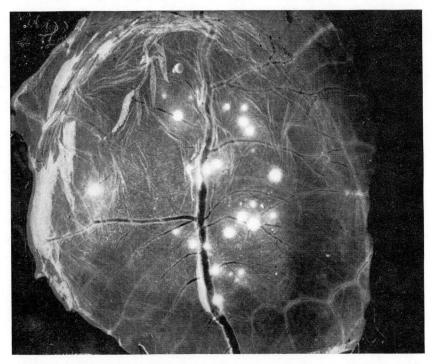

MEMBRANE OF CHICK EMBRYO shows white spots due to attack by adult-chicken lymphocytes implanted in egg. Technique isolates the 1 in 20,000 lymphocytes which apparently carries antibody pattern matching membrane antigen. Photograph was made by author.

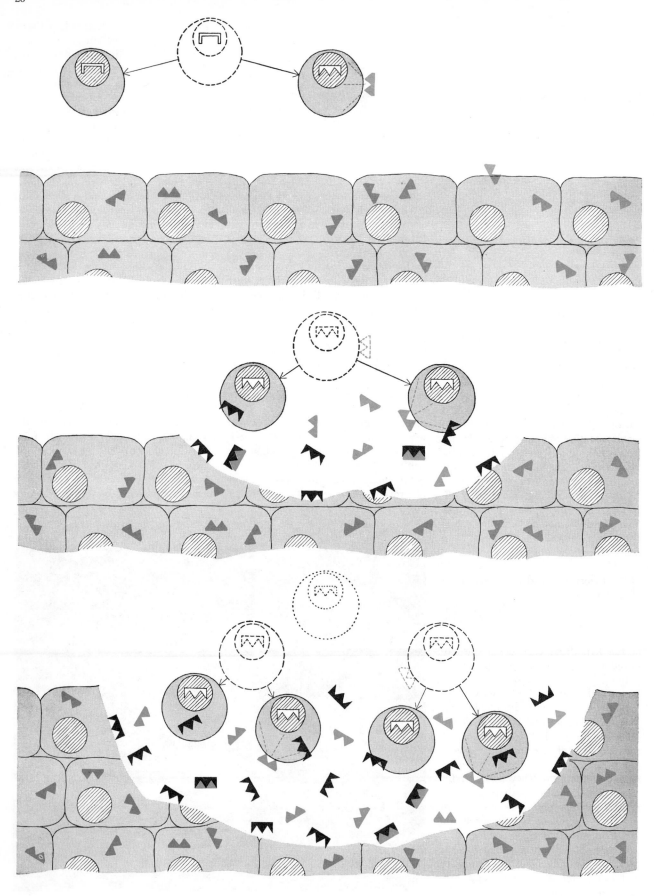

"VICIOUS CIRCLE" of autoimmune disease might start when immunological cell produces offspring (*top*) which by mutation has acquired a "forbidden" antibody pattern, matching a self-antigen. The antigen (*color*) stimulates proliferation of cell (*center*). Antibodies attack tissue which contains this antigen. More antigen is released, causing stepped-up attack (*bottom*).

sional interpretation is that this ratio of 1 to 20,000 reflects the proportion of the white cells with the preformed patterns that correspond to and react with antigens in the chick embryo not present in the chicken that provided the white cells.

The clonal-selection theory could be decisively disproved if it were possible to grow antibody-producing cells in tissue culture and show that from a very small initial population of cells any desired type of antibody could be produced by stimulation from a variety of antigens. So far no one has produced such a demonstration.

To me the most gratifying feature of the clonal-selection theory has been the way in which it can fit all the pieces into a reasonably self-consistent pattern. The explanation of the important auto-immune diseases was particularly obscure when the instructive theories of immunity were the only ones available. The selection theory allows these phenomena to fall easily into place. It postulates that a forbidden clone, through mutation or otherwise, enjoys an abnormal protection from destruction or inhibition by its corresponding antigen. There are difficult problems to be faced in some of the more severe autoimmune diseases, but in one group the process is more readily understood because the antigens concerned are normally of very limited accessibility in the body. They arise in such well-"insulated" tissues as those of the nervous system or the interior of the thyroid gland; they do not normally circulate in quantity in the blood and hence fail to eliminate the complementary clone during the embryonic selection period. Once the antibody-forming cells start to attack, they break down the cells and tissues containing the antigen, releasing more antigen. The antigen stimulates proliferation of the forbidden clone, which steps up the attack, and the vicious circle of autoimmune disease sets in [see illustration on opposite page].

At the other, theoretical, end of the conventional range of medicine is the central problem of biology—the way in which genetic information in the chromosomes of the cell nucleus is expressed in the specific geometric configuration of proteins such as enzymes. At this level, too, the idea of a preadapted pattern determined by the genetic material, which is the essence of the clonal-selection theory, seems to fit better with modern conceptions of protein synthesis than the rather crudely mechanical concept of the orthodox instructive theory.

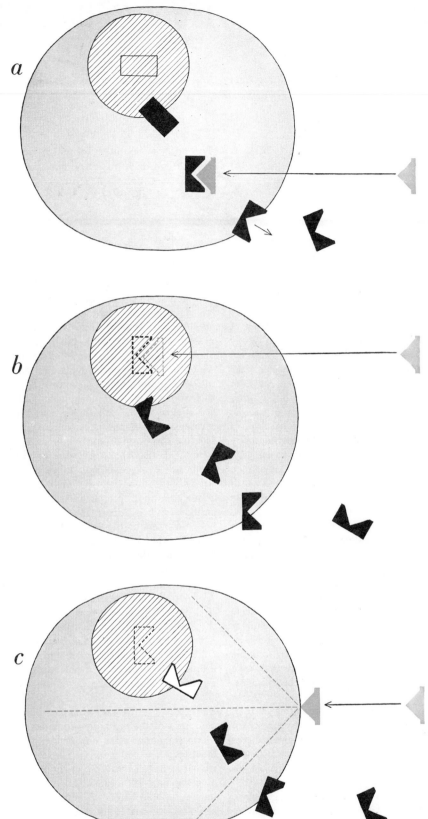

THREE THEORIES OF IMMUNITY are classical "instructive" hypothesis (a), the author's earlier indirect-template theory (b) and clonal selection (c). In the instructive theory antigen enters antibody-producing cell and becomes a direct template from which antibody takes its final, complementary form. In b the antigen somehow incorporates an image of itself in genetic mechanism of cell. Author's recent clonal-selection theory holds that the cell is "born" with pattern complementary to specific antigen, and that antigen does not enter the cell but simply selects and encourages proliferation of cell having right pattern.

2

How Cells Make Antibodies

by G. J. V. Nossal
December 1964

*The process has now been clarified by experiments
with single antibody-producing cells grown in culture.
These experiments indicate that antibody manufacture
is directed by the genes*

The human body is capable of producing on demand any one of thousands, possibly millions, of different antibodies, each specifically constructed to attack a specific antigen. How does it manage this complex task? Do the body's cells build antibodies in the same way that they build other proteins, under the direction of specific genes? If so, the cells must contain a very large number of different antibody genes and also an elaborate mechanism primed to switch on the right gene when the body is invaded by a particular antigen, be it a bacterium, a virus or some other foreign protein material.

At the Walter and Eliza Hall Institute of Medical Research in Melbourne we have been investigating these questions by means of special cell cultures. Conceptually the production of antibodies rather resembles a large industrial organization that manufactures a wide range of products in many different factories. The system offers three elements for analysis. First there are the factories themselves: the cells that make antibody. Then there are the products: the antibody molecules. Finally there are the specification-presenting customers, so to speak: the antigen molecules. We shall examine each of these in detail and attempt to show how the system is operated with such remarkable efficiency.

Until a couple of decades ago it was generally believed that antibodies were produced by the large antigen-devouring cells known as macrophages or "scavenger cells." Then in a classic study Astrid Fagraeus of Sweden brought forth evidence suggesting that the actual producers were a family of specialized cells called plasma cells, which show up in considerable numbers at the site of an infection as inflamma-

tion gets under way. She found that two days or so after she had injected a vaccine intravenously into an experimental animal "plasmablasts" began to appear in its spleen (a prime source of white cells). These young plasma cells divide rapidly, and after a few days their progeny become more specialized: the nucleus of the cell shrinks and the surrounding cytoplasm expands. The fact that this cytoplasm is rich in ribonucleic acid (RNA), which directs the synthesis of protein, was taken as a strong indication that the plasma cell actively produced protein—that is to say, antibody. Then Albert H. Coons and his co-workers at the Harvard Medical School added weight to this suspicion by showing that plasma cells actually contain antibody.

Work in our laboratory has now proved definitely that these cells do indeed manufacture antibody. We have been able to follow the process by culturing single plasma cells in tiny droplets. This procedure has made it possible to measure the production of antibody by living cells and to study the quality, purity and chemical characteristics of the antibody produced.

As the antigen for our first experiments we selected a protein extracted from the flagella, or "flippers," of Salmonella bacteria (which include the human typhoid bacilli). The flagella enable the bacteria to move about. Antiserum to this material (that is, serum containing antibody to its protein) will paralyze the flagella and rapidly immobilize the bacteria. Thus the organisms' reaction provides a ready test for the presence of the specific antibody.

We begin by injecting the flagella protein into a rat. After the rat has had time to react to the foreign protein

we remove the lymph nodes draining the site of the injection, tease the tissue apart into its individual cells and place each cell in a microdroplet of tissue-culture liquid, which we deposit as a hanging drop on the underside of a glass cover slip. The drop is covered with a film of paraffin oil to prevent its evaporation. All this is done with a micropipette and a micromanipulator under a phase-contrast microscope. We then incubate the cell in the drop for several hours at 37 degrees C. (the human body temperature). Having thus given the cell time to manufacture antibody, we finally inject three to 10 mobile Salmonella bacteria into the microdrop.

If the bacteria are of the right strain—that is, the same strain as the one from which the flagella protein, or antigen, was extracted—they stop moving promptly, often within a few seconds. On the other hand, bacteria of any other strain will go on swimming about indefinitely. The action is so specific that antibody that rapidly immobilizes *Salmonella typhi* has no effect whatever, even in high concentration, on the closely related *Salmonella paratyphi a*.

The lymph-node cells, for their part, show a similar specialization. Lymphocytes and scavenger cells give no evidence of having formed antibody; they fail to immobilize even the "right" bacteria. Plasma cells, on the other hand, frequently show the effect. In their young, plasmablast stage they produce relatively little antibody, but by the time they have matured they are loading the microdrop around them with so much antibody that the liquid will immobilize bacteria even when it is diluted 1,000 times. The immobilization test affords a measure of the amount of antibody produced by the cell, because the

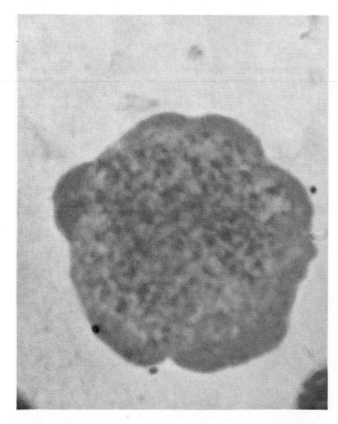

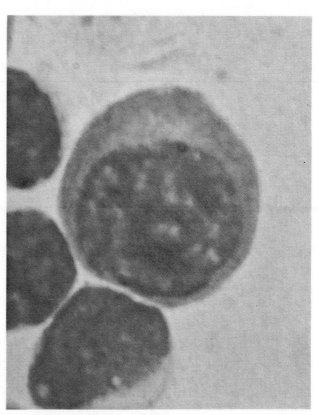

PLASMABLAST, the first type of cell induced by the introduction of an antigen, is shown in culture. The reddish cells that appear in these micrographs are not involved in antibody production.

IMMATURE PLASMA CELL is the offspring of the plasmablast. The cytoplasm (*blue outer region of the cell*) has expanded; the nucleus (*red interior*) and overall size of the cell have diminished.

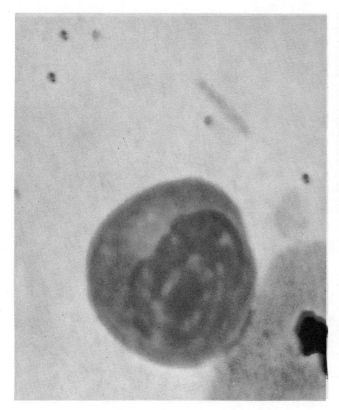

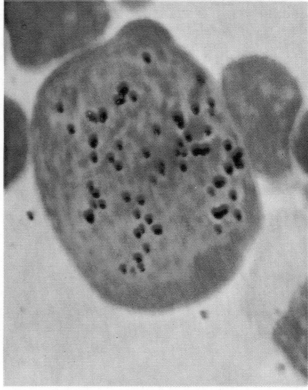

MATURE PLASMA CELL has an even more fully developed cytoplasm. Ribonucleic acid (RNA) located in the cytoplasm directs the synthesis of antibodies, the proteins that act to neutralize antigens.

RADIOAUTOGRAPH of plasmablast shows sites of deoxyribonucleic acid (DNA) synthesis. Precursor of DNA was labeled with radioactive atoms that on decaying made black dots in emulsion.

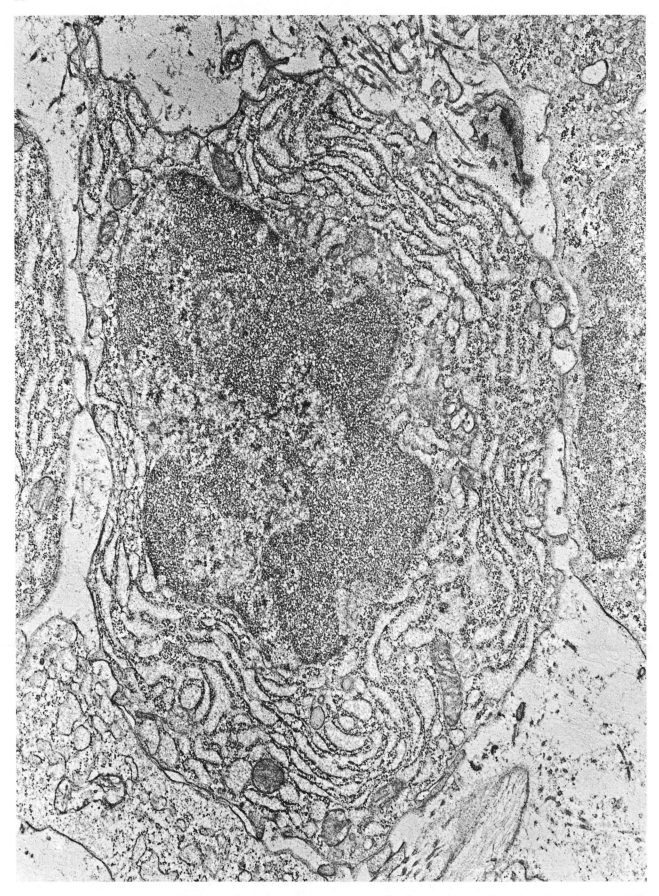

SITES OF ANTIBODY PRODUCTION, the ribosomes, appear as tiny black dots lining channels called the endoplasmic reticulum in this electron micrograph of a plasma cell enlarged some 28,000 diameters. The presence of an antigen has induced development of the endoplasmic reticulum to the point where the eccentrically shaped nucleus has been pushed into one region of the cell. The process by which antibodies, once made, are released from plasma cells is not known. The objects around the edges are other cells.

speed of immobilization depends on the concentration of the antibody. A mere few thousand molecules of antibody are enough to immobilize bacteria in a short time.

The evolution of the plasma cells again puts one in mind of the development of a large industrial plant. The young, primitive plasmablasts that emerge two or three days after the antigen has been injected represent the tooling-up stage. The plasmablast is a hive of activity; construction is proceeding apace. A few products are being turned out, but most of the energy is going into setting up the machinery and adjusting the assembly line. The mature plasma cell, on the other hand, is like a factory a decade after launching. This is the era of high production, regular dividends and little or no expansion. Nearly all the cell's energy is being put into its one specialized task: turning out a maximum of antibody for export and distribution.

How far does this specialization go? Is a given plasma cell restricted to making a single kind of antibody or can it synthesize more than one kind? We undertook experiments to find out whether or not a cell could produce various antibodies simultaneously. Although theoretical considerations had prepared us to expect fairly strict specialization, we were still somewhat surprised to learn how strict it actually was. With rare exceptions each cell made just one antibody, even when other plasma cells in the lymph nodes were equally busy making other antibodies. In other words, there was a sharp division of labor; the prevailing principle was one cell, one antibody. In about one case in 50 we found a cell making trace amounts of a second antibody, but this may have been accidental—the result, for example, of a tiny, undetectable shred of cytoplasm from another cell clinging to the cell in question.

As happens so frequently in present-day research, another group of workers had quite independently taken up the same investigation we had: the study of antibody production by single cells in microdroplets. A group headed by Melvin Cohn and Edwin S. Lennox that is now at the Salk Institute in La Jolla, Calif., used much the same technique, except that their antigens were virus proteins and the production of antibody was assayed by its neutralization of the virus's infectivity. To our dismay their findings differed in several important respects from our own. They concluded

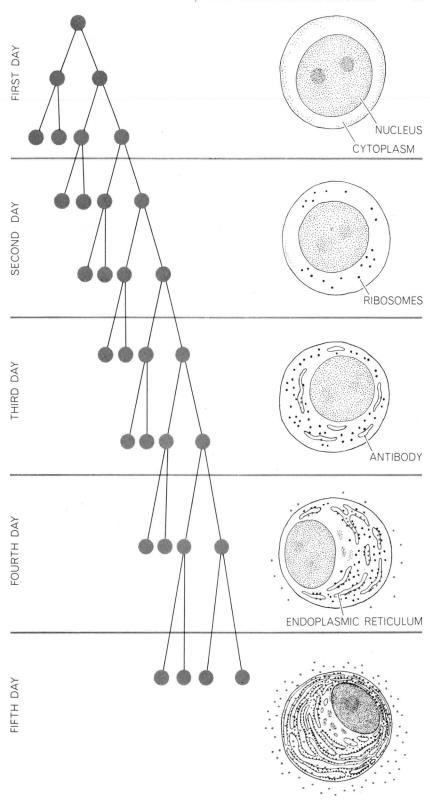

FIRST DAY
SECOND DAY
THIRD DAY
FOURTH DAY
FIFTH DAY

NUCLEUS
CYTOPLASM
RIBOSOMES
ANTIBODY
ENDOPLASMIC RETICULUM

CLONAL DEVELOPMENT of plasma cells is outlined in this representation of cells at five stages of maturity (*column at right*) and the generations to which they belong (*column at left*). After contact with an antigen the plasmablast takes some 10 hours to divide. The time of division grows successively longer; it is not until the fifth day after contact that mature plasma cells, members of the ninth generation, are producing a great deal of antibody (*colored dots*). Maturity can be seen to entail a shrinking of the nucleus and extension of the cytoplasm as the cell devotes itself to the task of making antibody. The nucleus consequently becomes dense and its two nucleoli (*dark spots in top cell*) seem invisible.

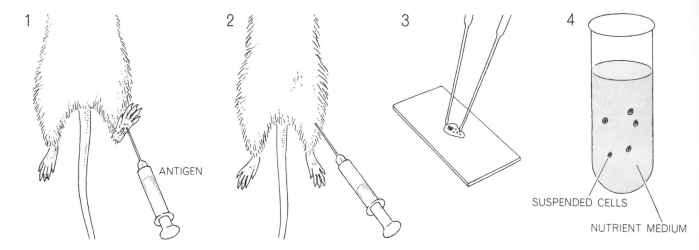

ISOLATING A PLASMA CELL was accomplished in the laboratory of the author as illustrated in this sequence of drawings. An antigen was injected into the footpad of a rat (*Step 1*). Five days later the draining lymph node was removed from the rat's leg (*Step 2*). Cells were teased out of the soft tissue with needles, spun in a centrifuge and suspended in a nutrient medium (*Step 3*). At right (*Step 5*) are a top view and side view of Step 4, in which a cell from the suspension is transferred by means of a

from their experiments that many plasma cells made two different antibodies simultaneously, and also that small lymphocytes, as well as plasma cells, often made antibody. We have been trying to find some reasonable explanation for this difference in results, but so far we have failed to do so. In our hands hundreds of experiments performed by members of our group in various laboratories on three continents have always yielded the same result: one cell, one antibody.

At all events, we begin to see the main outlines of the production picture. As the order for antibody comes in, by way of the arrival of an antigen, the white-cell construction centers (the lymph nodes, spleen or bone marrow as the case may be) commence to turn out the miniature factories that will produce the antibody. These units start as immature plasmablasts and take a little time—a matter of days—to tool up for full production as mature plasma cells. This leads us to the interesting question: What accounts for the great speeding up of antibody production that oc-

curs in a person who has already been exposed to a previous invasion by the same antigen?

"Immunological memory," as it is called, is by all odds the most remarkable feature of the immune response. A patient who has been vaccinated or has recovered from an infection responds to a second attack by the same antigen with so prompt and massive an outpouring of the appropriate antibody that the infection is stopped in its tracks. How is this stepped-up production accomplished? Do the plasma cells produce more antibody than they did the first time or does the new attack generate a greater number of these cells?

Investigating the question with further experiments, we found that both responses took place: in a reinfection there were more plasma cells and each cell formed more antibody. The multiplication of cells, however, was much more pronounced than the production increase by individual cells. It was as if the first exposure to the antigen had left the animal prepared with precursor cells that were ready to turn into plasma

cells of the right kind as soon as the original invader reappeared. We have named these precursors "memory" cells.

We next looked into another interesting feature of the immune response. It has been known for some time that the specific antibody produced by a mammal changes somewhat as the animal's response progresses. During the early stages of the response the animal produces an antibody molecule with a molecular weight of nearly one million; then it switches to making a lighter version of the same antibody with a molecular weight of only 160,000. The heavy and light versions of the molecule are respectively known as 19S and 7S; the "S" signifies Svedberg units, a measure of the rate of sedimentation of the molecules in a centrifugal field. Using the technique of analyzing antibody production by single cells, we established that the switchover occurred within each individual cell. At first the cell formed only the 19S antibody, then for a short period both 19S and 7S, and finally only 7S.

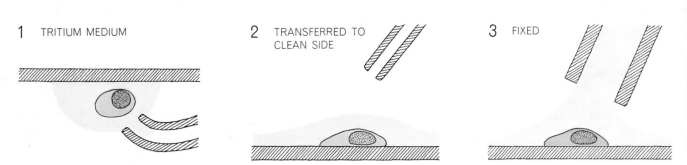

TRACING PROCESS begins with the introduction of tritium, the radioactive isotope of hydrogen, into the medium in which a plasmablast is suspended beneath the cover slip of a microscope slide. This labeled hydrogen is incorporated into thymidine and eventually appears in a constituent of the cellular DNA: thymine. The cell is transferred by a micropipette to a dry, clean slide (*Step*

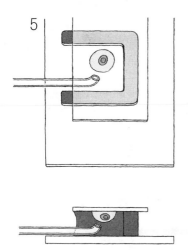

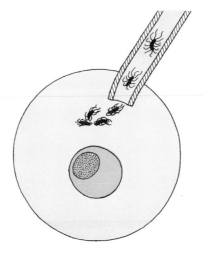

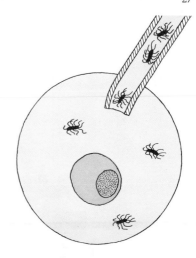

micropipette to the glass slip covering the well in a microscope slide. The droplet of nutrient medium containing the cell is suspended in paraffin oil at body temperature.

SPECIFICITY OF AN ANTIBODY was demonstrated by experiment in which an antigen that immobilizes *Salmonella typhi* bacilli was injected into a rat, and antibody-producing cells were isolated. When *Salmonella typhi* were put in contact with cells (*left*), they could not move. *Salmonella paratyphi* bacilli, a related strain, were unaffected (*right*).

To obtain more information about the workings of these factories it then became necessary to look into the chemical events taking place within them. The problem of finding out what is going on in a single cell of course calls for a technique of exquisite sensitivity. Fortunately such a technique is available. It is autoradiography, the procedure in which a cell is fed a substance labeled with radioactive atoms and the cell then records its metabolic uptake of this substance by its radioactive emissions; these are recorded in a photographic emulsion placed next to the cell [see "Autobiographies of Cells," by Renato Baserga and Walter E. Kisieleski; SCIENTIFIC AMERICAN Offprint 165].

We have used the technique to measure the rates at which our cells synthesize ribonucleic acid (RNA), deoxyribonucleic acid (DNA) and proteins. The radioactive label usually employed is tritium (hydrogen 3). For measurement of the manufacture of DNA, for example, the radioactive hydrogen is incorporated in thymidine, a precursor containing thymine, one of the building blocks

of DNA; for similar study of the synthesis of a protein the label is attached to an amino acid. The labeled substance is then added to the microdroplet containing our cell. After a certain measured time the cell is washed, dried on a glass slide, fixed, covered with a layer of photographic emulsion and put away in a dark place—all, of course, with a micromanipulator. Days or weeks later the slide is taken out and the photographic emulsion is developed and fixed in the usual way. This brings out the amount of darkening that has been produced by radioactive emissions from the cell. The radioactivity indicates how much labeled material the cell took up from the culture medium in the time that elapsed before the cell was fixed. Thus one can measure the rate at which the cell synthesized a given product (RNA, DNA or protein) simply by counting the number of darkened grains in the photographic emulsion.

A cell's production of DNA shows how fast cell division is taking place, because the cell doubles its content of this genetic material just before it di-

vides. Measuring DNA synthesis by means of autoradiography, we have found that the young plasmablasts divide about every 10 hours, which is about as fast as any mammalian cell can divide. After the offspring of these cells have reached the stage of full maturity as plasma cells, however, they apparently stop dividing. It appears that, starting with a single plasmablast, there are typically nine successive divisions, producing a "clone," or colony, of cells before division stops. The clone includes not only mature plasma cells but also a number of primitive "memory" cells that are prepared to react vigorously to any future encounter with the same antigen. Very likely these cells are able to organize themselves into "germinal centers."

In the plasmablast stage the cells produce a great deal of RNA and protein—mainly structural proteins and enzymes. The mature plasma cells, on the other hand, switch to synthesizing mainly antibodies: 90 to 95 percent of all the protein they produce is antibody. Curiously the mature plasma cells of rats,

PHOTOGRAPHIC EMULSION   5   DEVELOPED AND STAINED

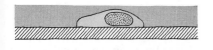

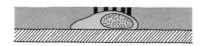

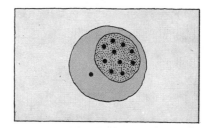

2) and fixed with methanol (*Step 3*). In Step 4 a photographic emulsion is placed on top of the microdroplet containing the cell. During the time the slide is stored in darkness (*Step 5*) rays

emitted as tritium decays mark the emulsion. The top view provided in the last step shows the sites at which radioactive substance was used. Such a view indicates where cell synthesized DNA.

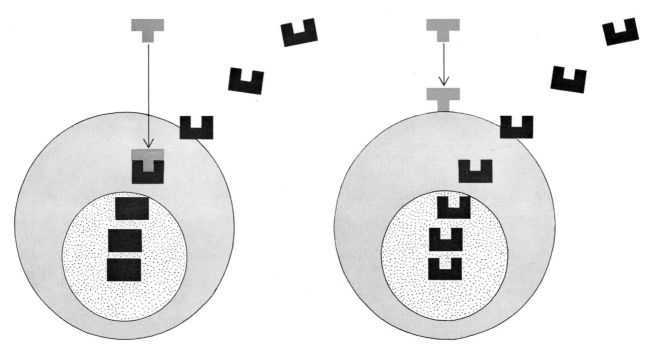

TWO THEORIES OF IMMUNITY are depicted. According to the classical "instructive" hypothesis (*left*) antigen enters a plasma cell and forms a template from which a complementary antibody is produced. The "clonal selection" theory (*right*) suggests that the mere contact of a given antigen and a given plasma cell signals DNA in the cell nucleus to start directing production of antibody.

which we used in our experiments, synthesize very little RNA, although RNA is usually required for protein synthesis. It seems that rats may be somewhat freakish in this respect; recent work has shown that human plasma cells make considerable amounts of RNA. Possibly in rats the cell reads the same RNA blueprints over and over in its manufacture of the antibody molecules.

The development of plasma cells has been studied not only by autoradiography but also by examination of the cells with the electron microscope. We have done little of this work ourselves, but many other groups have pursued intensive microscopic analyses of the cells' anatomy. The electron microscope can magnify the cell 100,000 times and resolve elements within the cell as small as two millionths of a millimeter in diameter.

At this magnification a mature plasma

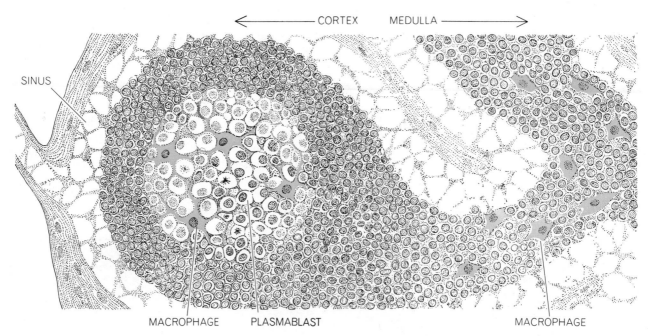

RESPONSE TO ANTIGEN in a lymph node is illustrated. The colored bodies are macrophages: free-swimming scavenger cells. Macrophages within a follicle, an elevation in the node, extend dendritic arms of cytoplasm that ensnare invading antigen while attracting plasmablasts. The multiplying plasmablasts form a cluster called the germinal center. Macrophages in the medulla, the inner region of the node, may also stimulate reproduction of plasma cells in their vicinity after engulfing (not ensnaring) antigen.

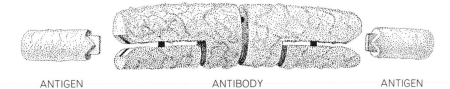

ANTIGEN   ANTIBODY   ANTIGEN

ANTIGEN CAPTURE by a 7S globulin antibody molecule is illustrated schematically. The antibody has two heavy and two light chains wound in flexible packets and bonded by sulfur atoms (*black bands*). The interaction of a heavy and a light chain at each extreme enables antibody to "open" in a manner conforming to shapes of a wide variety of antigens.

cell looks for all the world like the typical cells of a secretory gland. The cell cytoplasm contains a double membrane marked by an extensive network and studded with little black dots. These dots are the ribosomes—the tiny workshops that synthesize proteins. In many other types of cells ribosomes are strung together like a bead necklace in groups called polysomes. It is believed that the connecting string is "messenger" RNA, which contains the coded information for the construction of proteins, and that the ribosomes read the instructions on the string much as the output device of a business machine reads a punched tape. Certain electron micrographs of plasma cells suggest that perhaps the ribosomes in these cells also are organized into polysomes, but so far we have no conclusive evidence on this point.

A young plasmablast contains many free-floating ribosomes, but it shows no extensive network in its structure. The arrival of an antigen somehow sets in motion a complex series of changes that transforms the potential plasma cell from a relatively unspecialized unit into a highly organized, elaborately specialized system for producing and exporting proteins. The plasmablast begins to synthesize RNA at a high rate, forming messenger molecules and ribosomes in the process. When the factory is equipped for full production, the mature plasma cell not only synthesizes but also in some cases stores large quantities of antibody; occasionally these stores of protein actually become visible as crystals within the cell. How the antibody is released from the cell, or what controls the rate of export, is not known.

It is now high time we looked at the products of these factories: the antibody molecules. Unfortunately this is not at all a simple matter. The products of the plasma cells are about as diverse as the vast array of automobile models put out each year by General Motors. We can nonetheless learn something useful by concentrating our attention on the most common form—the Chevrolet of antibodies. It is the 7S molecule I have already touched on; its full name is 7S gamma globulin.

This molecule, it has recently been discovered, can be disassembled into four parts—four chains that are linked together in the full molecule by covalent sulfur links and hydrogen bonds. They come in two pairs: a pair of heavy chains each of molecular weight 50,000 to 60,000 and a pair of lighter ones of molecular weight 20,000. In each particular 7S antibody the two heavy chains (called *A* chains) are identical with each other and so are the two light ones (called *B*).

Now, it is known that an antibody neutralizes an antigen by somehow attaching itself to the antigen. Where in this four-part structure might we find the active combining site that locks on the antigen? Two different suggestions have emerged. Rodney R. Porter of the Wright-Fleming Institute in London has reported indications that the combining site is in the *A* chain. G. M. Edelman of the Rockefeller Institute, on the other hand, believes on the basis of his experiments that the combining site is shared between the *A* and *B* chains [*see illustration above*].

If Edelman's model is correct, it becomes unnecessary to suppose that the shape of the combining site in each specific antibody is determined by a different single gene, as the Porter scheme would imply. Assuming that this property actually is controlled by genes, a comparatively small number of genes, each specifying a variation of the *A* or *B* chain, would suffice. As few as 1,000 different versions of the *A* chain and 1,000 of the *B* chain could, in various combinations, produce at least a million different configurations to entrap a million different antigens.

Finally let us examine the antigens themselves. In a sense they can be called the managers of the antibody factories, because they direct what antibodies shall be produced. The arrival of a particular antigen on the scene starts

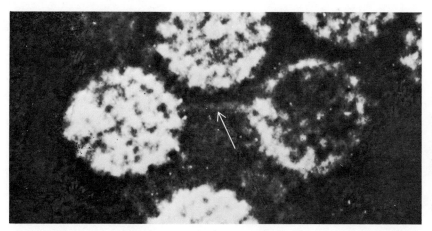

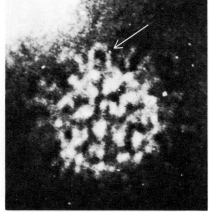

ANTIBODIES AND ANTIGENS appear in these electron micrographs. In the micrograph at left the antibody molecule (*strand indicated by arrow*) extends between two polyoma virus particles. In the micrograph at right an antibody molecule (*loop indicated by arrow*) attaches both combining sites to one antigen, a wart-virus particle. The micrographs have respective magnifications of 750,000 and 600,000. They were prepared by June Almeida, Bernhard Cinader and Allan Howatson of the University of Toronto.

a whole series of specific activities: the proliferation of plasmablasts, the synthesis of RNA and networks by these cells, their progressive differentiation toward mature plasma cells, the synthesis and assembly of A and B chains into antibody molecules, the creation of "memory cells" and so forth.

Seeking to find out how the antigen triggers all this, Gordon L. Ada and I, together with other workers in our Institute, have recently performed a series of experiments with radioactively labeled antigens. We labeled each antigen molecule with just one atom of radioactive iodine 125, firmly attached to a unit of the amino acid tyrosine in the molecule. At various intervals after the antigen had been injected into a rat we examined sections of the animal's organs by means of autoradiography to see where the antigen had gone. The technique enabled us to trace even single molecules of antigen to their destinations in the body.

We found, in the first place, that the antigen was very efficiently gobbled up by the large scavenger cells, or macrophages. The macrophages deep within the lymph nodes proved to be loaded, as expected, with the antigen. But we also found the antigen trapped in another system that had not been noted previously. In the outer part of the lymph node was a veritable web of fine strands of macrophage cytoplasm. This web captured antigen most actively. Thereafter it soon attracted primitive blast cells, including plasmablasts. These began to multiply and formed round collections of cells we call germinal centers. The exact function of these cells is not clear, but we believe they export both lymphocytes acting as memory cells and antibody-forming cells.

To our surprise we found that little or no antigen made its way into the antibody-producing cells themselves, at least as far as the autoradiographs showed. The plasmablasts occasionally seemed to contain a few molecules of antigen, but in the mature plasma cells there was so little of it that even if the antigen molecules had been broken into tiny pieces, there would not have been enough fragments to provide one for each ribosome or polysome in the cell. All this argued against the hypothesis that antibodies are shaped by contact with the antigen molecule or a fragment of it as the template.

What, then, does launch the plasma-cell system into activity and shape the production of the antibody? The only current theory that is consistent with all the observed facts is the "clonal selection" theory proposed by Sir Macfarlane Burnet [see "The Mechanism of Immunity," by Sir Macfarlane Burnet, the article beginning on page 12]. The essence of this theory is that the antibody-producing cells need no information from the antigen at all beyond the fact that it is present! The body is equipped with a variety of clones of cells of various capacities. Each group of cells has the potential to react to a particular antigen, and the arrival of that antigen simply triggers the already prepared cells to make the appropriate antibody. As we have seen, the plasmablasts that cluster around the antigen-laden web of the lymph node come into close contact with the antigen. Perhaps mere surface contact with the antigen is sufficient to launch the cells into activity.

Whether the clonal-selection theory is correct, or even partly correct, is still much debated. It seems clear, however, that antibodies are not molded on antigens as templates, and more and more the evidence points to the likelihood that they are constructed according to plans carried by the genes. One can imagine that through the ages the mutagenic processes of nature, working on a vulnerable area, or "hot spot," in the antibody genes (perhaps the two genes controlling the configurations of the A and B chains), have produced various mutations and thus have given rise to a varied assortment of such genes that persists in the body because of its value in coping with a variety of infections.

In terms of our industrial analogy, it appears that evolution has built an antibody-production system that would make any factory manager wide-eyed with envy. All the manager in this case (the antigen molecule) has to do is to walk up to the right building (an appropriate cell) and knock on the door. The knock sets off feverish activity inside the building: elaborate machines are speedily constructed and the number of workshops multiplies. Soon, without the manager having even crossed the threshold, there begins to come off the assembly line a steady stream of custom-built automobiles designed to suit him exactly. The manager himself did not design the car. Inside the initially empty factory building a very complex computer system (the cell's DNA) saw him coming, remembered all the mistakes and lessons of past ages in coping with his requirements and speedily arranged to greet him with the correct answer.

The Structure of Antibodies

3

by R. R. Porter
October 1967

*The basic pattern of the principal class of molecules
that neutralize antigens (foreign substances in the
body) is four cross-linked chains. This pattern is
modified so that antibodies can fit different antigens*

It has been known for millenniums that a person who survives a disease such as plague or smallpox is usually able to resist a second infection. Indeed, such immune people were often the only ones available to nurse the sick during severe epidemics. A general understanding of immunity had to await the discovery that microorganisms are the causative agents of infectious disease. Then progress was rapid. A key step was taken in 1890 by Emil Von Behring and Shibasaburo Kitasato, working in the Institute of Robert Koch in Berlin. They showed that an animal could be made immune to tetanus by an injection of the blood serum obtained from an animal that had survived the disease and had developed immunity to it. Serum is the clear fluid that is left behind when a blood clot forms; it contains most of the blood proteins. Thus immunity to tetanus is a function of a substance or substances in the blood. These substances were named antibodies.

Antibodies are produced by all vertebrates as a defense against invasion by certain foreign substances, known collectively as antigens. The most effective antigens are large molecules such as proteins or polysaccharides (and of course the microorganisms that contain these molecules). The demonstration of the appearance of antibodies in the blood is most dramatic if the antigen is a lethal toxin or a pathogenic microorganism: the immune animals live and the nonimmune die when injected with the antigen. Innocuous substances such as egg-white protein or the polysaccharide coat of bacteria, however, are equally effective as antigens. The antibodies formed against them can be detected by their ability to combine with antigen. This can be shown in many ways. Perhaps the simplest demonstration is provided by the precipitate that appears in a test tube when a soluble antigen combines with antibody contained in a sample of serum. The most remarkable aspect of this phenomenon is the specificity of the antibody for the antigen injected. That is, the antibody formed will combine only with the antigen injected

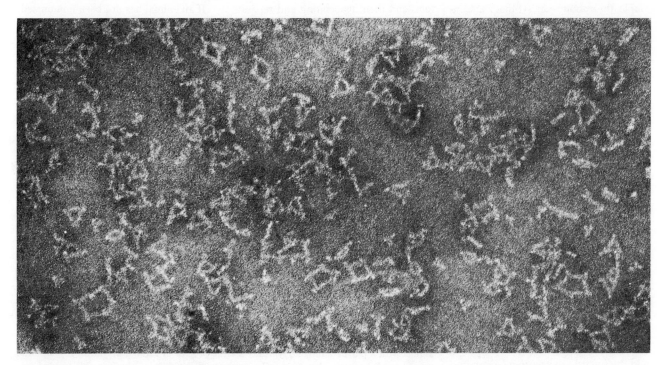

ANTIBODIES BOUND TO ANTIGENS are depicted in this electron micrograph made by Michael Green and Robin Valentine of the National Institute for Medical Research in London. The antigen itself is too small to be visible, but it evidently acts as the coupling agent that binds antibody molecules together to form the various multisided structures. The magnification is about 275,000 diameters.

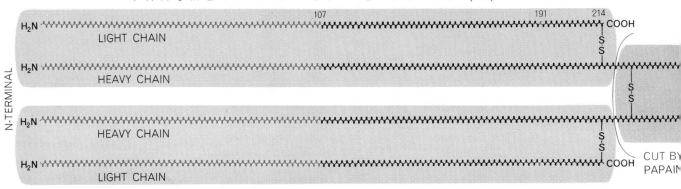

FRAGMENT ANTIGEN BINDING (Fab)

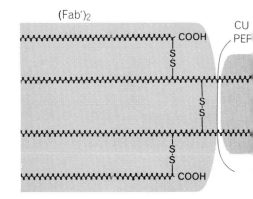

(Fab')₂

IMMUNOGLOBULIN GAMMA, the chief class of antibody, is a protein molecule consisting of four polypeptide chains held together by disulfide (S—S) bonds. The two light chains are identical, as are the two heavy chains. Depending on the source, the light chains contain from about 210 to 230 amino acid units; the heavy chains vary from about 420 to 440 units. Thus the lengths, the spacing between disulfide bonds and enzyme cleavage points shown here are approximate. The enzyme papain splits the molecule into three fragments (above): a fragment that forms crystals (Fc) and two fragments (Fab) that do not crystallize but contain the antigen binding sites. Approximately half of each Fab fragment (color) is variable in amino acid composition. Site 191 is genetically variable. When immunoglobulin gamma is split by the enzyme pepsin (right), the Fab fragments remain bonded together (Fab')₂ because the cleavage occurs on the other side of the central disulfide bond.

or with other substances whose structure is closely related.

Numerous different antibodies can be formed. Although an individual animal may respond poorly, or perhaps not at all, to a particular antigen, there is no known limit to the number of specific antibodies that one species, for example the rabbit, can synthesize. Conceptually there is a great difference between the capability of one species to synthesize a very large but limited number of antibodies and the capacity to synthesize an infinite number, but an experimental decision as to which is correct is not possible at present.

All antibodies are found in a group of related serum proteins known as immunoglobulins. The challenge to the protein chemist lies in the fact that antibody molecules are surprisingly similar even though they possess an enormous range of specific combining power. Although it is clear that there must be significant differences among antibodies, no chemical or physical property has yet been found that can distinguish between two antibody molecules: one able to combine specifically, say, with an aromatic compound such as a benzene derivative and the other with a sugar, although the benzene compound and the sugar have no common structural features. Antibodies of quite unrelated specificity appear to be identical,

within the limits of present experimental techniques, except, of course, in their specific combination with antigen.

An antibody can be isolated from the serum of an immunized animal only by using the special property of allowing it to combine with the antigen, freeing the complex from the other serum proteins and then dissociating and separating the antibody and antigen. This can be done by allowing a precipitate to form, washing the precipitate well with salt solution and then suspending the precipitate in weak acid. Under these

conditions the antibody-antigen precipitate will dissolve and dissociate, and the antibody and antigen can be separated from each other to yield the purified antibody. As we shall see, however, even this purified material usually contains a variety of antibody molecules that differ slightly in their molecular structure.

If an animal has not been immunized, it will still have a good concentration of immunoglobulin in its blood, usually about 1 percent by weight. This material is believed to be made up of many thousands of different antibodies

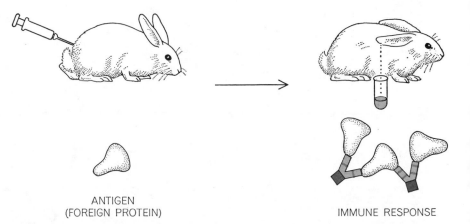

ANTIGEN
(FOREIGN PROTEIN)

IMMUNE RESPONSE

MIXTURE OF SIMILAR ANTIBODIES can be produced by injecting a rabbit or other animal with a purified antigen, typically a large protein of foreign origin. In response the animal produces antibodies, primarily immunoglobulin gamma, that are able to bind specifically to the antigen. Evidently a given antigen provides many different binding sites, thus giving rise to many different antibody molecules. If blood is removed from the animal

FRAGMENT CRYSTALLINE (Fc)

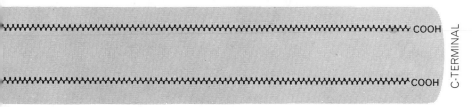

COOH

COOH

C-TERMINAL

Fc

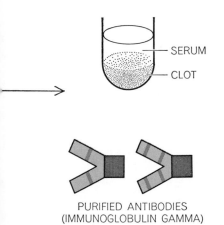

against microorganisms the animal has encountered during its lifetime or against other antigenic substances that accidentally entered its body. Evidence that this view is correct comes from experiments in which small animals have been born and raised in an entirely germ-free environment. Under these conditions the immunoglobulin content of the blood is much lower, perhaps only 10 percent of the immunoglobulin in the blood of a normal animal, suggesting that mild infections are the main source of antigens.

The immunoglobulins can be isolated from serum by the usual methods of protein separation. Hence the protein chemist has available for study two general kinds of immunoglobulin fraction: a complex mixture of many antibodies and purified antibodies that have been isolated by virtue of their specific affinity for the antigen. It would seem to be a relatively straightforward task, after the great progress made in the techniques of protein chemistry in recent years, to carry out detailed studies of such material and pinpoint the differences. Clearly structural differences responsible for the specific combining power of antibodies must exist among them and should become apparent.

Major difficulties have arisen, however, because the immunoglobulins have been found to be a very complex mixture of molecules and the complexity is not necessarily due to the presence of the many different kinds of antibody. One difficulty is that there are three main classes of immunoglobulins distinguished chemically from one another by size,

carbohydrate content and amino acid analysis. Antibodies of any specificity can be found in any of the classes; hence there is no correlation between class and specificity. The class present in the largest amounts in the blood and the most easily isolated is called immunoglobulin gamma. Since most of the work has been done with this material I shall limit my discussion to it.

Immunoglobulin gamma has a molecular weight of about 150,000, corresponding to some 23,000 atoms, of which a carbohydrate fraction forms no more than 2 or 3 percent. Chemical studies have shown that the immunoglobulin gamma molecule is built up of four polypeptide chains, which, as in all proteins, are formed from strings of amino acids joined to one another through peptide bonds. The four chains are paired so that the molecule consists of two identical halves, each consisting of one long, or heavy, chain and one short, or light, chain. The four chains are held to one another by the disulfide bonds of the amino acid cystine [see *illustration at top of these two pages*]. If the disulfide bonds are split, the heavy and light chains are still bound to each other. If, however, they are put in an acid solution or one containing a substance such as urea, they dissociate and can be separated by their difference in size.

Immunoglobulin gamma molecules can also be split by proteolytic enzymes such as papain, which breaks the molecule into three pieces of about equal size. Two, known as F*ab* (for "fragment antigen binding"), appear to be identical, and the third, known as F*c* (fragment crystalline), is quite different. F*ab* is so named because it will still combine with the antigen although it will not pre-

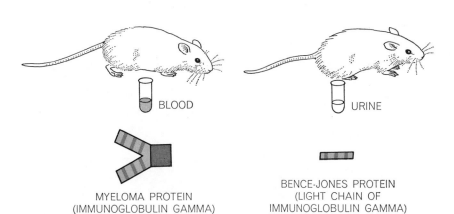

SERUM

CLOT

BLOOD

URINE

PURIFIED ANTIBODIES
(IMMUNOGLOBULIN GAMMA)

MYELOMA PROTEIN
(IMMUNOGLOBULIN GAMMA)

BENCE-JONES PROTEIN
(LIGHT CHAIN OF
IMMUNOGLOBULIN GAMMA)

and allowed to coagulate, antibodies can be isolated from the serum fraction. Even when purified by recombination with the original antigen, immunoglobulin gamma molecules produced in this way vary slightly.

IDENTICAL ANTIBODY-LIKE MOLECULES are produced in large numbers by mice and humans who suffer from myelomatosis, a cancer of the cells that synthesize immunoglobulin. These abnormal immunoglobulins, all alike, can be isolated from the animal's blood (*left*). Often an abnormal protein also appears in the urine (*right*). Called a Bence-Jones protein, it seems to be the light chain of the abnormal immunoglobulin.

cipitate with it. Each F*ab* fragment carries one combining site; thus the two fragments together account for the two combining sites that each antibody molecule had been deduced to possess. The F*c* fragment prepared from rabbit immunoglobulin gamma crystallizes readily, but neither the F*ab* fragments nor the whole molecule has ever been crystallized.

Since crystals form easily only from identical molecules, it was guessed that the halves of the heavy chain that comprise the F*c* fragment are probably the same in all molecules and that the complexity is mainly in the F*ab* fragments where the combining sites are found. The enzyme papain, which causes the split into three pieces, can hydrolyze a

great variety of peptide bonds, and yet only a few in the middle of the heavy chain are in fact split; it looks as if in the F*ab* and F*c* fragments the peptide chains are tightly coiled in such a way that the enzyme cannot gain access. This suggests a picture in which three compact parts of the molecule are joined by a short flexible section near the middle of the heavy chain.

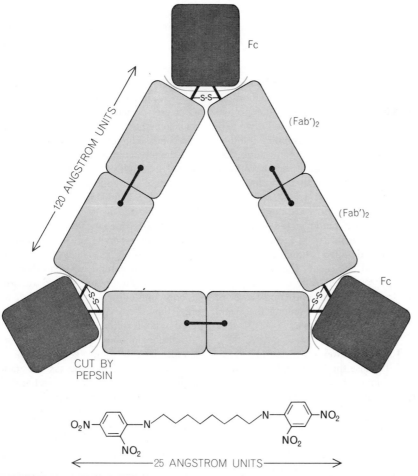

ANTIBODY-ANTIGEN COMPLEX seen in electron micrographs (*below and page 31*) is thought to have this triangular structure. Below it, drawn to a large scale, is the synthetic antigen: an eight-carbon chain with a dinitrophenyl group at each end. Three such antigen molecules appear able to bind together three immunoglobulin gamma molecules.

The full structure of a protein molecule showing the arrangement in space of the peptide chains and the positioning of the amino acids along them can at present only be achieved by X-ray crystallography. Such work has been started at Johns Hopkins University with the F*c* fragment. Electron microscopy, however, can provide much information about the shape of protein molecules, and successful electron microscope studies have been made recently with rabbit antibodies. When the antibodies are free, no clear pictures are obtained, which suggests that the molecules have a loose structure that is without definite shape. If they are combined with antigen, however, good pictures can be made. Michael Green and Robin Valentine of the National Institute for Medical Research in London prepared antibodies in rabbits that would combine with a benzene derivative known as a dinitrophenyl group. This can be done, as Karl Landsteiner showed many years ago, by injecting into the rabbit a protein on which dinitrophenyl groups have been substituted. Antibodies are formed, some of which combine specifically with the substituent dinitrophenyl coupled onto other proteins or into smaller molecules.

Green and Valentine investigated the smallest compound carrying two dinitrophenyl groups that would cross-link two or more antibody molecules. This proved to be an eight-carbon chain with a dinitrophenyl group at each end. This material does not form a precipitate with antibody, but with the electron microscope one can see ringlike structures that appear to contain three to five antibody molecules [*see illustrations on page 31 and at left*]. The small antigen molecule is not visible. The three-component structure is believed to consist of three antibody molecules linked by three molecules of invisible antigen. The lumps protruding from the corners are thought to be F*c* fragments. This interpretation is supported by using the proteolytic enzyme pepsin to digest off the F*c* fragment, leaving two F*ab* molecules held together by a disulfide bond and referred to as (F*ab'*)$_2$. When these (F*ab'*)$_2$ molecules are combined

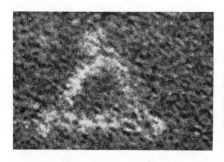
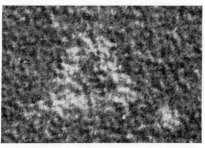

EFFECT OF PEPSIN COMPLEX is demonstrated in electron micrographs taken by Green and Valentine. In the normal complex formed by immunoglobulin gamma and the dinitrophenyl compound (*left*) a typical triangular structure contains a small lobe, or lump, at each corner, which is thought to be the F*c* part of the immunoglobulin molecule. If the antibody is first treated with pepsin, which splits off the F*c* fragment, the remaining (F*ab'*)$_2$ molecule still reacts with the antigen but the corner lobes are missing (*right*).

with antigen, rings are formed as before, but the lumps at the corners are now gone, confirming the idea that they were indeed the F*c* part of the molecule.

Since most interest centers on the antibody combining site, the next problem to solve is whether the site is to be found in the light chain, which is entirely in the F*ab* fragment, or in the half of the heavy chain that is also present, or whether the site is formed by both chains together. It has not been possible to get a clear answer to this problem because the chains cannot be separated except in acid or urea solutions; this causes a partial loss of the affinity for antigen, which is not recovered even after the acid or urea is removed. Present evidence suggests that the heavy chain is the most important but that the light chain plays a role. This may be because it actually forms a part of the site or because it helps to stabilize the shape that the heavy chain assumes and hence plays a secondary role that may be only partially specific.

In any case, the field is clear for a direct attempt at comparative studies of the chemical structure of the light chain as well as of the half of the heavy chain that lies in the F*ab* part of the molecule. The shape and hence the specificity of the combining site must depend on the configuration of the peptide chains of the F*ab* fragment; this is believed to be determined only by the sequence of the different amino acids in the chain. Therefore it is reasonable to expect that if the amino acid sequence is worked out for the F*ab* half of the heavy chain and perhaps also for the light chain, then in some sections sequences will be found that determine the configuration of the combining site and that will be characteristic for each antibody specificity. Attempts to carry out such sequence studies, however, seemed unattractive because of convincing evidence that all preparations of immunoglobulin gamma—even samples of purified antibodies obtained by precipitation with a specific antigen—were actually mixtures of many slightly different molecules with presumably different amino acid sequences.

Although the complexity of immunoglobulin gamma (and of the other classes of immunoglobulins) has presented investigators with a most difficult puzzle, considerable progress has now been made in solving much of it [*see illustration on this page*]. First, there are two kinds of light chain, named kappa and lambda, but in any one molecule both light chains are of the same type.

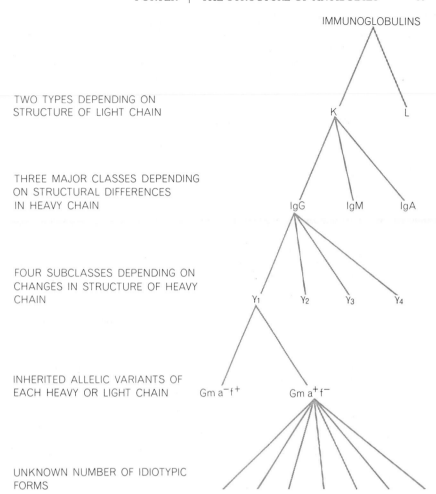

IMMUNOGLOBULINS

TWO TYPES DEPENDING ON STRUCTURE OF LIGHT CHAIN — K   L

THREE MAJOR CLASSES DEPENDING ON STRUCTURAL DIFFERENCES IN HEAVY CHAIN — IgG   IgM   IgA

FOUR SUBCLASSES DEPENDING ON CHANGES IN STRUCTURE OF HEAVY CHAIN — Y₁   Y₂   Y₃   Y₄

INHERITED ALLELIC VARIANTS OF EACH HEAVY OR LIGHT CHAIN — Gm a⁻f⁺   Gm a⁺f⁻

UNKNOWN NUMBER OF IDIOTYPIC FORMS

SUBDIVISIONS OF HUMAN IMMUNOGLOBULIN presented investigators with a difficult problem to unravel. For simplicity, subdivisions are shown for only one branch at each level. The abbreviation "*IgG*" stands for immunoglobulin gamma, the antibody found in largest amounts and the one most easily isolated. Idiotypic forms are apparently unique to individual animals and may involve alterations in both the light and the heavy chains.

The molecules containing kappa chains are known as *K* type and those with lambda chains as *L* type. Then in some species (probably in all) the immunoglobulin gamma class contains several subclasses; four have been identified in human gamma globulin. The subclasses differ in their heavy chains, which carry not only the characteristic features of the class but also small differences that distinguish the subclasses. In any one individual, molecules will be found of both *K* and *L* type, and they belong to all the subclasses. In addition each of the kinds of chain shows differences, known as allelic forms, that are inherited according to Mendelian principles. In an individual homozygous for this property only one allelic form of, say, the kappa chain will be present, but in a heterozygous individual there will be two forms of the kappa chain. It scarcely need be stressed that all these phenomena lead to a very complex mixture of molecules of immunoglobulin gamma in the serum of any

individual. Yet there is still another kind of complexity termed idiotypic. In certain circumstances it is possible for an animal to synthesize antibody molecules that are unique to itself, distinct from other antibody molecules of the same specificity in other individuals of the same species—and distinct from all other immunoglobulins in its own blood.

Perhaps the most remarkable aspect of all of this is that the complexity seems to bear no relation to the structure of the antibody combining site. As far as we know at present, any antibody specificity may be found on any of these many different kinds of molecule.

All such variations are likely to be based on differences in amino acid sequence, and already some differences relating to subclass and allelic changes have been identified. The structural differences are so small, however, that it is not possible to separate out single kinds of molecule by the methods available for the fractionation of proteins.

Thus it was a great step forward when it was recognized that in certain forms of cancer, immunoglobulin molecules of apparently a single variety appear in the blood. Such immunoglobulins have only one type of light chain and one subclass of heavy chain, and each chain belongs to one or the other allelic form. As far as we know each chain has only one amino acid sequence and therefore belongs to only one idiotypic form.

The disease responsible for this unique production of antibody is known as myelomatosis. Observed in both mice and men, it is a cancer of the cells that synthesize immunoglobulin, often those in the bone marrow. Apparently a single cell, one of the great number that synthesize immunoglobulins, starts to divide rapidly and leads to an excessive production of a single kind

of immunoglobulin. This provides evidence, incidentally, that the complexity of immunoglobulin molecules arises from their synthesis by many different kinds of cells. These abnormal immunoglobulins are known as myeloma proteins. Because they are often present in the blood in a concentration several times higher than all the other immunoglobulins together, they can be isolated rather easily.

Moreover, in about half of all myeloma patients an abnormal protein appears in the urine in large amounts. This substance was first observed by Henry Bence-Jones at Guy's Hospital in London in 1847 and has been known ever since as Bence-Jones protein. Its nature, however, was not recognized until five years ago, when Gerald M. Edelman and J. A. Gally of Rockefeller University and independently Frank W.

Putnam of the University of Florida showed that Bence-Jones protein is probably identical with the light chains of the myeloma protein in the serum of the same patient. Because Bence-Jones proteins can be obtained easily, without any inconvenience to the patient, they were the first materials used for amino-acid-sequence studies.

Although complete sequences have been worked out for only two Bence-Jones proteins in the mouse and only three human Bence-Jones proteins, perhaps 20 more have been partially analyzed. A remarkable fact has emerged. It seems that all Bence-Jones proteins of the same type have exactly the same sequence of amino acids in the half of the molecule that ends in the chemical group COOH (hence known as the C-terminal half) but show marked variation in the half that ends in the group

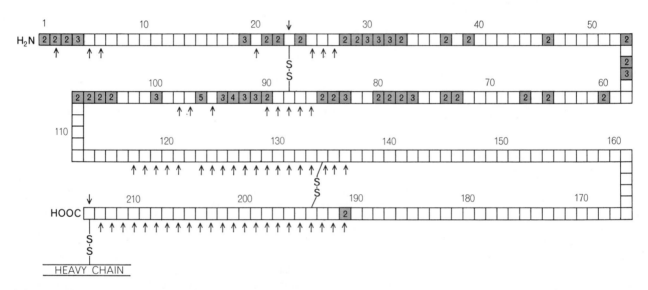

IMMUNOGLOBULIN LIGHT CHAIN, represented by analyses of human Bence-Jones proteins of the *K* type, has 214 amino acid units. Colored squares show where amino acids have been found to vary from one protein to another; blank squares show where no variation has yet been found. Numbers in the squares indicate how many different amino acids have been identified so far at a given site. Arrows mark positions where a particular amino acid has been found in at least five different proteins. Complete amino acid sequences are now known for three human Bence-Jones proteins and partial sequences for about 20 others. All variations occur in the first half of the chain with one exception, the variation at position 191. This is related to the allelic, or inherited, character of light *K* chains, hence differs from the alterations in the variable half of the chain. The diagram is based on one recently published by S. Cohen of Guy's Hospital Medical School in London and C. Milstein of the Laboratory of Molecular Biology in Cambridge.

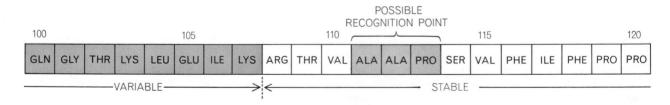

ALA	ALANINE	LYS	LYSINE
ARG	ARGININE	PHE	PHENYL-
GLN	GLUTAMINE		ALANINE
GLU	GLUTAMIC ACID	PRO	PROLINE
GLY	GLYCINE	SER	SERINE
ILE	ISOLEUCINE	THR	THREONINE
LEU	LEUCINE	VAL	VALINE

MIDDLE PART OF LIGHT CHAIN, as determined for one human Bence-Jones protein (*K* type), includes the amino acids at positions 111, 112 and 113 that are common to both *K*- and *L*-type Bence-Jones proteins of humans and to *K*-type Bence-Jones proteins of mice. It has been suggested that the section of the gene coding for this sequence may provide a special "recognition point" for the joining of two different genes responsible for the variable and stable sections of the light chain or, possibly, for bringing into play a mechanism to change the amino acid sequence in the variable section (*see illustration on page 38*).

NH₂ (the N-terminal half). Of 107 amino acid positions in this half, at least 40 have been found to vary. No two Bence-Jones proteins have yet been found to be identical in the N-terminal half, so that the possibility of molecular variation is clearly great. Given the possibility of variation at 40 sites and supposing that only two different amino acids can occupy these sites, it would be possible to construct 2^{40}, or more than 10 billion, different sequences. Actually as many as five different amino acids have been found to occupy one of the variable sites [*see upper illustration on opposite page*].

The amino acid sequence studies of the heavy chain are less advanced than those with the Bence-Jones proteins because the material is more difficult to obtain and is more than twice the length. Results with the heavy chain of two human myeloma proteins, however, have shown them to have many differences in sequence for more than 100 amino acids from the N-terminal end, whereas the remainder of the chain appears to be identical in both cases. Accordingly it seems certain that the heavy chains will show the same phenomena as the light chains; it is possible that the length of the variable section in both chains will be similar.

Inasmuch as both variable sections are in the F*ab* fragment of the molecule it seems obvious that these sections must participate in creating the many different antibody combining sites. All the work discussed here has been done with myeloma proteins, and since each has a single amino acid sequence in both heavy and light chains, it would follow that each will be a specific antibody against one of an untold number of different antigenic sites. The chances, therefore, of finding a myeloma protein in which antibody specificity is directed to a known, well-defined antigenic site seemed small. Nevertheless, several myeloma proteins have recently been found to possess antibody-like activity against known antigens. A comparison of the sequences of their heavy and light chains may give a lead as to where the combining site is located.

It has been believed with good reason that myeloma proteins are typical of normal molecules of immunoglobulin gamma, each being a homogeneous example of the many different forms present. It thus seemed likely that any attempt to determine the amino acid sequence of immunoglobulin gamma from a normal animal would be impossible, especially in the variable region that is

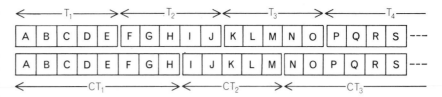

DETERMINATION OF AMINO ACID SEQUENCE in the polypeptide chains of proteins depends on the use of enzymes that cleave the chains into short fragments next to particular amino acids. The sequence in the resulting fragments can then be established. Thus trypsin might split a chain into fragments T_1, T_2, T_3 and T_4. Another enzyme, chymotrypsin, might split the same chain into fragments CT_1, CT_2 and CT_3. Since these fragments must overlap one can establish their order unequivocally and thereby the sequence of the entire chain.

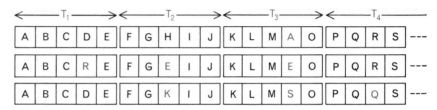

IMMUNOGLOBULIN SEQUENCE should be amenable to analysis even though a particular antibody sample might contain a variety of slightly different molecules. Slight variations at certain positions (*color*) should not prevent the ordering of similar fragments.

of particular interest. One would expect normal immunoglobulin gamma to be a mixture of many thousands of different molecules, each with a different sequence in the variable region.

Amino acid sequences of polypeptide chains are found by using enzymes to break the chains into pieces from 10 to 20 amino acids long. It is then possible to work out the sequence of each piece. By using different enzymes the original chain can be broken at different places, with the result that some pieces overlap. This provides enough clues for the whole sequence to be put together, rather like a one-dimensional jigsaw puzzle [*see upper illustration above*]. When the protein is pure, there is only one order of amino acids possible, and all the sequences of the individual fragments will fit into it.

One can see that if this method were attempted with a protein that was in fact a mixture of many slightly different proteins, each with a different sequence, a hopelessly confusing picture would probably result. The work with the myeloma protein suggested, however, that there would be a constant part as well as a variable part, and it seemed worthwhile to see what progress could be made in determining at least the constant part. Work at Duke University showed that the whole of the Fc section of the heavy chain of normal rabbit immunoglobulin gamma gave a coherent sequence and was therefore part of the stable section, as had been expected. Recent work in our laboratory has now

shown that the coherence continues well into the other half of the heavy chain. Although the work is far from complete, it seems possible that a full sequence will be established right through the entire heavy chain. Variations have been picked up in a number of positions and no doubt many more will be found, but the results are not completely confusing, as might have been expected if normal immunoglobulin gamma were a mixture of many thousands of myeloma proteins, each with substantially different sequences in the variable parts of the chain. The conflict between the results with the myeloma proteins and the recent results with normal rabbit immunoglobulin may be more apparent than real.

What does all this mean in terms of the structure of antibodies and their power to combine specifically with antigens? The phenomenon of a variable section and a stable section in both heavy and light chains is extraordinary and is unique to immunoglobulins; the variable section is in the part of the molecule known to contain the combining site. It therefore seems certain that this must be the basis of the specific configuration of the combining site.

It should be emphasized that all this work is very incomplete. In another year or so it will undoubtedly be much easier to see just how different one myeloma protein is from another in both the heavy and the light chains. It may be that the differences between any two

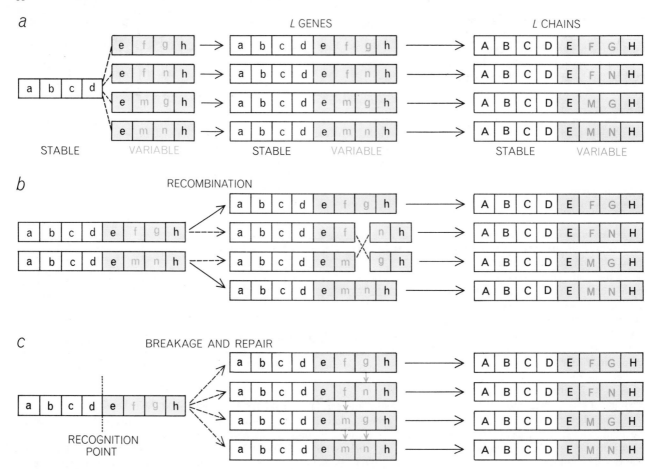

a

L GENES   L CHAINS

STABLE   VARIABLE   STABLE   VARIABLE   STABLE   VARIABLE

b   RECOMBINATION

c   BREAKAGE AND REPAIR

RECOGNITION POINT

VARIABILITY OF IMMUNOGLOBULIN MOLECULES has been explained by three principal hypotheses. The simplest (*a*) suggests that one gene codes for the stable section of each chain and that a great number, perhaps hundreds of thousands, code for the variable section. A second idea (*b*) is that several genes are divided into stable and variable sections and that the latter inter- change parts during cell division. A third proposal (*c*) suggests that there may be a recognition point in the gene (*see lower il- lustration on page 8*) and that an enzyme partially splits, or breaks, the gene on the variable side of that point. When repaired by other enzymes (*arrows*), mistakes are made, thus giving rise to many different amino acid sequences in the antibody molecule.

will on the average be small, so that for a mixture of many molecules the amino acid in any one position will be common to 80 or 90 percent of the molecules [*see lower illustration on page 37*]. Presum- ably this explains how it is possible to find a comprehensible amino acid sequence in normal immunoglobulin gamma.

It may also be, however, that myelo- ma proteins are not quite typical of nor- mal antibodies. Because they are the result of a disease they may exaggerate a normal phenomenon. Although they are invaluable in drawing attention to a fundamental mechanism, they may mis- lead us by exhibiting greater variability than is present in normal immunoglobu- lin gamma.

Whatever the answer, the existence of a stable section and a variable section, which has been shown so clearly in the Bence-Jones proteins and which also oc- curs in the heavy chains, is a remarkable phenomenon. The mechanism of its bio- logical origin has aroused intense in- terest. Many hypotheses have been put forward, but there are perhaps three

principal ones [*see illustration above*].

A straightforward mechanism would be to have a single gene coding for each stable section in the antibody molecule and as many genes as necessary (tens of thousands or hundreds of thousands) coding for the variable sections. The cell would also be provided with a means for fusing the product of the two kinds of gene to construct the complete immunoglobulin molecule. (In this as in the other suggestions, the presence of an antigen would somehow trigger pro- duction of the appropriate antibody.)

A second proposal invokes the con- cept of genetic recombination, which involves the exchange of parts of genes. One can imagine several genes that are divided into a stable portion and a vari- able portion. During cell division, when genes are pairing and duplicating, the variable portion would interchange sec- tions, thereby giving rise to many dif- ferent genes capable of coding the vari- able parts of the antibody molecule.

The third suggestion visualizes that the gene for, say, the light chain may

contain a "recognition point" midway in its structure [*see lower illustration on page 36*]. This might provide a specific attachment site for an enzyme that can split the nucleic acid of the gene only on the side coding for the variable section. When the broken portion is repaired by other enzymes, mistakes are made, there- by giving rise to many different se- quences of nucleotides—the nucleic acid building blocks that embody the genetic message. These differences are then translated into different amino acid se- quences in the variable portion of the antibody molecule.

There is no clear answer as to which methods, if any or all, are the operative mechanisms, but a continuation of the structural studies may provide a clearer understanding. When this understand- ing is attained, it should lead to ideas about how to change, stimulate or sup- press immune reactions as medical practice requires and therefore should be of great practical value as well as solving one of the most intriguing prob- lems in biology.

The Structure and Function of Antibodies

by Gerald M. Edelman
August 1970

The complete amino acid sequence of an immunoglobulin molecule has been determined, defining the structure of antibodies and providing information on their evolution and differentiation and how they work

"Immunity" is an everyday word, ordinarily applied to the elaborate set of responses by which the body defends itself against invading microorganisms or foreign tissues. There is much more to immunity than its clinical aspects, however. What we have come to know about the immune system and its key molecules, antibodies, makes it apparent that immunology bears directly on some very fundamental problems: the nature of the mechanisms whereby molecules recognize one another, the manner in which genes are expressed in higher organisms and the origin of a variety of disease states, including cancer. In one way or another the solution of these deep problems will require an understanding of the structure of antibody molecules.

Antibodies have been known since the classic studies of Emil von Behring in the late 19th century. Only recently, however, have we begun to understand how vertebrate organisms recognize the sometimes subtle chemical differences between their own molecules and foreign molecules, which are termed antigens. Our insights rest on three serial developments. The first was the demonstration by Karl Landsteiner in 1917 that animals could form antibodies against certain small organic chemicals of known structure. By manipulating and modifying these "haptens," Landsteiner and others showed that antibodies distinguish among different antigens by recognizing differences in their shape. Moreover, the early studies implied that the number of different antibodies any single animal can make must be very large indeed. If an animal could make antibodies that could specifically bind a synthetic hapten the animal or its ancestors had never encountered before in nature, it seemed likely that the animal could make antibodies to almost any foreign antigen. Further work has largely supported this inference: most vertebrates are indeed capable of making many thousands of different antibodies. The second fundamental development was the bold idea of selective immunity advanced in the late 1950's by Niels K. Jerne and Sir Macfarlane Burnet, who proposed that the body already has all the information for making any of its antibodies *before* it ever encounters an antigen. The third development was the analysis of the structure of antibodies, which has taken place largely in the past decade. Before discussing this last development in detail, it will be useful to outline the seminal idea of selective immunity and some of the advances made by cellular immunologists.

The main notion, as implied above, is that the cells of the antibody-forming system have among them all the information they need to make any antibody molecule before they ever encounter any antigen. The antigen molecule does not instruct antibody-producing cells to shape the antibody molecule to fit it. Instead it selects cells that are already making antibodies that happen to fit. Then it stimulates those cells to make large quantities of the antibodies.

Antibodies can be likened to ready-made suits. The antigen is a buyer who decides to pick a number of different suits that fit more or less well rather than instruct a tailor to make one suit to fit him to order. To be well satisfied, the buyer must patronize a store with a very large stock of suits in a great variety of sizes and styles. The immune system is like a store with an almost unlimited stock, one ready to please any possible customer. This analogy fails in one important respect: to be complete it should provide that after each somewhat different ready-made suit is picked the manufacturer would proceed to make thousands of exact copies of it.

In a simplified picture of the cellular mechanisms corresponding to this selective response, each cell makes only one kind of antibody, which has an antigen-binding site of a particular shape [*see top illustration on page 41*]. Presumably that antibody is located at the cell surface. An antigen injected into the body "tries on" different shapes. If a particular antibody "fits" more or less well, the cell making it divides and matures. Its progeny then make many more copies of the identical kinds of antibody, which may then be released into the blood to carry out their function of defense or of tissue rejection. Notice that this is a form of molecular recognition machine and that the specificity of recognition rests both on the presentation of a variety of antibodies and on the capacity of the cells to "amplify" the results of a recognition event. How are these requirements accomplished at a molecular level? In order to answer that question satisfactorily we must know a good deal about the structure of the antibody molecule itself.

A decade ago a number of experimental observations began to shed light on the details of antibody structure. The advance came when the results of sophisticated protein chemistry and genetic analysis fitted together with a classical observation about the products of a certain cancer. At the Rockefeller Institute in 1959 I found that antibody molecules consisted of polypeptide chains, or protein subunits, of more than one kind, and that the chains could be separated from one another by chemical means and studied in detail. These chains were called light chains and heavy chains because of the difference in their size, or molecular weight. At the same time R. R. Porter, now at the University of Oxford, showed that the antibody molecule could be cut into three different pieces by enzymes that cleave polypeptide chains. Two of them, termed "fragment antigen binding" (F*ab*), were identical and would still combine with antigen. The third, "fragment crystalline" (F*c*), was quite different: it would not combine with antigen but could be crystallized readily [see "The Structure of Antibodies," by R. R. Porter, the article beginning on page 31]. The observations on the two polypeptide chains and on the two fragments were the starting point for a series of investigations in many laboratories into the details of antibody structure.

Antibodies, it was known, were a family of proteins with a number of properties in common, found in the gamma globulin fraction of the blood. Unlike all proteins whose structure had been determined, antibody molecules were known to be very "heterogeneous": no single sequence of amino acids—the building blocks of proteins—could represent the polypeptide chains of antibodies, as can be done, for example, in the case of a "homogeneous" protein such as insulin or hemoglobin. This fact, together with the large size of antibody molecules, made it infeasible to carry out detailed chemical analyses of such molecules or to determine exactly how antibodies that

bound to different antigens differed from one another. Fortunately the structural studies of the polypeptide chains of the immunoglobulin molecule led to a clue that made it possible to bypass the problem raised by the intrinsic heterogeneity of antibodies. The clue had to do with the nature of certain homogeneous proteins made by tumors of plasma cells, the cells that ordinarily produce the most antibodies.

Knowledge of these tumors goes back to 1847, when Henry Bence Jones, physician at St. George's Hospital in London, published a paper titled "On a new substance occurring in the Urine of a patient with Mollities Ossium." It

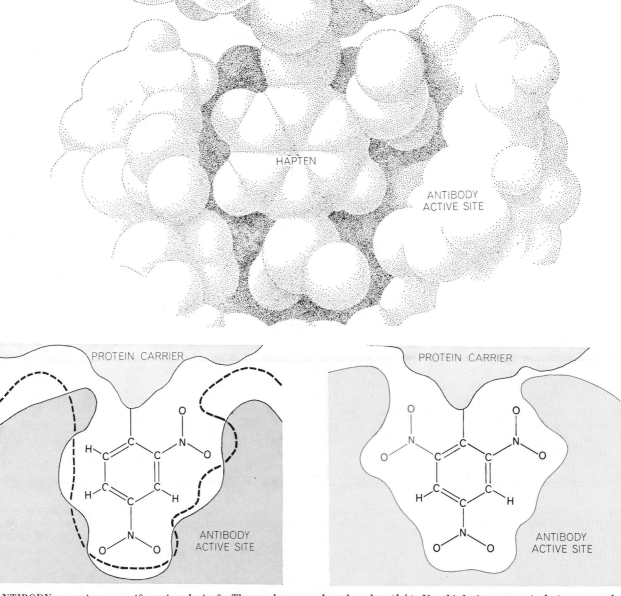

ANTIBODY recognizes a specific antigen by its fit. The top drawing shows the fit between the combining site on an antibody and a "hapten" antigen, a dinitrophenyl group, on a protein carrier. The bottom drawings show that two different antibody contours (*gray shape and black line*) can fit the dinitrophenyl group, one better than the other (*left*). If a third nitro group (*color*) were on the hapten (*right*), those two antibodies would not fit; a third antibody with a different antigen-combining site (*color*) would fit this picryl antigen. Because of picryl's similarity to dinitrophenyl, the third antibody would also fit the original hapten, but less precisely.

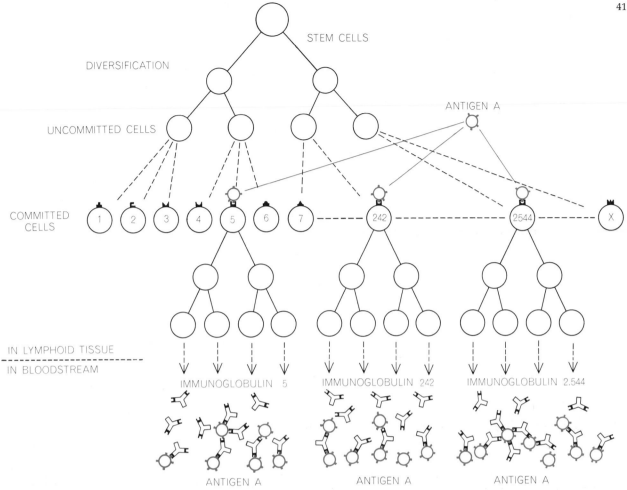

STEM CELLS

DIVERSIFICATION

UNCOMMITTED CELLS

ANTIGEN A

COMMITTED CELLS

1 2 3 4 5 6 7 242 2544 X

IN LYMPHOID TISSUE

IN BLOODSTREAM

IMMUNOGLOBULIN 5   IMMUNOGLOBULIN 242   IMMUNOGLOBULIN 2.544

ANTIGEN A   ANTIGEN A   ANTIGEN A

SELECTIVE-IMMUNITY THEORY holds that stem cells (precursors of antibody-producing cells) contain information for making all possible antibodies; at some point in embryonic development each is committed to producing a unique immunoglobulin (numbers). These receptor antibodies can interact with various antigens. A single antigen (color) may be recognized by more than one antibody-producing cell. Interaction of an antigen with a cell stimulates proliferation of the cell and the synthesis of antibody.

began as follows: "On the 1st of November 1845 I received from Dr. Watson the following note, with a test tube containing a thick, yellow, semi-solid substance:—'The tube contains urine of very high specific gravity; when boiled it becomes highly opake; on the addition of nitric acid it effervesces, assumes a reddish hue, becomes quite clear, but, as it cools, assumes the consistence and appearance which you see: heat reliquifies it. What is it?' "

Jones verified the peculiar thermosolubility properties of the protein, subjected it to a careful elementary analysis and concluded that it was the "hydrated deutoxide of albumin."

In succeeding years many attempts were made to answer Dr. Watson's question in a definitive way, but although some 700 papers on the subject appeared

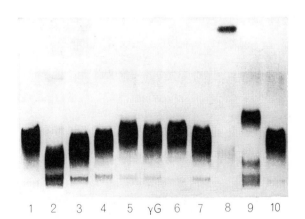

1 2 3 4 5 γG 6 7 8 9 10

MYELOMA PROTEINS from different patients are compared with a normal human immunoglobulin fraction by electrophoresis on a starch gel. The intact immunoglobulins migrate in approximately the same way (left). After dissociation into light and heavy chains

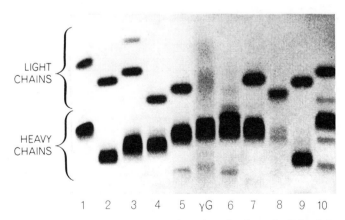

LIGHT CHAINS

HEAVY CHAINS

1 2 3 4 5 γG 6 7 8 9 10

(right) the myeloma proteins show sharp bands in the light-chain position but the normal protein shows a diffuse zone there because it is a heterogeneous mixture of immunoglobulins. Protein No. 8 is a Bence Jones protein and it therefore shows no heavy chain.

in the ensuing century, Bence Jones proteins remained a kind of medical and biochemical curiosity except in the domain of practical diagnosis: the demonstration of the protein in the urine called for a diagnosis of multiple myeloma, the malignant disease of plasma cells that was formerly called mollities ossium. This disease is usually associated with malignant proliferation of plasma cells, excessive production of serum gamma globulins called myeloma proteins, bone lesions, disturbances of calcium metabolism, kidney disorders and often, of course, excretion of the characteristic Bence Jones proteins.

It seemed that these proteins had something to do with immunoglobulins, but the exact relation remained obscure. The 1959 finding that immunoglobulins contained multiple polypeptide chains [see bottom illustration on preceding page] suggested that Bence Jones proteins were homogeneous light chains of the myeloma protein made by the tumor but not incorporated into whole molecules. This hypothesis was confirmed by my student Joseph A. Gally and me in 1962. Because different Bence Jones proteins had different amino acid compositions, we compared their properties with those of light chains of antibodies. These comparisons were instrumental in suggesting that antibodies with different antigen specificities differ from one another in the sequence of amino acids of which they are composed. Moreover, because the light chains produced by the myeloma tumors were pure, available in large amounts and smaller than a whole immunoglobulin molecule, it became possible to study the details of their chemical structure.

Once it had become apparent that these proteins might provide a clue to the nature of antibody variability, a number of laboratories undertook the task of determining their exact amino acid sequence. Since no two individuals produce the same Bence Jones proteins, each laboratory reported a different sequence, but from the first report of partial sequences by Norbert G. D. Hilschmann and Lyman C. Craig at Rockefeller University in 1965 it became clear that these proteins had a singular structure. Each molecule contained about 214 amino acids, linked together in a polypeptide chain. (The amino acids are numbered starting from the end of the molecule that is made first, the amino terminus.) From position 109 on various Bence Jones proteins had essentially the same sequence, and accordingly this part of the molecule was called the constant region. In striking contrast, the sequence of the first 108 amino acids differed markedly from one Bence Jones protein to another, and this first part of the chain was designated the variable region. Concurrent studies in several laboratories suggested that the heavy chains of myeloma proteins also had variable and constant regions. The homogeneity of the constant region enabled Robert L. Hill and his associates at Duke University to determine the amino acid sequence of the Fc fragment of rabbit immunoglobulin.

It was against this background that my colleagues and I decided to attempt the determination of the complete amino acid sequence of a whole immunoglobulin molecule. The earlier structural studies had suggested an overall picture and we wanted to confirm and extend it in detail so that we could apply it to an analysis of the origin and function of antibodies. We obtained a large amount of plasma from a patient with multiple myeloma, because it was essential to have enough of at least one myeloma protein. As a matter of fact, we obtained two different proteins from different patients for purposes of comparison. The difficulties of our project were related to the enormous size of the molecule, which has 19,996 atoms and is larger in terms of the number of unique amino acid sequences than any protein that had been determined up to that time. Our approach was based on the pioneering methods first developed by Frederick Sanger to analyze the insulin molecule, and the challenge, successfully met last year, was whether these methods would suffice.

The immunoglobulin molecule is about 25 times as large as insulin. If we could break the immunoglobulin molecule, its chains and its fragments into small pieces about the size of the insulin molecule itself, then we could use standard methods for determining amino acid sequence. A useful tool for such protein surgery had already been devised by Erhard Gross and Bernhard

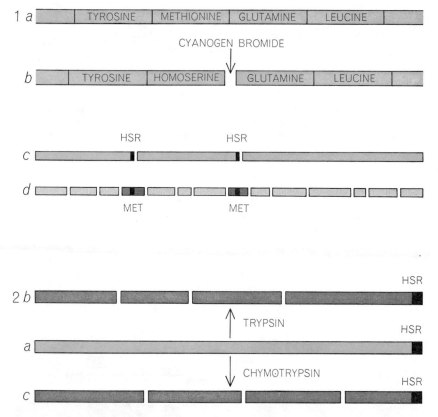

ANTIBODY CHAIN is cleaved by cyanogen bromide (CNBr) and the resulting fragments are ordered (1). The CNBr breaks a chain (a) at methionyl residues, which are converted into homoserine (b). To order CNBr fragments (c) the original chain is cleaved also with the enzyme trypsin, the tryptic fragments containing methionine are isolated (d) and their sequences are compared with those of the ends of the CNBr fragments. Then the amino acid sequence of each CNBr fragment must be determined (2). This is done by cleaving a CNBr fragment (a) with trypsin and determining the sequence of each tryptic peptide (b) by a chemical procedure. The tryptic peptides are ordered by comparison with the composition and partial sequences of different peptides (c) made by cleaving with chymotrypsin.

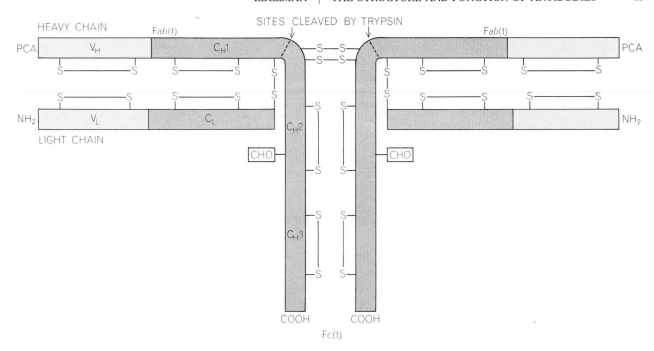

STRUCTURE of the immunoglobulin determined by the author and his colleagues shows two kinds of chain and regions in each. The protein can be cleaved into two antibody-binding fragments, Fab(t), and a "crystallizable" fragment, Fc(t). Sulfur-sulfur bonds are designated —S—S—. Light chains have variable and constant regions (V_L and C_L). Heavy chains have a variable region (V_H) and a constant region divisible into three homology regions (C_H1, C_H2 and C_H3). CHO indicates carbohydrate. Chains have amino (NH_2), carboxyl ($COOH$) and pyrollidonecarboxylic acid (PCA) ends. V_H and V_L are homologous, as are C_L, C_H1, C_H2 and C_H3.

Witkop of the National Institutes of Health. It depended on cyanogen bromide, a reagent that selectively cleaves polypeptide chains at the positions occupied by the sulfur-containing amino acid methionine; because there were just a small number of methionines in the molecule, we could expect a decently small number of pieces. With this reagent we were able to cleave the heavy chain of the immunoglobulin into seven pieces and the light chain into three pieces [*see illustration on preceding page*]. Each piece was then separated from the others by chromatography. A key procedure in these separations was molecular sieving on Sephadex, a technique developed largely by Jerker O. Porath of the University of Uppsala, which speeded up the thousands of separations required to determine the structure of immunoglobulin.

After the fractionation of the pieces the next step was to establish their order. This was done by cleaving the original chains not with cyanogen bromide but with enzymes that attack polypeptides at other specific sites. Those peptides that contained methionine and that would therefore overlap the cyanogen bromide fragments were then isolated. By comparing the two kinds of fragment we could see which ends of the cyanogen bromide fragments butted up against one another.

Each separate cyanogen bromide fragment could now be studied independently as if it were a separate small protein or polypeptide. Accordingly it was cleaved with enzymes into smaller peptides, which were separated. When small pure peptides were obtained, the sequence of their amino acids was determined directly by a chemical procedure. The order of the peptides was then established by breaking the whole cyanogen bromide fragment with a second enzyme that cleaved it at different sites and isolating a second set of peptides that overlapped the first set.

The sequence determination was thus a "two pass" procedure. In the first pass we obtained cyanogen bromide fragments and ordered them. In the second we treated each fragment as a separate protein, obtaining its peptides, ordering them and determining their amino acid sequence. When these tasks were finished, there remained the job of determining the location of the bonds between the sulfur atoms of the amino acid cysteine that helped to link the chains and parts of the chains together.

The completed structure showed that the antibody molecule differed from proteins that had been analyzed earlier not only in size but also in more unusual ways. Our molecule was what is classified as a γG, or gamma G, immunoglobulin molecule, an example of the most

prevalent class of immunoglobulins. As earlier studies had suggested, such a molecule consists of two identical light **and two identical heavy chains [*see illustration at top of page*]**. The structure is symmetrical, each half consisting of one light and one heavy chain. Although the actual shape or three-dimensional structure of the chains is not known, it is established that they are held together by weak forces and by interchain sulfur-sulfur bonds between corresponding pairs of cysteines; similar intrachain bonds are formed within each chain at approximately equal intervals. The most striking feature of the structure is its division into two kinds of region, variable regions and constant regions, whose disposition is related to these intervals. The length of the variable regions was determined by comparing the amino acid sequences of the light and the heavy chains to the sequences of Bence Jones proteins and to the sequence of another heavy chain that was analyzed concurrently. As in the Bence Jones proteins, the regions are so named because in different antibodies the variable regions differ in the sequence of amino acids that make up the chain, whereas the constant regions have the same sequence in each of the major classes of antibodies (except for a single variable amino acid at position 191). It has now been firmly established that it is the different sequences in the variable regions that give different shapes to various antigen-binding sites. The variety of shapes provides for a range of specific interactions with a great variety of antigens, including small molecules, other proteins, carbohydrates and even DNA itself.

There is another feature of the structure that merits notice. Detailed examination of the constant regions showed evidence of internal periodicity, which had already been hinted at by the distribution of the sulfur-sulfur bonds. Portions of the constant region of the heavy chain turn out to have homologous amino acid sequences, that is, sequences more similar than could occur by chance. These portions are designated C_H1, C_H2 and C_H3, and each is homologous also to the constant region of the light chain, C_L. It is these constant regions that carry out functions of the molecule other than the binding of antigens. For example, C_H2 is believed to be bound by members of a complex family of serum proteins known as complement, thus beginning the series of reactions that is capable of killing cells, one of the aspects of the immune response.

(The amino acid sequences of the variable and constant homology regions are presented below as a grid of three-letter codes. The following are best-effort readings.)

V_L (1 to 108):
ASP ILE GLN MET THR GLN SER PRO SER THR LEU SER ALA SER VAL GLY ASP ARG VAL THR ILE THR CYS ARG ALA SER GLN SER ILE SER ASN THR — — TRP LEU ALA TRP TYR GLN GLN LYS PRO GLY LYS ALA PRO LYS LEU LEU MET TYR LYS ALA SER —

V_H (1 to 114):
PCA VAL GLN LEU VAL GLN SER GLY — ALA GLY VAL LEU LEU PRO GLY SER SER VAL LEU VAL SER CYS LEU ALA SER GLY GLY THR PRO SER ALA SER ALA ILE ILE THR VAL ALA GLY ALA PRO GLY GLY GLY LEU GLY THR MET GLY GLY ILE VAL PRO MET PHE

C_L (109 to 214):
THR VAL ALA ALA PRO SER VAL PRO ILE PRO PRO PRO SER ALA GLY GLY — — LEU LEU SER GLY THR ALA SER VAL VAL CYS LEU LEU ALA ALA PRO THR PRO ALA GLY ALA LEU VAL — — GLY THR LEU VAL ALA ALA ALA LEU GLY SER GLY ALA SER GLY

C_H1 (119 to 220):
SER THR LEU GLY PRO SER VAL PRO PRO LEU ALA PRO SER SER LEU SER — — THR SER GLY GLY THR ALA ALA LEU GLY CYS LEU VAL LEU ALA THR PRO PRO GLY PRO VAL THR VAL — — SER THR ALA SER — GLY ALA LEU THR SER GLY — VAL HIS

C_H2 (234 to 341):
LEU LEU GLY GLY PRO SER VAL PRO LEU PRO PRO PRO LEU PRO LEU ALA THR LEU MET ILE SER ALA THR PRO GLY VAL THR CYS VAL VAL VAL ALA VAL SER HIS GLY ALA PRO GLY VAL LEU PRO ALA THR THR VAL ALA GLY — VAL GLY VAL HIS ALA ALA LYS

C_H3 (342 to 446):
GLY PRO ALA GLY PRO GLY VAL THR THR LEU PRO PRO PRO SER ALA GLY GLY — MET THR LEU ALA GLY VAL SER LEU THR CYS LEU VAL LEU GLY PRO THR PRO SER ALA ILE ALA VAL — — GLY THR GLY SER ALA ALA ASP — GLY GLY PRO GLY ALA THR LYS

AMINO ACID SEQUENCES of the variable regions (*top*) and of the constant homology regions (*bottom*) were fully determined. The extent of the homology between the two variable regions and among the four constant homology regions is indicated by the

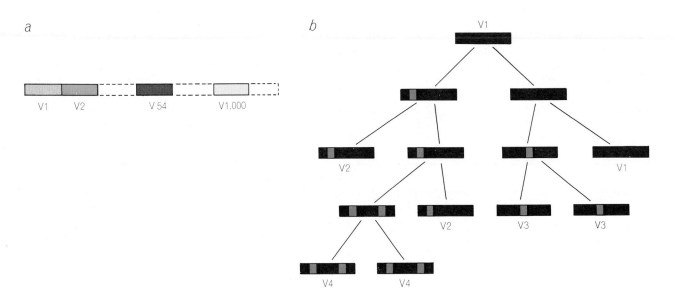

DIVERSITY of variable regions can be explained by three theories. A large number of genes, one for each variable region, could have arisen in the course of evolution (*a*). Alternatively, there could be one V gene, which mutates in an individual animal's body cells during development to produce the required variety (*b*). Finally, several V genes could evolve by mutation and be

The homology of the constant regions and the somewhat weaker homology of the variable regions to one another is demonstrated by directly comparing their amino acid sequences [*see chart at right and diagram just below*]. This is an unusual finding, and it means that the regions must be related in their evolutionary origins. It is likely that present-day antibodies have evolved by a process

ALA	ALANINE		LEU	LEUCINE
ARG	ARGININE		LYS	LYSINE
ASN	ASPARAGINE		MET	METHIONINE
ASP	ASPARTIC ACID		PCA	PYROLLIDONECARBOXYLIC ACID
CYS	CYSTEINE		PHE	PHENYLALANINE
GLN	GLUTAMINE		PRO	PROLINE
GLU	GLUTAMIC ACID		SER	SERINE
GLY	GLYCINE		THR	THREONINE
HIS	HISTIDINE		TRP	TRYPTOPHAN
ILE	ISOLEUCINE		TYR	TYROSINE
			VAL	VALINE

[Amino acid sequence comparison charts with residue positions numbered 60, 70, 80, 90, 100 (upper set) and 170, 180, 190, 200, 210 (lower set).]

coloring or shading of identical residues in each position; dark and light shading indicates identities that occur in pairs at one position.

Gaps have been introduced to maximize the homology. The numbering across the top is that of positions of residues in light chains.

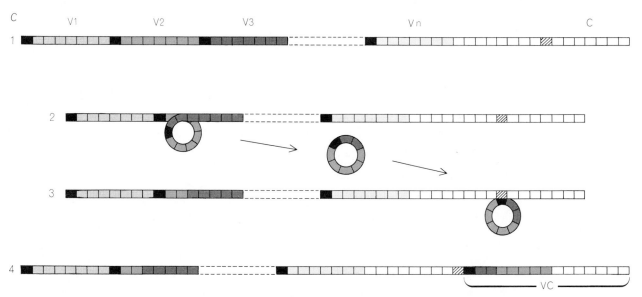

selected during evolution, and then be recombined in many different ways in the animal (*c*). In this process the evolved genes (*1*) might recombine to form a ring-shaped V-gene episome (*2*), a variant gene composed of sequences from adjacent V genes. The episome might be translocated and become integrated with the C gene (*3*) to form the complete VC gene that is expressed (*4*).

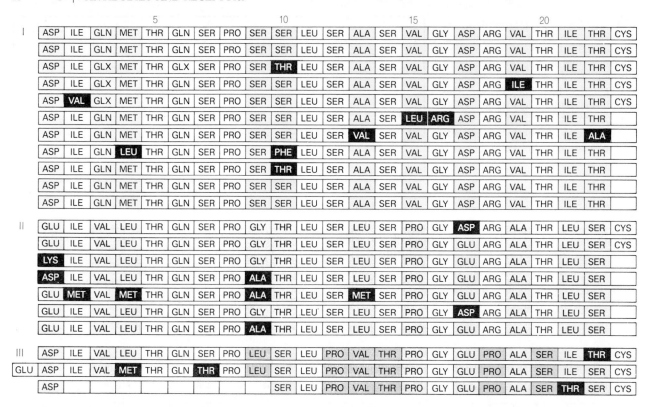

PATTERN OF VARIATION of three different subgroups of one class of light-chain variable regions yields clues to their genetic origin. Each line represents a partial sequence (the first 23 residues) determined in the laboratories of H. D. Niall and P. Edman, C. Milstein, Norbert G. D. Hilschmann, Frank W. Putnam or Lee Hood. Each subgroup (*roman numerals*) has a characteristic sequence, indicated in each case by a dominant color or shade of gray. Within each subgroup there are variations (*black*) that arose from mutations. (*GLX* refers to positions where it was not yet definitely established whether the residue was glutamic acid or glutamine.)

known as gene duplication. A primitive gene of a size sufficient to specify one homology region must have doubled and tripled, thereby forming a larger gene whose segments then became somewhat different from one another, as reflected in the sequences. By a similar process the genes for the two kinds of chain, heavy and light, appear to have had a common ancestor. This hypothesis, which was first suggested by Hill at Duke and S. Jonathan Singer of the University of California at San Diego, is strongly supported by the structure of the whole molecule.

A comparison of the variable regions with the four constant homology regions shows that although they have roughly the same length, they have few sequences in common. Did they also arise from the same original gene? Probably, far back in evolution, but if so, they must have diverged rapidly as they carried out different functions of the antibody. Indeed, studies by C. Milstein of the Medical Research Council in England and by Lee Hood of the National Institutes of Health indicate that in each individual there must be more than one gene for each variable (V) region. Earli-

er, pioneering genetic investigations by Jacques Oudin of the Pasteur Institute and by Rune Grubb of the University of Lund had laid the groundwork for the conclusion that there is only one gene for each constant (C) region. Since the polypeptide chains of antibodies appear to be made in one piece, as are other proteins, it seems that information from two genes is required to specify a single polypeptide chain. This is a unique situation, because in all proteins that have so far been investigated a single gene is enough to specify a single polypeptide chain.

The analysis of antibodies, then, poses two special problems: How can the V genes vary so that many different V regions are made in each individual? And how can such a V gene, which evolved to give the antibody system a range of different combining sites, be joined with a C gene that evolved to specify the constant portions of the chains and thus carry out effector functions?

Before attempting to suggest answers to these questions, let us look at the actual variation seen in V regions [*see illustration at top of page*]. The varia-

tion has several important characteristics. First, the genetic-code dictionary (in which each amino acid is coded for by a triplet of three DNA nucleotides) reveals that the variation arises from onebase changes in the code words for the amino acids in each variable position. This means that the variations were caused by mutations, just as in the case of other proteins. Second, not every position in the V region varies. For example, no one has ever observed that any of the cysteines that contribute to the sulfur bonds are missing or replaced by another amino acid. Third, certain positions seem to have more variations than others, although the number of examples is still too small for one to be completely sure of this. These last two observations mean that the variation is not random but is the result of some kind of selection. We can conclude that, as in other proteins, both mutation and selection are responsible for antibody variation.

The question about the origin of variability can be resolved into two more pointed questions. They are: Where and when do these processes occur? How many V genes are required? One theory suggests that the variation and selection occur during evolution, so that in an animal each different V region has a corresponding V gene. This would require a very large number of V genes in the germ cells. Another theory states that there is one V gene, which mutates not during evolution but somatically—in the body cells of the individual animal—and that the mutant cells are somehow selected. A third theory, which I favor, is that there are a few V genes, which have mutated and have been selected in evolution but which then recombine somatically in the cells of the animal to provide the broad variational pattern. This last theory has the advantage that the same processes that recombine the V genes could also accomplish the fusion of V and C genes that is required to make a single antibody chain; one can thus account with one mechanism for the two questions: How is antibody diversity created? How are V and C genes joined?

The mechanism may be one that is somewhat similar to mechanisms that have already been described for infection of the bacterium *Escherichia coli* by the bacterial virus lambda. A piece of DNA (a V gene) could be removed from a row of V genes (each having evolved to be slightly different) and could then be inserted and fused with a C gene. If the DNA is removed as a ring, the process would effectively permute the sequence, leading to variation [*see bottom illustration on pages 44 and 45*]. As mentioned above, the alternative somatic theory is that a single V gene is mutated and then translocated, following which the cell making the VC product is selected for or against within the body. Which of these theories is correct remains to be defined, but both theories require a process of assembly of a VC gene from separate V and C genes. This requirement suggests that it may be by the translocation of genes that the cell achieves its goal of making just one kind of immunoglobulin. Molecular differentiation of this type is so far unique to the immune system, but it may in fact turn out to be important in other systems of differentiation among higher organisms.

Although the molecular details of the mechanism of translocation and recombination remain hypothetical, there is some recent evidence that we are on the right track in concluding that antibody variation is somatic in origin. The evidence comes from studies of the genetics of mouse immunoglobulins done with my student Paul D. Gottlieb. These

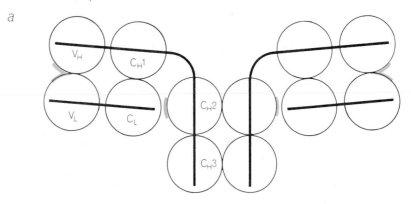

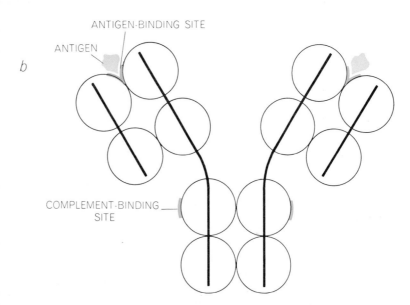

BINDING OF ANTIGEN may stabilize a change in the shape of the antibody that triggers a series of immune reactions. Here the antibody is drawn as a flexible grouping of compact domains, with the chain structure suggested by the heavy black lines (*a*). The antigen is bound by the variable regions, perhaps facilitating a pivoting movement of the molecule that exposes effector sites, such as the complement-binding site, in the C regions (*b*).

experiments are still in their early stages, however, and the actual mechanism of variation has so far not been demonstrated.

The origin of the required diversity and the restriction of that diversity to one kind of antibody for each cell seem to be mirrored in the structure of the antibody molecule. What does antibody structure tell us about how these molecules actually carry out their functions? It is clear that antibodies have two kinds of task: first, recognizing the antigen, and second, doing something to the antigen or initiating a chain of cellular responses. The task of antigen-binding is delegated to the V regions. The more dynamic role of influencing cellular responses, the binding of complement and the initiation of processes that alter the antigen appears to be the function of the

C regions. In some sense the antibody molecule must behave as a switch: binding the antigen must change the antibody's state in such a way as to "turn on" its effector functions. It is known that protein molecules can act as switches by changing their shape. There is now a hint that this may be the case for antibodies. When antibodies are viewed in the electron microscope after combination with antigens, their dimensions appear to be smaller than those of unbound immunoglobulins measured by X-ray scattering in solution. This raises the possibility that the binding of the antigen causes a rearrangement of the structure of the antibody molecule, which is known to be somewhat flexible. The rearrangement might consist, for example, of a pivoting movement involving part of the constant region of the heavy chains [*see illustration on preceding page*]. Binding sites for complement might be exposed by this pivoting, as well as other sites for different effector functions. Similar mechanisms may be involved in triggering the antibody-producing cell to divide and mature.

As these hypotheses indicate, much remains to be done in the field of antibody structure. What has been learned indicates that the antibody system is special and that it may have evolved to solve its problem of molecular recognition in a unique way. There remains the intriguing possibility, however, that the special genetic mechanisms hinted at by the differentiation of antibody-producing cells will be found in other systems of cellular differentiation; certainly there are at least conceptual similarities to some other systems of pattern recognition, such as those of the central nervous system. In any event, whether the immune system turns out to be unique or representative of a more general type of evolutionary development, we can expect practical consequences of great significance for fields of study such as immune tolerance, organ transplantation and autoimmune disease to flow from a continuing analysis of the structure of antibodies.

The Immune System

by Niels Kaj Jerne
July 1973

This diffuse organ has the assignment of monitoring the identity of the body. Its basic constituents are lymphocytes and antibody molecules, which recognize both foreign molecules and one another

The immune system is comparable in the complexity of its functions to the nervous system. Both systems are diffuse organs that are dispersed through most of the tissues of the body. In man the immune system weighs about two pounds. It consists of about a trillion (10^{12}) cells called lymphocytes and about 100 million trillion (10^{20}) molecules called antibodies that are produced and secreted by the lymphocytes. The special capability of the immune system is pattern recognition and its assignment is to patrol the body and guard its identity.

The cells and molecules of the immune system reach most tissues through the bloodstream, entering the tissues by penetrating the walls of the capillaries. After moving about they make their way to a return vascular system of their own, the lymphatic system [*see illustration on page 51*]. The tree of lymphatic vessels collects lymphocytes and antibodies, along with other cells and molecules and the interstitial fluid that bathes all the body's tissues, and pours its contents back into the bloodstream by joining the subclavian veins behind the collarbone. Lymphocytes are found in high concentrations in the lymph nodes, way stations along the lymphatic vessels, and at the sites where they are manufactured and processed: the bone marrow, the thymus and the spleen.

The immune system is subject to continuous decay and renewal. During the few moments it took you to read this far your body produced 10 million new lymphocytes and a million billion new antibody molecules. This might not be so astonishing if all these antibody molecules were identical. They are not. Millions of different molecules are required to cope with the task of pattern recognition, just as millions of different keys are required to fit millions of different locks.

The specific patterns that are recognized by antibody molecules are epitopes: patches on the surface of large molecules such as proteins, polysaccharides and nucleic acids. Molecules that display epitopes are called antigens. It is hardly possible to name a large molecule that is not an antigen. Let us consider protein molecules, which include enzymes, hormones, transport molecules such as hemoglobin and the great variety of molecules that are incorporated in cellular membranes or form the outer coat of viruses or bacteria.

Antigens and Antibodies

Each of the innumerable protein molecules is made up of polypeptide chains: linear strings of a few hundred amino acids chosen from a set of 20 amino acids. The number of amino acids in a large protein molecule is about equal to the number of letters in the column of text you are now reading, which is a linear string of letters chosen from an alphabet of 26 letters. Different protein molecules have different amino acid sequences just as different texts have different letter sequences. The string of letters in this column of text has been neatly "folded" into successive lines. The polypeptide chains of a protein molecule are also folded, although not so neatly. Their structure looks more like what you would obtain by haphazardly compressing a few yards of rope between your hands. There is nothing haphazard, however, about the folding of a particular polypeptide chain; the folding, and thus the ultimate conformation of the protein molecule, is precisely dictated by the amino acid sequence.

The parts of the folded chains that lie at the surface of a protein molecule make up its surface relief. An epitope (or "antigenic determinant") is a very small patch

of this surface: about 10 amino acids may contribute to the pattern of the epitope. As Emanuel Margoliash of the Abbott Laboratories and Alfred Nisonoff of the University of Illinois College of Medicine showed for different molecules of cytochrome *c*, the replacement of just one amino acid by another in a polypeptide chain of a protein frequently leads to the display of a different epitope. The immune system recognizes that difference and is able to check on mutant cells that make mistakes in protein synthesis. Not only can an individual immune system recognize epitopes on any protein or other antigen produced by any of the millions of species of animals, plants and microorganisms but also it can distinguish "foreign" epitopes from epitopes that belong to the molecules of its own body. This recognition is a crucial event, since antibody molecules attach to the epitopes they recognize and thereby earmark the antigens (or the cells that carry them) for destruction or removal by other mechanisms available to the body.

Epitopes are recognized by the combining sites of antibody molecules. An antibody is itself a protein molecule consisting of more than 20,000 atoms. It is made up of four polypeptide chains: two identical light chains and two identical heavy chains. A light chain consists of 214 amino acids and a heavy chain of about twice as many. Antibody molecules are alike except for the amino acids at about 50 "variable" positions among the first 110 positions, which constitute what is called the variable region of both the light and the heavy chains. At the tip of each variable region there is a concave combining site whose three-dimensional relief enables it to recognize a complementary epitope and make the antibody molecule stick to the molecule displaying that epitope. Whether a combining site will recognize one epitope or a different one depends on which amino acids are located at the variable positions. If at each of 50 positions of both chains there were an independent choice between just two amino acids, there would be 2^{100} (or 10^{30}) potentially different molecules! The situation is not that simple, however. The chains fall into subgroups, within each of which there are far fewer than 50 variable positions. On the other hand, at some of those variable positions, clustered in so-called hot spots, the choice is actually among more than two alternative amino acids. There is general agreement that the differences in amino acid sequence among antibody molecules derive from mutations that have occurred in the genes encoding antibody structure.

The Recognition Problem

Smallpox being the nasty disease it is, one might expect nature to have de-signed antibody molecules with combining sites that specifically recognize the epitopes on smallpox virus. Nature differs from technology in its approach to problem solving, however: it thinks nothing of wastefulness. (For example, rather than improving the chance that a spermatozoon will meet an egg cell, nature finds it easier to produce millions of spermatozoa.) Instead of designing antibody molecules to fit the smallpox virus and other noxious agents, it is easier to make millions of different antibody molecules, some of which may fit. By way of analogy, suppose someone makes gloves in 1,000 different sizes and shapes: he would have a sufficiently well-fitting glove for almost any hand. Now imagine that hands were a great deal more variable; for example, the length of the fingers on a hand might vary independently from one inch to six inches. By making, say, 10 million gloves of different shapes the manufacturer would never-theless be able to fit practically any hand—at the expense of efficiency, to be sure, since most of the gloves might never find a customer to fit them. Now be more wasteful still: have a factory with machines capable of turning out gloves of a billion different shapes, but turn off 99 percent of the machines, so that the factory actually turns out a random collection of 10 million of the potential billion shapes. You would still be doing all right. So would your colleague running a similar factory. Although the two sets of gloves you and he would make would show only a 1 percent overlap, each set would serve its purpose well enough.

That is how some of us think the immune system solves its recognition problem. By a more or less random replacement of amino acids in the hot-spot positions of the variable regions of antibody polypeptide chains, a set of millions of antibody molecules is generated with

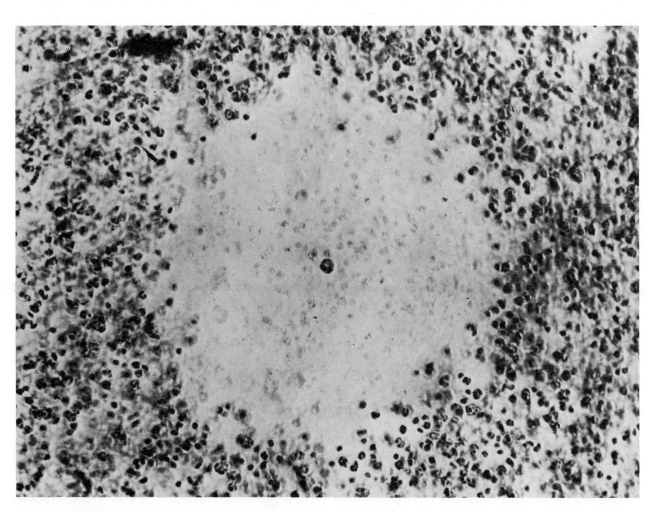

EFFECT OF ANTIBODY on an antigen is illustrated dramatically in a photomicrograph made by the author and Albert Nordin. The cell in the center is a plasma cell, an antibody-secreting lymphocyte of the immune system. It was embedded in a layer of culture medium along with millions of sheep red blood cells. The plasma cell is one that makes antibody against the sheep cells, specifically against epitopes, or small surface patches, on molecules in the surface membrane of the cells. Antibodies secreted by the plasma cell have destroyed the red blood cells in the area into which the antibodies have diffused; the radius of the area of destruction is about 1/5 millimeter. The technique illustrated here has become a standard one for measuring the immune response to an antigen.

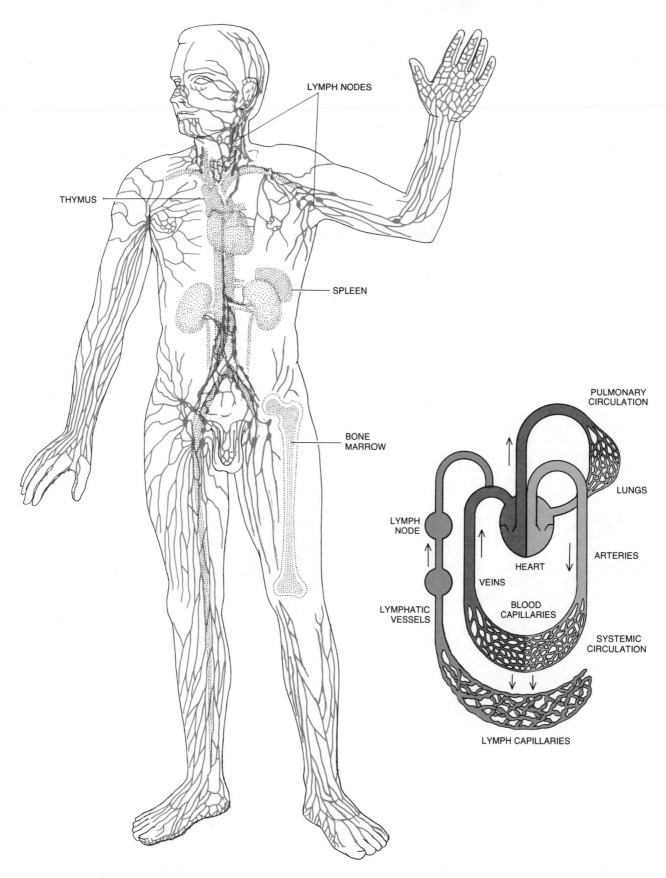

IMMUNE SYSTEM consists of the lymphocytes and the antibody molecules they secrete. The cells and antibodies pervade most of the tissues, to which they are delivered by the bloodstream, but are concentrated in the tissues shown in color: the tree of lymphatic vessels and the lymph nodes stationed along them, the bone marrow (which is in the long bones, only one of which is illustrated), the thymus and the spleen. The lymphatic vessels collect the cells and antibodies from the tissue and return them to the bloodstream at the subclavian veins. Lymphocytes are manufactured in the bone marrow and multiply by cell division in the thymus, the spleen and the lymph nodes. The relation of the blood vessels and the lymphatic vessels is shown highly schematically in the illustration at right.

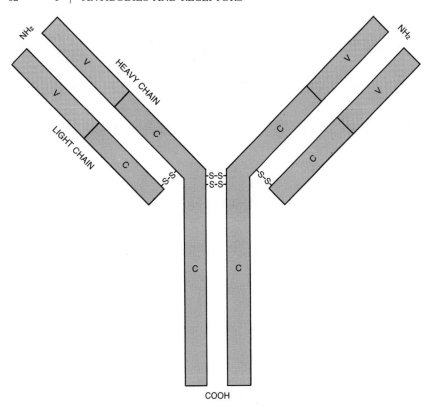

LINEAR STRUCTURE of an antibody molecule is shown schematically. The two heavy chains and two light ones are connected by disulfide bridges. Each chain has an amino end (NH$_2$) and a carboxyl end (COOH). Chains are divided into variable (V) regions (color), in which the amino acid sequence varies in different antibodies, and constant (C) regions.

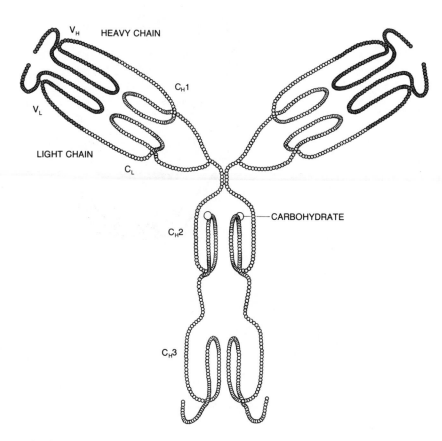

FOLDING OF THE FOUR CHAINS is suggested in this drawing based on a bead model of the antibody molecule made by Gerald M. Edelman and his colleagues. Each bead represents an amino acid, of which there are more than 1,200. The variable regions are in color.

different combining sites that will fit practically any epitope well enough. As has been demonstrated by Jacques Oudin of the Pasteur Institute and by Andrew Kelus and Philipp G. H. Gell of the University of Birmingham for rabbits and by Brigitte A. Askonas, Allan Williamson, Brian Wright and Wolfgang Kreth of the National Institute for Medical Research in London for mice, individual animals make use of entirely different sets of antibodies capable of recognizing a given epitope.

There is one serious snag in all of this, to which I alluded above: one's immune system does not seem to recognize the epitopes on molecules and cells that are part of one's own body. This property, which Sir Macfarlane Burnet called the discrimination between self and not-self, is often referred to as self-tolerance. You might think that self-tolerance derived from nature's being wise enough to construct the genes coding for your antibodies in such a way as not to give rise to combining sites that would fit epitopes occurring in your own body. It can easily be shown, however, that this is not so. For example, your father's antibodies could recognize epitopes occurring in your mother; some antibody genes inherited from your father should therefore code for antibodies recognizing epitopes inherited from your mother.

Self-tolerance, then, is not innate. It is something the immune system "learned" in embryonic life by either eliminating or "paralyzing" all lymphocytes that would produce self-recognizing antibodies. An original observation of this phenomenon by Ray D. Owen of the California Institute of Technology was generalized in a theoretical framework by Burnet and received experimental confirmation by P. B. Medawar in the 1950's, bringing Nobel prizes to Burnet and Medawar in 1960.

The Lymphocyte

Emil von Behring and Shibasaburo Kitazato discovered the existence of antibodies in Germany in 1890, but it was not until the 1960's that the structure of antibodies was determined, through the investigations initiated by R. R. Porter of the University of Oxford and Gerald M. Edelman of Rockefeller University [see "The Structure of Antibodies," by R. R. Porter, beginning on page 31 in this volume, and "The Structure and Function of Antibodies," by Gerald M. Edelman, the article beginning on page 39]. The two men shared a Nobel prize last year for that work. Long before the structure of antibodies was known, however, antibodies had been the subject of detailed studies. And yet it was not known that antibodies are produced by activated lymphocytes. Even 20 years ago lymphocytes were not thought to have anything to do with the immune system, something that seems odd now that they are known to constitute the immune system! It was only in the early 1960's that the involvement of lymphocytes was proved by James L. Gowans and Douglas McGregor of the University of Oxford.

Most lymphocytes (about 98 percent of them) do not actually secrete antibody. They are the "small" lymphocytes, spherical cells measuring about a hundredth of a millimeter in diameter, and they are said to be in a resting state. In order to secrete antibody a small lymphocyte must first become enlarged. In that state it can not only secrete antibody molecules but also divide and become two cells, which in turn can become four cells and so on. The offspring cells constitute the clone, or cell line, derived from one small lymphocyte.

As was originally postulated by Burnet in 1957, the antibody molecules produced by a lymphocyte and by the cells of its clone all have identical combining sites [see "The Mechanism of Immunity," by Sir Macfarlane Burnet, the article beginning on page 12]. G. J. V. Nossal, Burnet's successor as director of the Walter and Eliza Hall Institute of Medical Research in Melbourne, and his co-workers have accumulated much of the experimental evidence that now firmly supports this "single commitment" of the lymphocyte [see "How Cells Make Antibodies," by G. J. V. Nossal, the article beginning on page 22]. The cells of one lymphocyte clone are committed to the expression of two particular genes coding for particular variants of the variable regions of the light chain and the heavy chain. Already in its resting, nonsecreting state a small lymphocyte produces a relatively small number of its particular antibody molecules, which it displays on the surface of its outer membrane. These antibody molecules are the "receptors" of the cell. A small lymphocyte displays about 100,000 receptors with identical combining sites, which are waiting, so to speak, for an encounter with an epitope that fits them.

When such an epitope makes contact, the lymphocyte can either become "stimulated" (respond positively) or become "paralyzed" (respond negatively), which is to say it is no longer capable of being stimulated. Investigations in progress by David S. Rowe of the World Health

Organization, working in Lausanne, and Benvenuto Pernis at our Basel Institute for Immunology suggest that the distinction between excitatory and inhibitory signals may reside in differences in the constant regions of the lymphocyte's receptor antibody molecules. Whether a lymphocyte will choose to respond positively or negatively can be shown to depend on several conditions: the concentration of the recognized epitopes, the degree to which those epitopes fit the combining sites of the receptors, the way the epitopes are presented (for example whether they are presented on molecules or on cell surfaces) and the presence or absence of other lymphocytes that can "help" or "suppress" a response. Much current experimentation aims at clarifying these complex matters.

A stimulated lymphocyte faces two tasks: it must produce antibody molecules for secretion and it must divide in order to expand into a clone of progeny cells representing its commitment. Progeny cells that go all out into the production and secretion of antibody molecules are called plasma cells. Each of them must transcribe its antibody genes into 20,000 messenger-RNA molecules that serve 200,000 ribosomes, enabling the cell to produce and secrete 2,000 identical antibody molecules per second. Other cells of the clone do not go that far; they revert to the resting state and represent the "memory" of the occurrence, ready to respond if the epitope should reappear. The immunological memory of what Stephen Fazekas de St. Groth of

the University of Sydney, who is now working in our laboratory in Basel, has called "original antigenic sin" is remarkably persistent. People who are now 90 years old, for example, and had influenza in the 1890's still possess circulating antibodies to the epitopes of the influenza virus strains that were prevalent at that time.

If a lymphocyte that recognizes an epitope does not become stimulated, it may become paralyzed. Paralysis can occur when a lymphocyte is confronted by very high concentrations of epitope; this is called high-zone tolerance. David W. Dresser and N. Avrion Mitchison, who were working at the National Institute for Medical Research, have shown that paralysis can also result from the continuous presence of extremely small epitope concentrations, below the threshold required for stimulation; this is called low-zone tolerance. We need more knowledge of the mechanisms leading to paralysis, not only in order to understand how the immune system learns to tolerate self-epitopes but also to be able to induce the system to tolerate organ transplants.

Germ-Line and Soma Theories

The enormous diversity of antibodies raises the question of the origin of the genes that code for the variable regions of antibody molecules. Essentially two answers have been proposed to this question. They are the germ-line theory and the somatic theory. The argument of the germ-line theory is straightforward: All the cells of the body, including lym-

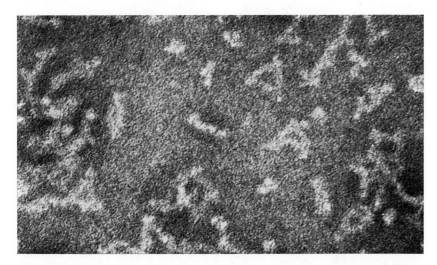

ANTIBODY MOLECULES are visible in an electron microscope when they are linked to antigens and one another in antigen-antibody complexes. In this micrograph, made by N. M. Green and the late Robin Valentine of the National Institute for Medical Research in London, rabbit antibodies are enlarged 500,000 diameters. The antigen is a short polypeptide chain with a dinitrophenyl group at each end; the antibodies are from a rabbit that was immunized against dinitrophenyl epitopes. The antigens (too small to be visible) link antibodies to form polygonal complexes whose geometry derives from antibody structure.

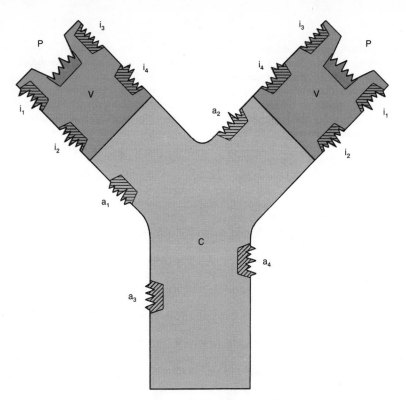

FUNCTIONAL TOPOGRAPHY of the antibody molecule is mapped. The end of each arm of the Y has a combining site (*p*) that recognizes epitopes on antigen molecules. The antibody also has its own epitopes, which can be recognized by other antibodies' combining sites. These include allotopes (*a*) in constant regions and idiotopes (*i*) in variable regions.

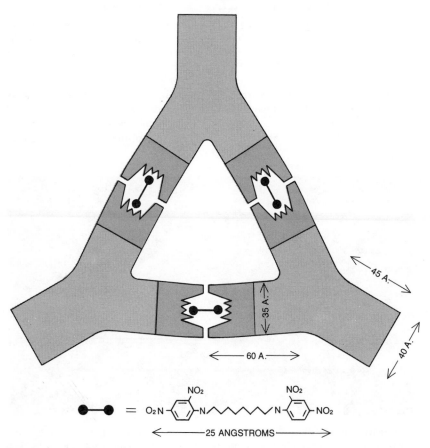

TRIANGULAR STRUCTURES in the micrograph on the preceding page are trimers, or complexes of three antibody molecules, linked by three double-ended dinitrophenyl antigens. The dimensions were worked out by Green and Valentine from electron micrographs.

phocytes, have the same set of genes, namely those in the fertilized egg from which the individual arose. Therefore genes for any antibody that an individual can make must already have been present in the fertilized egg cell. They are all transmitted to the individual's children through the germ-cell line: egg and spermatozoa and their precursors.

The somatic theory does not accept this approach. It is argued that the immune system needs millions of different antibodies for epitope recognition. Individual mice of an inbred strain, all having the same germ-line genes, have been shown to make use of entirely different sets of antibody molecules. The germ-line theory implies that the set of all these sets is represented in the genes of every single mouse of that strain. In that case, however, many of the genes would seem to have no survival value for the mouse, so that such a large number of genes cannot arise or be maintained in Darwinian evolution. Most antibody genes must therefore have arisen in the course of the somatic development of the individual by modification of a smaller number of germ-line genes. That is the point of departure for several variants of the somatic theory.

I have proposed that an inherited set of germ-line genes code for antibodies against certain self-epitopes. The clones of cells expressing these genes become suppressed except for mutant cells that, by an amino acid replacement, display new combining sites on their antibody receptor molecules. These mutant cells represent the enormous repertoire of antibodies that recognize foreign epitopes. An organ that could breed such mutant cells is the thymus gland. More than 10^{10} new lymphocytes arise in the thymus every day; the vast majority of these cells are killed in the thymus or immediately after they leave it.

It is not possible here to discuss the merits of these theories. That would require consideration of a large body of experimental results, such as the explorations of the genetics of immune responsiveness by Baruj Benacerraf of the Harvard Medical School, Hugh O. McDevitt of the Stanford University Medical Center and Michael Sela of the Weizmann Institute of Science in Israel.

T Cell and *B* Cell

All the lymphocytes that circulate in the tissues have arisen from precursor cells in the bone marrow. About half of these lymphocytes, the *T* cells, have passed through the thymus on their way to the tissues; the other half, the *B* cells, have not. This dichotomy was first discovered by Henry N. Claman of the University of Colorado Medical School and was characterized by Jacques F. A. P. Miller and Graham Mitchell, both of whom are now working with us in Basel. It has been the subject of thousands of investigations during the past five years. *T* cells and *B* cells cannot be distinguished by their form. Only *B* cells and their progeny cells secrete antibody molecules. One might think that this leaves little scope for *T*-cell function. On the contrary, *T* cells appear to be all-important. They too can recognize epitopes and must therefore, almost by definition, possess antibody molecules as surface receptors, although these receptor molecules have been much harder to demonstrate experimentally than those on *B* cells.

T cells can kill other cells, such as cancer cells, and transplanted tissues that display foreign epitopes. *T* cells can also suppress *B* cells or alternatively can help *B* cells to become stimulated by epitopes. This "helper" function of *T* cells has been repeatedly demonstrated both in animal experiments and in experiments with cells in culture. In the cell-culture experiments, based on a technique developed by Richard W. Dutton and Robert I. Mishell at the University of California at San Diego, lymphocytes taken from the spleen of an untreated animal are grown in a plastic dish together with molecules or cells that display foreign epitopes. After a few days' incubation lymphocytes that produce and secrete antibody molecules against the foreign epitopes can be shown to be present in the culture by the assay method for single antibody-producing cells [*see illustration on page 50*]. These antibody molecules are made by *B* cells, but the experiment will not work if only *B* cells are present. As soon as *T* cells are added to the culture dish, however, the *B* cells begin to respond and to produce antibody.

The dichotomy of the immune system into *T* and *B* lymphocytes adds a further dimension to the conceptual framework needed for the system's comprehension. That is not only an intellectual need but also a practical one, since the immune system is now known to be crucially involved in a vast number of diseases ranging from microbial infections and allergies to cancer, rheumatism, autoimmunity and many other degenerative disorders of aging.

The Lymphocyte Network

I have mentioned two striking dualisms within the immune system. One is the dichotomy of the lymphocytes into *T* cells and *B* cells, with functions that are partly synergistic and partly antagonistic. The second is the duality of the potential response of a lymphocyte when its receptors recognize an epitope: it can either respond positively (become stimulated) or respond negatively (become paralyzed). It is important to realize that the immune system displays a third dualism, namely that antibody molecules

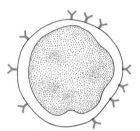 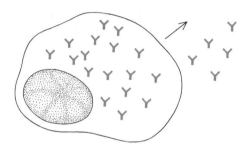

can recognize and can also be recognized. They not only have combining sites enabling them to recognize epitopes but also display epitopes enabling them to be recognized by the combining sites of other antibody molecules. That is true for the antibody molecules attached to the outer membranes of lymphocytes and serving as receptors as well as for the freely circulating antibody molecules, which can be regarded as messages released by lymphocytes.

Epitopes occur on both the constant and the variable regions of an antibody molecule. Since the patterns of the vari-

LYMPHOCYTES, the cells of the immune system, produce antibodies. Each cell is committed in advance to the production of one specific antibody. In its resting state, as a small lymphocyte (*left*), the cell displays such antibody molecules (*color*) on its surface as "receptors." The advent of an antigen with an epitope that fits the combining site of this particular antibody molecule may stimulate the lymphocyte to grow, change in structure and divide, eventually giving rise to a large number of plasma cells (*right*): lymphocytes specialized for the rapid synthesis and secretion of this cell line's specific antibody molecules.

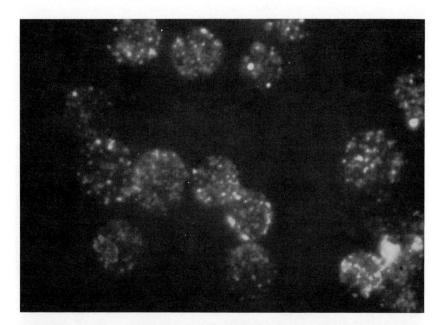

RECEPTOR ANTIBODY MOLECULES are demonstrated by a fluorescent stain in a photomicrograph made by Benvenuto Pernis. The cells are small lymphocytes from a patient with lymphocytic leukemia, in which a line of lymphocytes proliferates out of control. The receptor antibodies on the cell surfaces have epitopes in their constant regions (allotopes) characteristic of human antibody molecules. An antibody directed against those allotopes is prepared by injecting human serum into a rabbit. Rhodamine, a fluorescent dye, is coupled to the antibodies, which are added to a suspension of the lymphocytes. The bright spots on the cells represent fluorescent antibody bound to receptor molecules they "recognize."

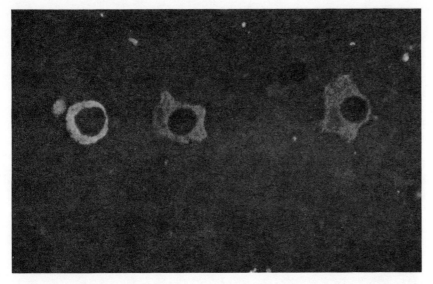

INTERNAL ANTIBODY MOLECULES, being produced by plasma cells for secretion, are stained in this photomicrograph and the one at the bottom of the page, also made by Pernis. The plasma cells are from a rabbit that is heterozygous for the structural gene that determines the constant region of the antibody molecule and therefore its set of allotypes, or its allotype; that is, the rabbit inherited paternal and maternal chromosomes containing two different determining genes. The plasma cells have been stained with two preparations of fluorescent antibodies: one, to which a green-fluorescing stain has been coupled, is directed against the paternal allotype (call it allotype *A*) and the other is directed against the maternal allotype (*B*). The internal antibodies in some of the plasma cells bind to the green-staining preparation, indicating that they are antibody molecules carrying allotype *A*.

able-region epitopes are determined by the variable amino acid sequences of the polypeptide chains, there are millions of different epitopes. The set of such epitopes on a given antibody molecule was named the idiotype of that molecule by Oudin. When antibodies produced by animal *A* are injected into animal *B*, animal *B* will produce antibodies against the idiotypic epitopes ("idiotopes") of the injected antibody molecules. That is also true when *A* and *B* belong to the same animal species and even when they

are of the same inbred strain, that is, when they are genetically identical. Evidence is emerging that, within one animal, the idiotopes occurring on one antibody molecule are recognized by combining sites on a set of other antibody molecules, and that the idiotopes on the receptor molecules of one lymphocyte are recognized by the combining sites of the receptor molecules of a set of other lymphocytes. We thus have a network of lymphocytes and antibody molecules that recognize other lymphocytes

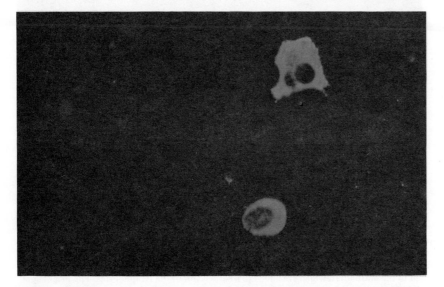

OTHER INTERNAL ANTIBODIES, in other plasma cells from the same field of the preparation as the micrograph at the top of the page, stain red. They are molecules with allotype *B*. Although all the rabbit's lymphocytes and plasma cells contain both the paternal and the maternal chromosomes, each cell expresses only one or the other constant-region gene.

and antibody molecules, which in turn recognize still others.

I am convinced that the description of the immune system as a functional network of lymphocytes and antibody molecules is essential to its understanding, and that the network as a whole functions in a way that is peculiar to and characteristic of the internal interactions of the elements of the immune system itself: it displays what I call an eigen-behavior. (Eigen in German means peculiar to, or characteristic of. Eigen-behavior is analogous to such concepts as the eigenvalue or eigenfrequency of certain physical systems.) There is an increasing body of evidence for this view.

Antibody molecules are normally present in the blood in a concentration of about 5×10^{16} molecules per milliliter. The total concentration of combining sites and idiotopes is therefore of the order of 10^{17} per milliliter. If the immune system made use of 10 million different combining sites and 10 million different idiotopes, each single variant of these elements would be present, on the average, in a concentration of about 10^{10} per milliliter. Mitchison at the National Institute for Medical Research and Nossal, Gordon L. Ada and their colleagues at the Walter and Eliza Hall Institute and the Australian National University, experimenting with low-zone tolerance, have shown that epitope concentrations ranging for different antigens from a million to 10^{12} epitopes per milliliter suffice either to suppress or to paralyze lymphocytes that can recognize the epitopes. Nisonoff and his co-workers at the University of Illinois College of Medicine and Humberto Cosenza and Heinz Köhler at the University of Chicago have shown that injecting into an animal antibodies against an idiotype suppresses lymphocytes that have receptors with idiotopes recognized by those antibodies. Leonard A. Herzenberg of the Stanford University Medical Center and Ethel Jacobson in our laboratory in Basel find that *T* lymphocytes recognizing epitopes on the receptors of *B* lymphocytes can suppress those *B* lymphocytes.

What this adds up to is that lymphocytes are subject to continuous suppression by other lymphocytes and by antibody molecules with idiotopes or combining sites that fit. Some lymphocytes escape from suppression and divide. New lymphocytes emerge. Others remain suppressed or decay. The eigen-behavior is the dynamic steady state of the system as its elements interact. As the system expands in the course of development and later life, new idiotopes and new combining sites emerge. The "self"-epitopes of other tissues impinge on the network and cause certain elements to become more numerous and others less numerous. In this way each individual develops a different immune system.

Invading foreign antigens modulate the network; early imprints leave the deepest traces. A given foreign epitope will be recognized, with various degrees of precision, by the combining sites of a set of antibody molecules, and lymphocytes that are committed to producing antibody molecules of that set are then stimulated and become more numerous. That is not, however, the only imprint made by the foreign epitope. The set of combining sites that recognized the epitope also recognizes a set of idiotopes *within* the system, a set of idiotopes that constitutes the "internal image" of the foreign epitope. The lymphocytes representing the internal image will therefore be affected secondarily, and so forth in successive recognition waves throughout the network [*see illustration below*].

The structural properties of the immune system and its eigen-behavior reside in these complex ramifications.

Immune System and Nervous System

The immune system and the nervous system are unique among the organs of the body in their ability to respond adequately to an enormous variety of signals. Both systems display dichotomies: their cells can both receive and transmit signals, and the signals can be either excitatory or inhibitory. The two systems penetrate most other tissues of the body, but they seem to avoid each other: the "blood-brain barrier" prevents lymphocytes from coming into contact with nerve cells.

The nerve cells, or neurons, are in fixed positions in the brain, the spinal cord and the ganglia, and their long processes, the axons, connect them to form a network. The ability of the axon

of one neuron to form synapses with the correct set of other neurons must require something akin to epitope recognition. Lymphocytes are 100 times more numerous than nerve cells and, unlike nerve cells, they move about freely. They too interact, however, either by direct encounters or through the antibody molecules they release. These elements can recognize as well as be recognized, and in so doing they too form a network. As in the case of the nervous system, the modulation of the network by foreign signals represents its adaptation to the outside world. Both systems thereby learn from experience and build up a memory, a memory that is sustained by reinforcement but cannot be transmitted to the next generation. These striking analogies in the expression of the two systems may result from similarities in the sets of genes that encode their structure and that control their development and function.

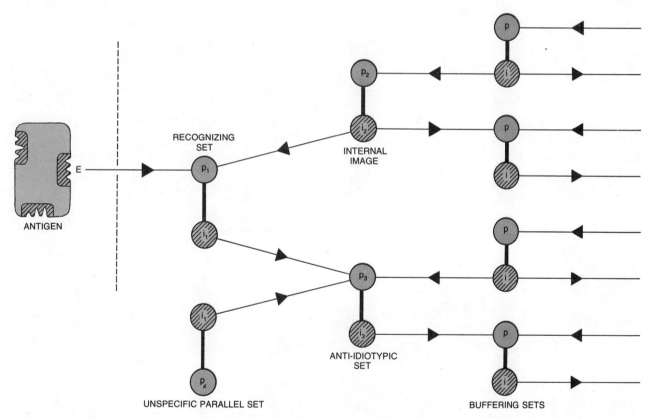

LYMPHOCYTE NETWORK is diagrammed in an effort to indicate how its steady-state ("eigen") behavior is established and how the network responds to an antigen. An epitope (E) on the antigen is recognized by a set (p_1) of combining sites on antibody molecules, both circulating antibody and cell-surface receptors. Cells with receptors of the recognizing set p_1 are potentially capable of responding to the antigenic stimulus (*arrowhead*) of epitope E, but there are constraints. The same molecules that carry combining sites p_1 carry a set of idiotopes (i_1). These are recognized within the system by a set of combining sites (p_3), called the anti-idiotypic set because they tend to suppress (*reverse arrowhead*) the cells of set i_1. (These idiotypes i_1 are also found on molecules with com-

bining sites that do not belong to the recognizing set p_1 but rather are unspecific with regard to epitope E.) On the other hand, the set p_1 also recognizes internal epitopes i_2, which therefore constitute an internal image of the foreign epitope E. In the steady state, molecules of the internal image tend to stimulate cells of set p_1 and thus to balance the suppressive tendency of the anti-idiotypic set. When the foreign antigen enters the system, its stimulatory effect on recognizing set p_1 allows cells of that set to escape from suppression. (The same thing happens to unspecific cells of the parallel set p_x.) The resulting immune response to the antigen is modulated by the buffering effects of many more sets of combining sites and idiotopes (*right*), which have a controlling influence on the response.

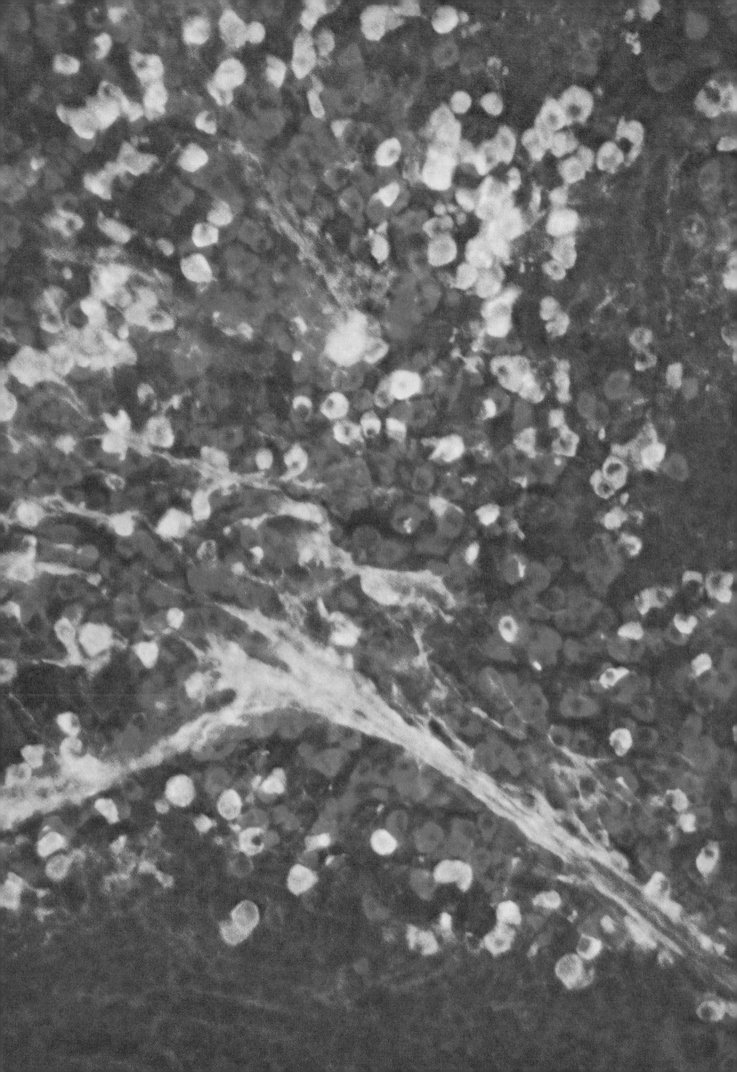

6

The Development of the Immune System

by Max D. Cooper and Alexander R. Lawton III
November 1974

*The highly diversified cells that defend the body
against foreign substances derive from a single kind
of precursor. Differentiation of the cells is controlled
by the environment in which they mature*

Two systems of immunity protect the body from the hazards of infection and cancer. One is the cell-mediated immune response, which combats fungi and viruses and initiates the rejection of tumors and foreign tissues, such as transplanted organs. The other is humoral immunity, which is effective against bacterial infections and viral reinfections. Although the two mechanisms are not entirely independent, and cooperation between them is sometimes important, they are distinct.

The ultimate basis for this division of labor in the immune system lies in two populations of cells native to lymphoid tissue but also found in other parts of the body, particularly in the blood. During development the two lines of lymphoid cells look alike; they cannot be distinguished by mere inspection. Moreover, both derive from the same primitive precursors: the hemopoietic stem cells, which also give rise to several other kinds of blood cells. In spite of their common origin and superficial resemblance the cells do differ; they play dissimilar roles in the body's response to foreign materials and tumor cells.

In addition to the division of the immune system into two classes of lymphoid cells, there is great diversity within each class. In both classes each cell is capable of recognizing a particular antigenic determinant: one of the chemical groupings by which biological substances such as proteins communicate their identity. There are millions of possible antigenic determinants, and apparently there are immunologically active cells capable of recognizing each of them.

Investigations of how this diversity springs from the apparent uniformity of the stem cells may help us to discover how the immune system is constructed and how it works. We may also gain a better understanding of cell differentiation in general, one of the principal challenges of modern biology. Finally, a working knowledge of these mechanisms is needed if we are to devise ways of correcting disorders of the immune system, many of which seem to arise from flaws in cell differentiation.

Thymus and Bursa

The twofold nature of the immune system was delineated in a series of experiments performed by Merrill W. Chase and Karl Landsteiner of the Rockefeller Institute for Medical Research. (Landsteiner is better known for an earlier discovery: in 1900 he established the A, B and O blood types.)

Chase and Landsteiner demonstrated that some kinds of immune reaction could be transferred from one animal to another only by the exchange of living cells, whereas others could be transmitted by blood serum. The cells required in the former experiment are lymphocytes: small, unpigmented cells included with several other types among the leukocytes, or white blood cells. Up to that time the function of lymphocytes had been unknown.

The serum component capable of transferring immunity consists of the protein molecules called antibodies, which combine with foreign substances. A few years earlier it had been discovered that the antibodies belong to that part of the blood serum called the gamma-globulin fraction. Antibodies are secreted by plasma cells, which are descendants of lymphocytes, but not the same lymphocytes, it was eventually discovered, that effect cell-mediated immunity [see "How Cells Make Antibodies," by G. J. V. Nossal, beginning on page 22].

That the functional duality of the immune system might have a developmental basis was suggested by the discovery of certain immunodeficiency diseases; the disorders might be considered experiments of nature. Ogden C. Bruton, a pediatrician at the Walter Reed Army Medical Center, identified the first—an impairment of humoral immunity—in a young boy afflicted with multiple bacterial infections. The disease is characterized by a lack of plasma cells and a consequent inability to make antibodies. Lymphocytes of the cell-mediated system, on the other hand, are abundant, and they enable the patient to resist viral and fungal infections quite well.

SPECIFICITY OF CELLS in the immune system is illustrated by the stained section of tissue from the spleen of a mouse that is shown in the illustration on the opposite page. The tissue was stained with two fluorescent dyes attached to antibodies to specific classes of immunoglobulins. Antibodies to immunoglobulin M were labeled with the green dye fluorescein, those to immunoglobulin G with the red dye rhodamine. The labeled antibodies bind selectively to plasma cells bearing the appropriate immunoglobulins on their surface. The fact that none of the cells were stained with both of the dyes indicates that each mature plasma cell produces only one class of immunoglobulins. The photomicrograph, which enlarges the section of tissue about 2,500 diameters, was made by one of the authors (Lawton).

The obverse pattern of immunodeficiency—an impairment of cell-mediated immunity—has also been detected. Individuals with this condition, who are vulnerable to viruses and fungi, have fewer than the normal number of lymphocytes, but they have plasma cells and produce circulating antibodies. Some children are born lacking both lymphocytes and plasma cells; without either system of immunity they quickly succumb to infection by a variety of microorganisms.

The explanation of these conditions has been achieved mainly through experiments with mice and chickens. In 1961 Jacques F. A. P. Miller, then at the Chester Beatty Research Institute in London, and Robert A. Good and his colleagues, then at the University of Minnesota Medical School, simultaneously discovered that removal of the thymus gland from newborn mice and rabbits prevents normal development of the immune system. Branislav D. Jankovic, Barry G. W. Arnason and Byron H. Waksman, then at the Harvard Medical School, showed that the thymus plays a similar role in rats. The immunodeficiency produced by neonatal thymectomy is particularly severe in mice because the immune system of the mouse is comparatively immature at birth.

The thymus is a gland that in man lies in the chest just below the sternum; its function had long been a puzzle to biologists. A solution to the puzzle began to emerge when it was demonstrated that mice deprived of a thymus have reduced numbers of lymphocytes and a marked deficiency in cell-mediated immunity, as revealed by their impaired ability to reject grafts of skin and other tissue from unrelated mice. In mice thymectomy also inhibits the production of antibodies to most antigens. For this reason it was at first thought that the mammalian thymus controls the development of precursor cells for both cell-mediated and humoral immunity. The theory had to be modified, however, when it was found that mice without a thymus have an abundance of plasma cells and display a vigorous antibody response to certain antigens.

Immunologists were led to a more precise definition of the role of the thymus by an earlier (and for a time generally ignored) observation made by Bruce Glick, who was then a graduate student at Ohio State University. Glick and his associates had discovered that the development of humoral immunity in chickens could be severely stunted by the removal shortly after hatching of a lymphoid organ called the bursa of Fabricius. The bursa is a small pouch found only in birds, attached to the intestine near the cloaca; it is named for the 16th-century Paduan anatomist Hieronymus Fabricius ab Aquapendente, who first described it [see illustration on this page].

It was later shown that another technique that inhibits the development of the bursa, treatment of chick embryos with the male sex hormone testosterone, also depresses antibody production, usually without diminishing the animals' capacity to reject foreign skin grafts. A small proportion of chicks subjected to this "hormonal bursectomy," however, are tolerant of foreign skin, an anomaly first noted by Noel L. Warner and Aleksander Szenberg of the Walter and Eliza Hall Institute of Medical Research in Melbourne. In these birds, they discovered, the thymus as well as the bursa is poorly developed. Because testosterone has multiple deleterious effects on embryos the treated chicks are sickly and usually die soon after hatching. In order to clarify the results of their experiments Warner and Szenberg excised the thymuses of chicks; the result was lymphocyte deficiency and feeble graft rejection. Their conclusion, that in birds the thymus and the bursa exert different influences on immunological development, was the first suggestion of a developmental division of the immune system [see "The Thymus Gland," by Sir Macfarlane Burnet, the article beginning on page 88].

The polarity thus established in chickens could not, however, be immediately extended to mammals. Some aspects of the separation of cell-mediated and humoral immunity in chickens were not in accord with those seen in human immunodeficiencies; in addition the mouse thymus seemed to govern all cell-mediated immune functions, whereas the chicken thymus seemed to exercise only partial control. Refined techniques were necessary to resolve these discrepancies.

Neither of the methods employed previously was entirely satisfactory. Removing an organ at birth or at hatching cannot ensure the elimination of its influence, since it may have produced immunologically competent cells during embryonic life. Hormones, on the other

IMMUNE SYSTEM OF BIRDS is centered in two organs, the thymus and the bursa of Fabricius. The thymus, which consists of seven pairs of lobes alongside the trachea, controls the development of cell-mediated immunity. The bursa, a pouch that is found only in birds and that is attached to the intestine near the cloaca, influences the immunoglobulin-secreting cells that effect humoral immunity. The lymphocytes that pass through the thymus are called *T* cells, those from the bursa are called *B* cells. Lymphocytes also colonize the bone marrow and the spleen, but only after their residence in either the thymus or the bursa.

hand, even when they are applied to the fertilized egg early enough to suppress immunological functions, affect both bursa and thymus and thereby allow only imperfect discrimination between the two systems. In order to avoid these difficulties one of us (Cooper), working with Good and Raymond D. A. Peterson at the University of Minnesota Medical School, employed another approach. Either the thymus or the bursa was surgically removed from newly hatched chicks; then, to destroy any cells influenced earlier by these organs, the birds were exposed to X rays. After the animals had recovered from the irradiation the structure and function of their immune systems were examined.

These experiments made plain several parallels between avian and mammalian immunology. The effects of thymectomy and irradiation on the immune system of chickens were remarkably similar to those of thymectomy alone in mice. The treated birds were runty and deficient in lymphocytes; all cell-mediated immune functions were suppressed. In addition they were unable to produce antibodies as well as control birds with intact thymuses. Birds subjected to bursectomy and irradiation, on the other hand, like the antibody-deficient boy described by Bruton, had plenty of lymphocytes and normal cell-mediated immune responses but lacked plasma cells and their products: the circulating antibodies. Plasma-cell function could be restored by the injection of lymphocytes from the bursa of an untreated bird. It had been shown earlier in mice that grafts of thymus tissue or injections of large numbers of lymphocytes taken from the thymus could restore cell-mediated immunity to mice lacking thymuses.

T Cells and B Cells

The view of the separate developmental pathways followed by thymic and bursal lymphocytes provided by these experiments accorded well with the observations of other investigators. E. C. Ford and his colleagues at the Harwell Radiation Research Institute in England had employed chromosomal markers to trace the migration of precursor cells in mice from the bone marrow to the thymus and thence to the spleen and peripheral lymph nodes. Their results implied that the precursors of a second population of lymphocytes, made up of cells that do not pass through the thymus, are also present in the bone marrow of mice. Other studies, in particular those of James E. Till and E. A. McCullough of the Ontario Cancer

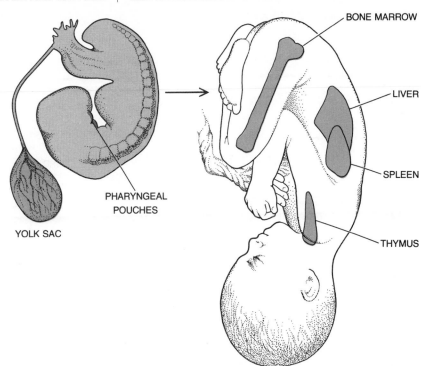

MAMMALIAN IMMUNOLOGICAL DEVELOPMENT can be illustrated through the anatomy of the human fetus. The precursors of lymphocytes originate early in embryonic life in the yolk sac and subsequently migrate through the spleen and liver to the bone marrow. Also early in development, cells from two of the embryonic structures called pharyngeal pouches migrate into the chest to form the thymus, which in mammals as in birds controls cell-mediated immunity. Mammals have no bursa of Fabricius, however; in mammals immunoglobulin-secreting cells may develop in the fetal liver and possibly in the spleen.

Institute and John J. Trentin of the Baylor College of Medicine, revealed that the descendants of a single stem cell can include both kinds of lymphocytes as well as other blood cells.

Several years earlier Jacob Furth of the Oak Ridge National Laboratory had discovered that early removal of the thymus prevents the development of a lymphoma (a cancer of lymphoid tissue) that appears spontaneously in a certain strain of mice. Many other mouse lymphomas proved to be dependent on the thymus, apparently because the thymus is the sole source of cells susceptible to the lymphoma-producing effects of certain viruses and chemicals. A related effect was reported in chickens by Peterson and Ben R. Burmester, who were working at the Department of Agriculture Regional Poultry Research Laboratory in East Lansing, Mich.; they found that bursectomy, but not thymectomy, prevents the development of a virus-induced lymphoma in chickens. In this case the virus is one that can infect many types of cells and replicate in them; only in the bursa, however, does it encounter lymphoid cells at a stage of differentiation where they are susceptible to malignant transformation.

By 1965 it was possible to construct

a model of the development of the immune system in chickens and mice based on the differentiation of cells into thymic and bursal lines [see illustrations on next two pages]. The model implied that immunodeficiency diseases could be viewed as the consequences of defects in stem cells or of the failure of the cells to develop along one or the other pathway. The model also suggested that lymphoid malignancies could be regarded as abnormalities in the differentiation of cells belonging to either the thymic or the bursal system.

That the model could be extended to the human immune system was soon confirmed by Angelo M. Di George, a pediatrician at the Temple University School of Medicine, who discovered that children born without a thymus are deficient in lymphocytes and lack cell-mediated immune functions. Plasma cells and circulating antibodies are present in such children, suggesting that in man antibody-producing cells do not originate in the thymus. In mice additional support for the theory was obtained in further experiments with animals subjected to thymectomy and irradiation. The mice were given infusions of stem cells bearing genetic markers different from those of the host animal.

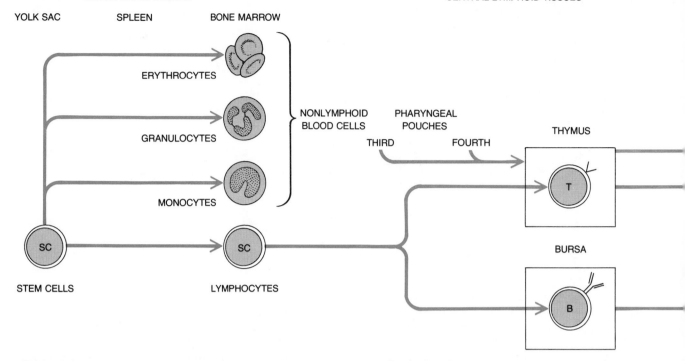

HEMOPOIETIC TISSUES

YOLK SAC   SPLEEN   BONE MARROW

ERYTHROCYTES

CENTRAL LYMPHOID TISSUES

NONLYMPHOID
BLOOD CELLS

PHARYNGEAL
POUCHES
THIRD   FOURTH

THYMUS

GRANULOCYTES

MONOCYTES

SC

STEM CELLS

SC

LYMPHOCYTES

T

BURSA

B

DIFFERENTIATION OF LYMPHOCYTES in birds follows a pathway discovered mainly through experiments with chickens. In the embryo the precursor cells called hemopoietic stem cells migrate from the yolk sac through the spleen to the bone marrow, where they divide and diversify, producing many kinds of blood cells. Those that are eventually to become lymphocytes must undergo further differentiation outside the bone marrow. Some pass

through the thymus and are transformed into *T* cells; when activated by an antigen, they secrete molecules called lymphokines, which participate in an attack on the antigenic material. Stem cells that migrate to the bursa of Fabricius instead of the thymus are induced to become antibody-making *B* cells; when these are stimulated by an antigen, they divide repeatedly, giving rise to a clone of plasma cells that secrete large quantities of antibody. *T* cells

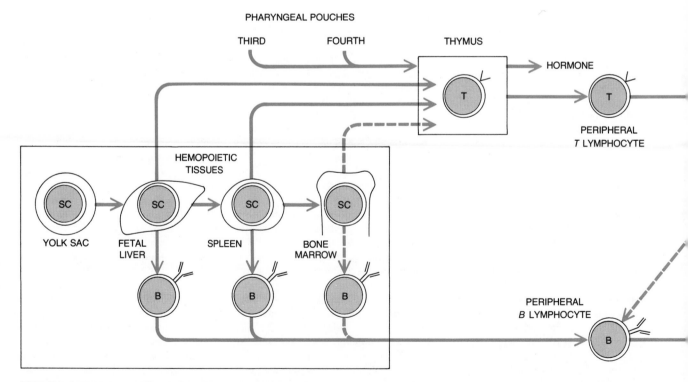

PHARYNGEAL POUCHES

THIRD   FOURTH   THYMUS

HORMONE

T

T

PERIPHERAL
T LYMPHOCYTE

HEMOPOIETIC
TISSUES

SC   SC   SC   SC

YOLK SAC   FETAL   SPLEEN   BONE
            LIVER   MARROW

B   B   B

PERIPHERAL
B LYMPHOCYTE

B

DEVELOPMENT AND DIVERSIFICATION of mammalian lymphocytes follows a program similar to but not identical with that in birds. The ultimate source of immunologically active cells is again the yolk sac, but stem cells from that embryonic structure travel through the fetal liver as well as the spleen before taking up

residence in the bone marrow. As in birds, the influence of the thymus is essential to the generation of *T* cells, but the site at which stem cells are induced to become *B* cells has not been unambiguously identified. The fetal liver may be the first organ in which immunoglobulin-bearing cells appear. Mammalian stem

CIRCULATION AND PERIPHERAL
LYMPHOID TISSUES

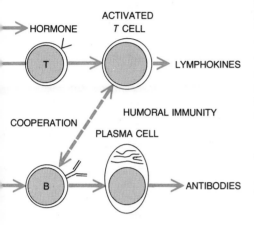

may be influenced by a thymic hormone
after they have left the gland itself, and they
may cooperate in stimulating B cells to proliferate. The symbols on the surface of the
lymphocytes represent antigen receptors;
in B cells these are immunoglobulins; the
nature of the receptor on T cells is unknown.

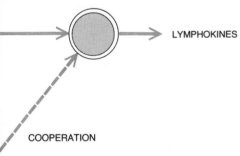

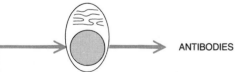

cells, like those of birds, are the precursors
of other kinds of blood cells in addition to
the lymphocytes. Cooperation between the
two classes of lymphocytes in the response
to certain antigens has been demonstrated.

The markers could be detected later in
antibody-producing cells and their products, indicating that the humoral immune system had been reconstituted in
the absence of the thymus.

The formulation of a model of immunological development based on the
notion that there are two distinct lines
of lymphoid cells offered numerous insights into the behavior of the immune
system. Many observations remained to
be explained, however, such as the fact
that in mice and chickens deprived of a
thymus the humoral immune system is
apparently insensitive to certain antigens, even though plasma cells and antibodies are present. The observation
could be accounted for by postulating
the need for thymus-derived cells to cooperate with cells from the bursa. That
there is such cooperation was demonstrated in a classic series of experiments
performed by Henry N. Claman, E. A.
Chaperon and R. F. Triplett of the University of Colorado School of Medicine,
A. J. S. Davies of the Chester Beatty Research Institute and Graham F. Mitchell
and Jacques Miller, then working at the
Walter and Eliza Hall Institute. They
found that in the presence of an antigen
thymus lymphocytes promote the transformation of thymus-independent lymphocytes into plasma cells.

This model of lymphocyte differentiation has dominated immunology during
the past 10 years. All the tenets of the
doctrine have been confirmed repeatedly by experiment. The elucidation of the
mechanisms by which lymphoid cells
diversify and through which the two
classes interact has become a central
problem in immunology.

For convenience lymphocytes developing in the thymus are designated T
cells; antibody-producing cells, develop-
mentally dependent on the avian bursa
or its mammalian equivalent, are called
B cells. As we have mentioned, the two
types of cell are identical in appearance,
but they can be distinguished by an
array of markers that have been discovered on their surfaces. Some of these
markers are antigens roughly analogous
to the blood-group antigens found on
the surface of red blood cells. Because
their expression is confined to certain
cell types they are called differentiation
antigens, a term coined by Edward A.
Boyse and Lloyd J. Old of the Sloan-
Kettering Institute for Cancer Research.
The theta antigen in mice, for example
(there is a similar antigen in humans), is
present on both mature and immature T
cells but not on B cells, and thus it
serves as a convenient marker for one
cell line. B cells possess other surface an-

tigens, such as the "mouse-specific B
lymphocyte antigen." Martin C. Raff,
then working at the National Institute
for Medical Research in England, was
the first to demonstrate that B cells and
T cells can be discriminated by markers
such as these.

Since both B cells and T cells (and
other cell types as well) have a common
ancestry in the hemopoietic stem cells, it
seems probable that their differentiation
is controlled at least in part by factors
external to the cell. In birds and mammals stem cells first appear in the yolk
sac, a membranous structure connected
with the intestinal cavity of the embryo.
Later in embryonic development they
migrate through the bloodstream to colonize the liver (in mammals) and spleen
(in both birds and mammals) before
moving on to settle permanently in the
bone marrow. The pattern of differentiation that a stem cell eventually assumes
is thought to depend on influences exerted within the microenvironment of
the site to which it migrates. There is
some evidence to suggest, however, that
the stem cells ancestral to lymphocytes
may be committed to the production of
either T cells or B cells before they migrate to the organs in which these cells
are formed.

The Development of T Cells

In considering the development of T
cells the central question is: How do a
relatively few stem cells give rise to a
large and heterogeneous population of T
lymphocytes? This question has so far
defied attempts to provide a precise answer because the nature of the antigen
receptor on T cells has not yet been defined. Without knowledge of the receptor the functioning of the T cell cannot
be adequately described. Nevertheless,
much information on the development
and functioning of T cells has been
gained; the evidence to date suggests
that the heterogeneity of the cells arises
primarily in the thymus.

The structural framework of the thymus (but not of the lymphocytes the
gland contains) is formed from epithelial
cells that initially line the third and
fourth pharyngeal pouches, which are
embryonic structures in the region that
eventually becomes the throat. Early in
the embryonic development of most
mammals these epithelial cells begin to
specialize and migrate down the neck
into the chest, where some of them complete their development to form the
thymus. It was once thought that thymus epithelial cells were themselves
transformed into lymphocytes, but stud-

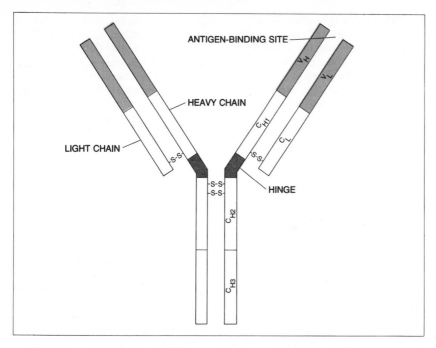

ANTIGEN-BINDING SITE

V_H

V_L

HEAVY CHAIN

LIGHT CHAIN

C_{H1}

C_L

-S-S-

-S-S-

-S-S-
-S-S-

HINGE

C_{H2}

C_{H3}

IMMUNOGLOBULIN MOLECULE consists of four polypeptide chains, each made up of many amino acid units. Two of the chains are longer and are designated heavy chains; the smaller ones are called light chains. The molecule is held together by disulfide bonds (-S-S-) but can flex in the region of the hinge. In part of each chain the amino acid sequence is the same in all molecules of the same type; this is called the constant region. There are three or four constant domains in each heavy chain (C_{H1}, C_{H2}, C_{H3}) and one in each light chain (C_L). The genes specifying the constant region may have evolved through the duplication of a primordial gene the size of a single domain. In the variable regions (*color*) the amino acid sequence differs from molecule to molecule. The immunoglobulin binds antigens at clefts formed by folds in the variable regions of the heavy and light chains.

IMMUNO-GLOBULIN	LIGHT CHAIN	HEAVY CHAIN	OTHER CHAINS	STRUCTURE
IgM	KAPPA OR LAMBDA	MU	J	
IgG	KAPPA OR LAMBDA	GAMMA₁ GAMMA₂ GAMMA₃ GAMMA₄		
IgA	KAPPA OR LAMBDA	ALPHA₁ ALPHA₂	J, SC	
IgD	KAPPA OR LAMBDA	DELTA		
IgE	KAPPA OR LAMBDA	EPSILON		

CLASS OF AN IMMUNOGLOBULIN is determined by the type of heavy chain in the molecule. There are five types—mu, gamma, alpha, delta and epsilon—and subclasses of gamma and alpha. In addition each immunoglobulin can have either of two kinds of light chain: kappa or lambda. Some of the immunoglobulins form oligomers, or associations of a few subunits in a single molecule. IgM is ordinarily a pentamer, with five subunits and with an additional "joining" chain, or *J* chain, shown here as a black dot. IgA occurs as a monomer, dimer and trimer, with respectively one, two and three subunits. The *J* chain is present in oligomeric forms, and the dimer, when found in secretions such as saliva and tears, is bonded to yet another polypeptide: the secretory component (*SC*), shown here as a gray disk.

ies by Malcolm A. S. Moore and John J. T. Owen at the University of Oxford have since proved that the provenance of *T* cells is in the yolk sac.

At a time when only a few primitive precursor cells have entered the thymus, the gland can be removed and the tissue grown in culture. When that is done, each stem cell gives rise to thousands of *T* lymphocytes. Thymus lymphocytes are among the most rapidly proliferating cells in the body, dividing about three times in a day. One possible factor favoring the high rate of lymphocyte production is the need to supply the rest of the body with *T* cells. Another is the need to provide conditions suitable for the generation of diversity.

There is a considerable body of evidence suggesting that stem cells must actually pass through the thymus in order to become *T* lymphocytes. The thymic epithelium could influence stem cells by direct contact or by hormones active within its tissues. Hormones from the thymus have been shown to promote the maturation of *T* cells after they have left the thymus, thus providing a mechanism by which the parent (or foster-parent) organ can maintain control over its wandering offspring. Evidence obtained recently suggests that thymic hormones may even be able to influence the differentiation of cells that have not yet entered the gland.

Lymphocytes found within the thymus are called thymocytes, to distinguish them from the *T* cells released by the thymus to the peripheral tissues. Most thymocytes are functionally immature, but a small subpopulation is capable of recognizing and responding to antigens. If these cells are confronted with cells from another individual, they are activated; they enlarge, divide and release large molecules called lymphokines that participate in the elimination of the foreign material. *T* cells can also enlist the aid of macrophages, large digestive cells, in destroying pathogens, and mature thymocytes may release factors that stimulate *B* cells to respond by increasing the production of antibodies. The specificity of thymus lymphocytes can be readily demonstrated. If an antigen is rendered highly radioactive, *T* cells recognizing it are killed in the encounter, but other *T* cells, which presumably recognize other antigens, are not harmed. By this phenomenon of "antigen suicide" Anthony Basten and his co-workers at the Walter and Eliza Hall Institute showed that thymus cells propagate in diverse clones, lines of cells that are genetically identical.

T cells leave the thymus by way of

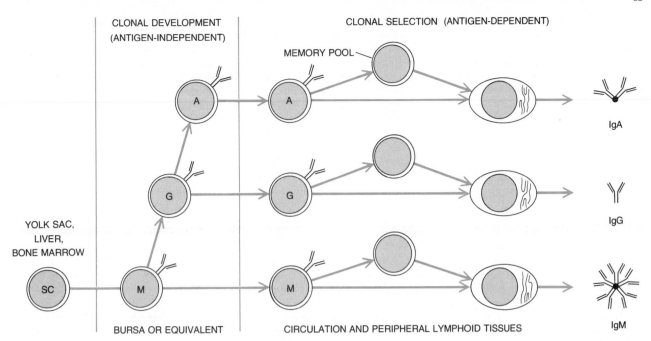

CLONAL DEVELOPMENT
(ANTIGEN-INDEPENDENT)

CLONAL SELECTION (ANTIGEN-DEPENDENT)

MEMORY POOL

YOLK SAC,
LIVER,
BONE MARROW

BURSA OR EQUIVALENT

CIRCULATION AND PERIPHERAL LYMPHOID TISSUES

IgA

IgG

IgM

MATURATION OF B CELLS takes place in two stages. The first requires an inductive microenvironment, such as that of the bursa, but does not require stimulation by antigens. The "virgin" B cells initially synthesize immunoglobulin of a particular light-chain type and antigen specificity; the heavy-chain class is at first invariably mu, and the immunoglobulin is therefore IgM. Most of the progeny of these cells migrate to the peripheral lymphoid tissues, but some remain behind to develop further. They stop making the mu heavy chain and begin to make the gamma chain, and thus switch from IgM to IgG synthesis. The light-chain type and the specificity of the molecules are not altered. These IgG-making cells also have many descendants, some of which later switch from IgG to IgA synthesis by the same mechanism. In the second stage of development a clone of B cells is "selected" by an encounter with the antigen for which it is specific. The selected clone proliferates, and some of the progeny develop into plasma cells, which secrete antibody copiously. Others serve as memory cells, which can reinforce the immunological response in subsequent encounters with the same antigen.

the bloodstream and seldom return to their birthplace. Their main route of migration has been elucidated by James L. Gowans of Oxford. The *T* cells slip between the epithelial cells that line the venules (the small blood vessels on the venous side of the capillary bed) and enter special regions of the lymph nodes and the spleen called thymus-dependent zones. Here a cell that has encountered an antigen that corresponds to its receptor will divide repeatedly, expanding the clone of cells responsive to the same antigen. After temporary residence in the thymus-dependent zones the *T* cells make their way into the lymphatic circulation and reenter the bloodstream in the neck, where the main lymphatic vessel, the thoracic duct, empties into the subclavian vein. The circulation of the cells through the body greatly increases the probability that they will encounter any foreign substance or malignant cells present.

The Development of *B* Cells

Tracing the life history of the *B* cell is made easier by the availability of its products: the humoral antibodies. After a *B* cell completes its terminal differentiation and becomes a plasma cell it synthesizes and secretes about 2,000 identi-

cal antibody molecules per second until it dies, usually within a few days after reaching maturity.

The determination of the structure of antibody molecules was an important achievement that has made possible many of the subsequent advances in immunology [see "The Structure of Antibodies," by R. R. Porter, the article beginning on page 31, and "The Structure and Function of Antibodies," by Gerald M. Edelman, the article beginning on page 39]. Antibodies belong to the family of proteins collectively called the immunoglobulins (Ig). Each antibody molecule consists of two pairs of polypeptide chains (chains of amino acid units); because the chains of one pair are longer and have a higher molecular weight than those of the other, the chains are classified as heavy and light. In the molecule the four chains are related by bilateral symmetry [see *top illustration on opposite page*].

The light chains can be either of two types, kappa or lambda, although in any one molecule both light chains are always of the same type. There are five types of heavy chain (mu, gamma, alpha, delta and epsilon), which determine the immunoglobulin class of the antibody (IgM, IgG, IgA, IgD and IgE). Some immunoglobulins also have addi-

tional polypeptides, and some form oligomeric associations of from two to five units (each unit consisting of paired light and heavy chains). In addition there are within some of the classes multiple subclasses, and there are allelic variations, that is, alternative forms of genes at a particular locus on a chromosome. Several alleles may be present in a population, and an individual may inherit different ones from his mother and father [see *bottom illustration on opposite page*].

Both the light and the heavy chains of the antibody molecule can be subdivided into constant regions (C_L and C_H), in which the amino acid sequence is essentially invariant, and variable regions (V_L and V_H). Much of the variability in the *V* regions is found in three small areas, which are called hypervariable. X-ray-crystallographic studies by L. M. Amzel and his colleagues at the National Institutes of Health have shown that the polypeptide chains fold in such a way that the hypervariable regions of each V_L and V_H chain interact to form a cleft or pocket. It is these clefts—there are two per molecule—that bind to antigens. The amino acid sequence of the constant regions thus determines the class of an immunoglobulin, and therefore its biological role, whereas the variable regions determine its specificity. These characteristics of the molecule are in turn determined by genetic events in the *B* cell that synthesizes it, and the diversity of immunoglobulins merely reflects the remarkable genetic diversity of *B* cells. With certain exceptions each *B* cell is confined to the production of antibody of a single class, subclass, light-chain type, allelic type and specificity.

In chickens, and probably in all birds, stem cells are induced to become *B* cells in the bursa of Fabricius. Moore and Owen have shown that stem cells begin migrating into the bursal epithelium by the 13th day of embryonation, which is about eight days before chicks hatch. By the next day some of the immigrant stem cells have been transformed into lymphoid cells producing IgM. A few days later a smaller proportion of bursa lymphocytes begin to synthesize IgG, and just before the time of hatching still fewer begin making IgA. *B* cells at this time are rich in polyribosomes, the intracellular bodies on which proteins are synthesized, but they lack the well-developed secretory organelles that characterize mature plasma cells. The relatively small amounts of immunoglobulins produced by the rapidly dividing cells are not yet secreted but are incorporated into the cell membrane.

In the peripheral lymphoid tissue the sequence in which plasma cells develop recapitulates that of cells in the bursa: first IgM is synthesized and secreted, then IgG and finally IgA. (The events controlling the production of IgD and IgE are less well understood.) Each type of plasma cell ordinarily does not appear, however, until several days after the corresponding *B* cell. Exposure to high concentrations of antigens hastens the maturation of plasma cells in peripheral areas, and maintaining the experimental animal in a germ-free environment retards it. Inside the bursa neither condition has much effect on the initiation of lymphocyte formation.

That the bursa controls the capacity of chickens to produce the several classes of immunoglobulins was learned by studying the effects of bursectomy at various times during embryonic development. Removal of the organ on the 16th or 17th day of development frequently results in the permanent absence of all *B* cells and their mature plasma-cell progeny. The result is often complete and permanent agammaglobulinemia: a lack of the gamma-globulin fraction of the blood serum, which contains the antibodies. When the bursa is removed at about the 19th day, IgM is usually present in the mature bird, but IgG and IgA are not. When bursectomy is performed at hatching (21 days), IgM and IgG are

delayed in reaching normal concentration but may eventually exceed normal levels; IgA, on the other hand, is often permanently lacking. The effect of these procedures is to arrest the development of the bursal line of lymphocytes at intermediate stages of differentiation. They can tell us two things about the development of humoral immunity: first, in chickens the bursa appears to be the exclusive site for the formation of *B* cells and, second, individual *B* lymphocytes are irrevocably committed to the synthesis of IgM, IgG or IgA when, in that order, they leave the parent organ.

Two competing theories could explain the generation of class diversity among *B* lymphocytes. Within the bursal environment different stem cells might be induced to begin synthesizing the immunoglobulins IgM, IgG and IgA, or lymphocytes that initially express IgM could be made to switch to IgG and later to IgA. In a series of experiments in our laboratory at the University of Alabama in Birmingham Medical Center, Paul W. Kincade demonstrated that the latter is the more likely explanation. He found that in the bursa the cells containing IgG frequently contain IgM as well (a situation that is not common in any other part of the body). This pattern suggested that while a cell is in the bursa it can change products; it was confirmed

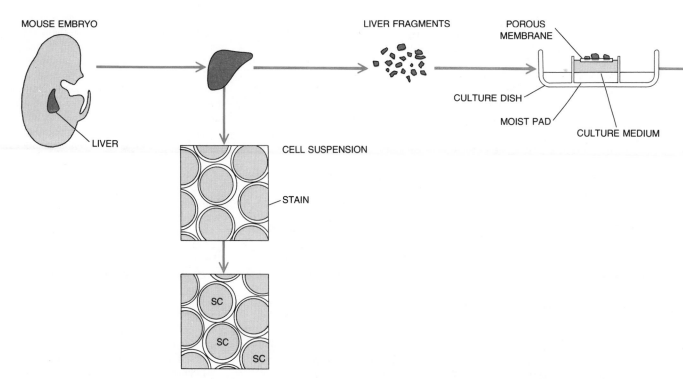

POSSIBLE MAMMALIAN EQUIVALENT of the avian bursa of Fabricius was identified in an experiment showing that *B* cells (lymphocytes bearing immunoglobulins) can develop from stem cells in the fetal liver. Livers were removed from mouse embryos 12 to 15 days old, cut into fragments and grown in a culture dish. *B* cells were not present initially, but they could be detected after a week's growth. Their presence was revealed by staining a suspension of cells with labeled antibodies specific for the heavy chains of immunoglobulins; the stained cells were then examined under a microscope. The *B* cells developed in the same sequence that is obby experiments in which chick embryos were treated with foreign antibodies capable of recognizing the heavy chain of IgM as an antigen. (Since that is the mu chain, the antibodies are called anti-mu antibodies.) Anti-mu antibodies temporarily suppressed not only IgM-containing cells but also all B lymphocytes, a result consistent with the theory that IgG and IgA cells are merely the progeny of IgM cells. Subsequent removal of the bursa permanently obliterated all traces of the entire B-cell line, again indicating that there is only one population of bursa-derived lymphocytes, which manufactures the immunoglobulins in the sequence IgM, IgG, IgA.

A further conclusion about the development of humoral immunity could be drawn from these observations. It appears that the signals controlling the generation of lymphocytes within the bursa are different in kind from those mediating the further differentiation of the cells once they leave the bursa. The former are intrinsic to the bursa, whereas the latter must include the influence of exogenous antigens. From these concepts we derived a general model for B-cell differentiation [see illustration on page 65]. It is an elaboration of the clonal selection theory proposed by Sir Macfarlane Burnet, in which antigens select preexisting cells bearing the ap-

A Model of Cell Differentiation

Before a cell can be selected by an antigen it must be generated from an undifferentiated precursor and induced to manifest the appropriate antibody. In our model this process begins with the migration of a stem cell into a particular environment: the avian bursa of Fabricius or its mammalian equivalent. The first detectable step in differentiation is the synthesis of IgM antibodies, most of which are incorporated into the cell membrane, where they serve as receptors for a single antigen.

Still under the influence of the inductive microenvironment, the clonal precursor undergoes a series of mitotic divisions, producing from one cell a great many identical offspring. The majority of the daughter cells migrate to the peripheral tissues, but at some point one or more of those remaining in the bursa (or its equivalent) take a second step in differentiation by switching from IgM synthesis to IgG synthesis. The change is believed to involve only the expression of the two genes that specify the constant regions of the mu and gamma heavy chains; the cell merely stops manufacturing the mu chain and begins making the gamma chain. The light-chain type of the clone is not altered, nor are the variable regions of either chain, so that the specificity of the molecule for its antigen does not change. It is proposed that precursor cells committed to IgA synthesis arise from a similar mechanism in which the cell switches from gamma to alpha heavy chains. Precursor cells for IgD and IgE and the various subclasses could develop in the same way, but too little is known of their origin for them to be explicitly included in the model.

Further B-cell differentiation is initiated by external factors, primarily environmental antigens, in most cases with the cooperation of other types of cells, such as T lymphocytes and macrophages. The second stage begins when immunologically competent "virgin" B lymphocytes are stimulated by contact with an antigen to proliferate and thereby form either plasma cells or additional B lymphocytes called memory cells. The production of memory cells is a mechanism for the expansion of selected clones; it enables an individual who has

propriate receptors and stimulate them to proliferate, thereby increasing production of the antibody specific to that antigen [see "The Mechanism of Immunity," by Sir Macfarlane Burnet, beginning on page 12].

been exposed to an antigen once to respond more promptly and vigorously in a second encounter. B cells are transformed into plasma cells through an intermediate form called a lymphoblast. The large quantities of antibody secreted by the mature plasma cell initiate the elimination of the antigens, usually by activating the group of enzymes collectively called complement [see "The Complement System," by Manfred M. Mayer, the article beginning on page 143].

The way in which antigens induce B cells to divide and mature is not entirely clear, but two types of signal are thought to be involved. One is the direct interaction of antigens with antibodies on the surface of the lymphocyte, presumably through some correspondence of shape. Antigens with closely spaced, repeating antigenic determinants, such as polysaccharides (chains of sugar units), are most efficient in this mode of stimulation. Another signal is communicated by activated T cells, and factors from T cells may reach B lymphocytes by way of the surface of macrophages. A secondary stimulus augmenting the antigen seems to be more important for triggering the terminal differentiation of B cells into plasma cells than it is for inducing the formation of memory cells. The requirement for T-cell cooperation also varies with the class of immunoglobulins. IgM immune responses are the least dependent on thymus-derived cells, and IgA responses are the most dependent.

A final stage in the control of the humoral immune response is the prevention of excessive proliferation of B cells and the overproduction of specific antibodies. This is accomplished by a feedback mechanism in which an antibody inhibits the proliferation of the clone of cells that produced it. Recent evidence suggests that a special class of "suppressor" T cells may also be important in modulating the immune reaction.

Because mammals have no identifiable bursa, it is not now possible in experiments with mice to surgically remove the source of newly formed B cells. Many of the experiments that helped to elucidate the development of the immune system in birds can therefore be carried out in mammals only with modified techniques. One of these techniques consists in attacking the B cells in situ by repeated injections of foreign antibodies beginning at birth; the antibodies are specific for antigenic determinants on the heavy chains of immunoglobulins.

With Richard M. Asofsky of the National Institutes of Health, we found that anti-mu antibodies given to newborn

ONE WEEK

LIVER FRAGMENTS AND GROWTH

CELL SUSPENSION

STAIN

B
B
B

served in living animals: first to appear were those bearing IgM, then IgG and finally IgA. The experiment was performed at University College London by John J. T. Owen, Martin C. Raff and one of the authors (Cooper).

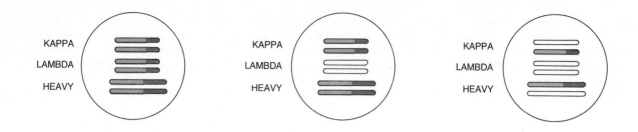

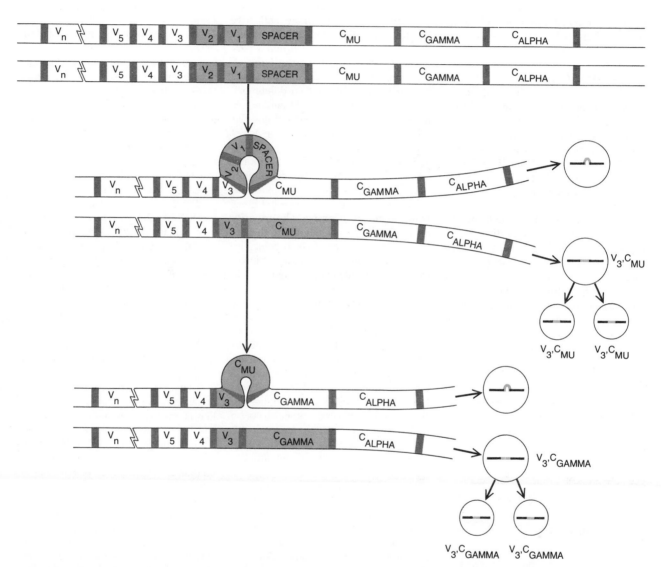

HYPOTHETICAL GENETIC MECHANISM for the generation of diversity among *B* cells postulates the repression of certain genes and, the formation of loops in DNA. Three independent families of genes specify the polypeptide chains of immunoglobulin molecules (*circled diagrams at top*). One family codes for kappa light chains, another for lambda light chains and a third for the various classes of heavy chains. Each family consists of genes in tandem on a pair of chromosomes for constant regions (*black*) and variable regions (*color*). The first stage in the differentiation of the cells is the repression of the genes for one light chain; here the lambda chain is deleted. Next, one set of genes in each remaining family is repressed. The information expressed by the cell thus consists of a set of genes for one kind of light chain, in this case kappa, and a complement of genes for all the heavy chains. In the lower illustration the heavy-chain genes are shown in detail. They can be considered domains in tandem array on a long sequence of DNA; the genes for variable regions are separated from those for constant regions by a spacer, and each of the genes is bounded by zones called recognition units (*black bands*). The constant-region genes are arranged in the order mu, gamma, alpha. A variable-region gene is selected for expression when a loop forms in the DNA (*colored segment*), bringing the gene for the third variable region (V_3) into contact with the one for the mu-chain constant region (C_{mu}). The loop is stabilized by the recognition units of the two genes. When this segment of the DNA replicates during cell division, the genetic information in the loop is deleted, and the daughter cells therefore produce immunoglobulins with the mu heavy chain (IgM) and of specificity determined by variable-region gene V_3. In a later generation another loop forms, this time excising the mu-chain genes and leading to progeny cells that make IgG. Loops formed in later generations could explain the development of IgA-secreting cells and the expression of all the remaining variable-region genes.

mice led to the almost complete elimination of B-cell activity, whereas T-cell development and function were unimpaired. After the treatment fewer than 2 percent of all spleen cells were found to bear the surface marker for B cells, compared with about 45 percent in control mice. Serum concentrations of all classes of immunoglobulins were depressed. Even when challenged with potent antigens, the treated animals were incapable of producing antibodies. The results of this investigation and similar results obtained independently by Dean W. Manning and John W. Jutila of Montana State University were entirely consistent with those of experiments in birds.

If the proposed mu-gamma-alpha sequence of gene expression for the constant regions of the heavy chains is correct, then elimination of IgG precursors as they first appear should block IgA synthesis as well. An experiment testing this hypothesis was complicated by the fact that during gestation maternal IgG is transferred across the placenta to the fetus, making it difficult to suppress IgG synthesis. In only one of several experiments did repeated injections of antigamma antibody completely eliminate IgG production. IgA-producing cells were suppressed in the IgG-deficient mice, but they were present in those mice making normal amounts of IgG. In all the animals IgM production was unimpaired. Inhibition of IgA synthesis by injections of anti-alpha antibodies had no effect on either IgM or IgG. Because the experiment in which IgG synthesis was suppressed has been so difficult to reproduce, the mu-gamma-alpha sequence cannot be considered proved. It is clear, however, that all B cells are the progeny of cells that have synthesized IgM at an earlier stage of development.

There is other evidence in mammals indicating that a change in the expression of genes for the constant regions of the heavy immunoglobulin chains (C_H) is responsible for the change in the class of immunoglobulins synthesized by B cells. In studies of a man with a myeloma (a cancer of the bone marrow) that resulted in excessive proliferation of cells producing IgM and IgG, An-Chuan Wang and H. Hugh Fudenberg and their colleagues at the School of Medicine of the University of California at San Francisco found that only the constant regions of the heavy chains distinguished the products of the two kinds of cancerous cells. The light chains and the variable regions of both heavy and light chains were identical in amino acid composition, even though the two classes of immunoglobulins were being manufactured by separate populations of malignant plasma cells. These and other observations indicate that a C_H gene switch is at least possible.

The Mammalian Bursa Equivalent

One of the principal impediments to the study of B-cell development in mammals has been our ignorance of where the development takes place. In the search for a mammalian equivalent of the bursa of Fabricius many kinds of tissue have been considered—for example the bone marrow and the spleen. One theory that for a time seemed promising was proposed by one of us (Cooper), Good and our colleagues; it held that the appendix and certain other intestinal lymphoepithelial tissues were the mammalian sites of B-cell induction. The theory has since turned out to be wrong, at least to the extent that these regions cannot be the only sites of B-lymphocyte formation.

In mammalian embryos lymphocytes bearing surface immunoglobulins appear first in the blood-forming organs. In mice having a gestation period of 20 days B cells appear in the liver and the spleen at 16 or 17 days. Several days earlier hemopoietic stem cells stream from the yolk sac into the liver and then the spleen. Recently Owen, Raff and one of us (Cooper), working at University College London, have shown in an organ-culture study that B cells arise *de novo* in these hemopoietic tissues [*see illustration on pages 66 and 67*].

Livers were removed from mouse fetuses between the 12th day and the 15th day of gestation, cut into small fragments and floated in a culture medium atop a porous membrane. Receiving nutrients from below and oxygen from above, liver fragments will grow in such an environment for several days. During the first week in culture B cells appeared in the same sequence as the one in which they emerge in the living fetus. IgM- and IgG-bearing cells were detected at almost the same time; they were followed by IgA cells. As in chick embryos and newborn mice, anti-mu antibodies blocked the development of all B lymphocytes.

Whole spleens can also give rise to immunoglobulin-bearing lymphocytes. Whether or not the lymphoid stem cells in the spleen have already been influenced by passage through the liver is for now not known. The primacy of the liver as a B-cell induction site does seem to be a possibility, in part because its origin, like that of the avian bursa, is in epithelial tissue; the spleen, on the other hand, is derived from embryonic mesenchyme.

As is predicted by our model, the various immunoglobulin classes of B cells develop as well in media free of exogenous antigens as they do in culture media containing antigenic materials, such as calf-serum proteins. Class diversity also develops normally whether or not T lymphocytes are present in the culture. These factors would be expected to influence only the second phase of B-cell differentiation: that which takes place as a response to an antigen.

Other investigations of the influence of antigens on B-cell diversity have approached the question differently. Joan L. Press and Norman R. Klinman of the University of Pennsylvania School of Medicine have shown that the precursors of cells bearing antibodies to a specific antigen appear with comparable frequency in the spleens of fetal mice and mature mice. Because the antigen would not be encountered in fetal life, their findings support the view that clonal diversity in B cells arises independent of contact with antigens. Patricia G. Spear and her colleagues at Rockefeller University have reached a similar conclusion through experiments employing a different technique for detecting antigen-reactive B lymphocytes in fetal and adult animals. For now it cannot be stated with certainty that "intrinsic" antigens (such as the histocompatibility antigens that are the major determinants of self-recognition) play no role in the ontogeny of B cells, but there is an abundance of evidence to suggest that the development of diversity in B lymphocytes is not a response to random contacts with antigens from the external environment.

The Genetics of Immunity

As the experiments recounted above imply, there is every reason to believe that the primary differentiation of stem cells into a diverse population of B cells and other cells follows an orderly program encoded in the genes, and that the program operates without prompting from the external environment. For this reason it is essential that an explanation of immunological development be based ultimately on genetic principles.

In most proteins a single gene encodes all the information for the synthesis of a single polypeptide chain; this is not so in the case of the immunoglobulins, as was first suggested by William J. Dreyer and J. Claude Bennett of the California Institute of Technology. Hereditary studies and the amino acid sequences of immunoglobulins both suggest that the constant and the variable regions of each polypeptide chain are specified by different genes, and that there are in fact three distinct families of structural genes for antibody molecules. Each family consists of a number of genes in tandem array coding for the variable regions of heavy or light chains and, nearby on the same chromosome, a smaller number of genes for the constant regions. One family specifies kappa light chains, the second lambda light chains and the third the various classes and subclasses of heavy chains. The genes within each family are linked, but the three families are not; they are probably located on separate chromosomes.

The chromosomes are of course paired, but information from only one chromosome of each pair is expressed. The repression of one set of genes in each pair is necessary if the model is to account for the observed behavior of plasma cells; even in an individual that is heterozygous for a genetic marker on an immunoglobulin, each plasma cell expresses only one of the alleles, a phenomenon called allelic exclusion.

The first step in constructing an immunoglobulin from this genetic program is therefore the functional repression of the immunoglobulin genes on one of the paired chromosomes bearing each gene family. The mechanism must then select which light-chain family, kappa or lambda, is to be expressed. Two families of genes then remain: one family for light chains and one for heavy chains; the latter determines the class of the immunoglobulin.

The next decision is the selection of a particular set of variable-region genes for both the heavy and the light chains; these will together determine the specificity of the antibody. The number of inherited variable genes remains a matter of controversy, but most investigators agree that it must be fairly large, and it could be enormous. Advocates of one theory, called the germ-line theory, argue that all the necessary variable-region genes are inherited. Others hold that much of the variability of the molecule is generated by somatic mutation or recombination of genes, in which case they would not be passed on to offspring. There is evidence suggesting that the genes specifying the variable and constant regions are joined in the DNA in the cell nucleus, and that a single RNA message is transcribed from the DNA and employed to direct the synthesis of each polypeptide strand in the antibody molecule.

Several models for the splicing together of variable-region and constant-region genes have been proposed. One that might account for both the joining of V and C genes and for the sequential switch from one class of immunoglobulins to another assumes that the C_H genes are linked in the order mu, gamma, alpha. Loops formed in the DNA would excise each of these genes in sequence; when the looped DNA was transcribed or replicated, the information in the loop would be deleted, so that separate clones of cells making each class of antibody would be created in turn. The same mechanism could also account for the selection of one gene for the variable regions from the pool of many genes, thereby determining the specificity of the molecule [see illustration on page 68].

One potential method of choosing between the various theories of gene splicing and selection is through the study of apparent exceptions to the rule that a single B cell can produce only one class of antibodies at a given time. Benvenuto Pernis of the Basel Institute for Immunology has demonstrated that rabbit B cells producing IgG may have IgM on their surface; with David S. Rowe of the World Health Organization labora-

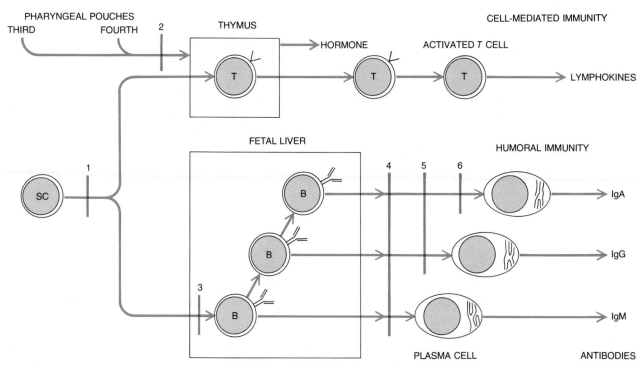

IMMUNODEFICIENCY DISEASES can be considered defects in the differentiation of lymphocytes and lymphoid tissues. The absence of both B cells and T cells suggests a failure of lymphocyte precursors and can be repaired by transplanting stem cells (1) from the fetal liver or the bone marrow. Individuals born without a thymus (2) lack cell-mediated immunity; the functions of this system can be restored by the transplantation of a fetal thymus. The failure of stem cells to develop into B lymphocytes (3) is a congenital, sex-linked disorder first described by Ogden C. Bruton; presumably it derives from a defect of the B-cell-induction site, probably the fetal liver. In other disorders of antibody production B cells are present but they are not stimulated by antigens to divide and develop into mature plasma cells. The arrest of differentiation may be absolute, and therefore lead to a deficiency of all classes of immunoglobulins (4); it may involve cells making IgG and IgA (5), or it may be confined to IgA-secreting cells only (6).

tory in Lausanne he has gone on to show that human *B* lymphocytes may apparently make IgM and IgD simultaneously.

Pernis' findings in rabbits could be explained by the presence of a long-lived messenger molecule for mu chains, which might remain active after the transcription of DNA had switched from the mu-chain to the gamma-chain gene. The second case is more difficult to explain and may represent an instance of simultaneous transcription of genes for antibodies that are of different classes but share the same specificity. Pernis and Maxime Seligmann of the Hôpital Saint-Louis in Paris have discovered in a patient with a *B*-lymphocyte malignancy IgM and IgD molecules on the cell surface that share activity against IgG. The expression of specificity to the same antigen can be interpreted to mean that the variable regions of the heavy chains of both immunoglobulins are identical. If it can be unequivocally demonstrated that the same V_H gene can be transcribed simultaneously with two C_H genes, the model presented here would be excluded in favor of one that makes provision for more than one copy of each V_H gene. Deciphering nature's solution to the problem of generating diversity in the immune system should be of tremendous importance in understanding the differentiation of other kinds of cells.

Abnormal Development

Knowledge of how lymphoid cells differentiate also offers insight into disorders of the immune system, and in some cases it may reveal at what point the system has gone awry. Markers that can be employed to detect *B* lymphocytes, for example, have helped to show that most boys with Bruton's disease (the sex-linked congenital deficiency in plasma cells and circulating antibodies) are virtually devoid of *B* cells in all stages of differentiation. This observation suggests that the disease might be caused by a flaw in the organ of *B*-cell generation, perhaps the fetal liver. Patients who develop a deficiency in plasma cells and antibodies later in life, on the other hand, often have normal numbers of *B* lymphocytes bearing immunoglobulins of all classes. In this case it appears that the defect is in the later stages of differentiation and prevents the maturation of *B* cells into plasma cells.

In other immunodeficient individuals the development of one class or more but not all classes of antibody-producing cells is arrested. In isolated IgA deficiency, a condition in which only that class of immunoglobulins is lacking, *B* cells bearing IgA are almost always found in the bloodstream. The defect is present in one of every 500 people of European ancestry. L. Y. Frank Wu of our laboratory has found that *B* cells from some IgA-deficient patients can be stimulated to mature and secrete antibodies by growing them in a culture with an extract from pokeweed, a plant that contains several substances that influence the behavior of lymphoid cells. The pokeweed extract can also stimulate the differentiation of lymphocytes from some individuals who are deficient in all classes of immunoglobulins. Such discoveries inspire hope that in the future it may be possible to correct life-threatening immune disorders. Infants born without a thymus have already been successfully treated with thymus grafts, and infants lacking both *T* and *B* cells have been immunologically repaired through transplants of bone marrow and fetal liver.

Markers peculiar to *T* and *B* cells also make it possible to identify the cells involved in lymphoid cancers. Some cases of acute lymphocytic leukemia, for example, appear to be *T*-cell malignancies. Malignant proliferation of *B* cells occurs at several stages of differentiation. Myelomas are characterized by uncontrolled growth of clones of mature plasma cells, whereas chronic lymphocytic leukemia and Burkitt's lymphoma involve *B* lymphocytes. The macroglobulinemias of Waldenström, named for Jan Waldenström of the General Hospital at Malmö in Sweden, represent an accumulation of cells in transition from *B* lymphocytes to antibody-secreting cells.

The virus-induced lymphoma of bursal cells in chickens resembles Burkitt's lymphoma in man, a malignant disease that also appears to be caused by a virus. The tumorous lymphocytes invariably produce IgM, regardless of their location in the body. It therefore seems plausible that the virus that precipitates the cancer transforms the cells during clonal differentiation, interrupting the usual course of gene expression at the time when the cell would ordinarily change from the synthesis of IgM to the synthesis of IgG. Because the cells seem to be susceptible to the oncogenic effects of the virus only at a particular stage of differentiation, it appears that the development of the malignancy depends on what part of the host-cell genome is being expressed. Whether or not these speculations prove to be correct, they hint at potentially valuable concepts that may be refined through further study of developmental processes in the immune system.

II

CELL-MEDIATED IMMUNITY

CELL-MEDIATED IMMUNITY

II

INTRODUCTION

By 1960 it was clear that out of the mass of phenomena that could be looked on as immunological one could sort out one very large set in which antibody production was clearly concerned. In addition to the serological reactions directly produced by antibody, the phenomena of this set included several types of skin tests and other manifestations of tissue reactivity, among which were the positive reactions following tests for allergic reactivity to pollens and the like in persons subject to hay fever, and the Arthus reaction to soluble proteins. Both types of sensitization can be transferred to an initially nonsensitive individual by general or local injection of serum from a positive reactor. Interaction of antigen and antibody in the tissue, usually with complement, produces one or more pharmacologically active agents, giving rise to a rapidly appearing inflammatory or necrotic response.

A second category of reactions to antigens in sensitized or immune subjects is separated from the first under the general label of delayed hypersensitivity (DH) reactions. The prototype of these reactions is the response to tubercle bacillus protein (PPD—purified protein derivative) when this is injected into the skin of people or animals who are or have been infected with tuberculosis. Reactivity from a sensitized animal, usually a guinea pig, can be transferred to normal animals by cells from the spleen, lymph nodes, or peritoneal exudate, but not by serum. In Alfred J. Crowle's 1960 article there is a clear account of the contrasts between acute and delayed hypersensitivity and the significance of these for medicine, which is still reasonably adequate. A present-day reader, however, will recognize at once that Crowle's article was written just before immunologists became interested in the thymus.

In this group of articles on cell-mediated immunity, the central feature is the demarcation and function of T and B cells, just as it remains the most active field of current immunological research. The earliest work in this field and a number of the early misconceptions are reported in my 1962 article. The most exciting news at that time was, first, the discovery by Jacques Miller of the effects of neonatal thymectomy in mice, and second, the work by Warner and Szenberg in the Walter and Eliza Hall Institute at the Royal Melbourne Hospital in differentiating the immunological functions of thymus and bursa in the chicken. Not very long afterwards it was found that for most types of antibody production in the mouse the cooperation of T cells with B cells was necessary. This third major discovery in the field is one for which Graham Mitchell and Jacques Miller should receive most credit. Taken together, these three seminal discoveries set the ground rules for many of the activities that have taken place in cellular immunology since the early 1960s. Like any other scientific article or lecture reviewing a newly opened field, the 1962 article on the thymus is badly off the mark at certain points. Miller's neonatally thymectomized mice produced much-reduced titers of antibody against most antigens, and it was thought that in the mammal the thymus would fill the functions served by both bursa and thymus in the chicken. As a logical implication of this it was assumed that the development of natural tolerance took place almost entirely in the thymus. Neither of these assumptions has stood the test of continued study in the intervening years, but it can also be confessed that no simply stated and satisfying alternative interpretation has yet come to light.

It is generally accepted that in the adult mammal B cells derive from stem cells in the bone marrow, only small but perhaps not wholly insignificant numbers being present in the thymus in the form of memory cells. The interpretation of natural tolerance has metaphorically been placed in cold storage until unanimity can be reached on the nature of the T-cell receptors. Cooper and Lawton express this by saying that without knowledge of the receptor the functioning of the T cell cannot be adequately described. This holds not only for tolerance but almost equally for the helper function of T cells in antibody production and the production of graft-versus-host reactions like the cellular foci produced on chorioallantoic membranes. Even though all immunologists agree that the answer is not yet to hand, it is a reasonable prediction that what we shall probably agree is a provisionally satisfying answer will be available before 1980. As long as it is recognized for what it is, a critical look at the problem of T-cell receptors and the main alternative solutions would seem a wholly appropriate topic for this anthology.

T-CELL RECEPTORS

When T cells are needed in quantity so that a serious attempt can be made to isolate and characterize a specific receptor, several problems confront the experimenter immediately. The first is that for practical purposes a T cell is negatively defined by the fact that it has no immunoglobulin visible by standard immunological tests on its surface. With refined tests all workers are agreed that there is some Ig present but very much less than on B cells. It is also known that T cells, human or murine, can be extremely heterogeneous when tested either for their capacity to respond specifically to various antigens or by their executive functions as helpers, cytotoxic cells, lymphokine producers, and so on. Everyone in the field dreams of a way by which a single T cell could be cloned, i.e., isolated under conditions where it could multiply and eventually produce an unlimited population of identical cells. Unfortunately this has not yet been achieved for any normal lymphocyte. B cells infected by Epstein-Barr virus will produce monoclonal cell lines, but the only continuing culture lines of T cells are from malignant conditions and are therefore quite unsuitable for physiological study. In default of a satisfactory monoclonal population, the experimenter can only attempt to remove from a mixed population of lymphocytes all those that carry significant amounts of immunoglobulin. Under good conditions the residual lymphocytes will have only 1 or 2 percent of B cells and perhaps 95 percent of cells giving an appropriate, positive identification as T cells. Such a population may not be quite "pure" enough.

The reason for studying the T receptors is to learn what is the basis of the specific reactivity of T cells: what sort of receptors do they carry that recognize the particular pattern of an antigen—what Jerne calls the epitope—to which the cell will respond? Broadly speaking, the main points to be considered as evidence are, first, that to function as helper cells, T cells must be able to respond to the same antigen that stimulates the cooperating B cell to produce an antibody and, second, that allowing for many minor differences

DONOR CELLS FROM MOUSE SPLEENS	IRRADIATED RECIPIENTS OF DONOR CELLS	
	MOUSE OF STRAIN *A*	MOUSE OF STRAIN *B*
MOUSE OF STRAIN *A* MOUSE OF STRAIN *B*	UNENLARGED SPLEEN ENLARGED SPLEEN	ENLARGED SPLEEN UNENLARGED SPLEEN

GRAFT-VERSUS-HOST REACTIONS IN MICE can be measured by weighing the mouse spleens. Two strains of mice, *A* and *B*, differing in major histocompatibility antigens, are used as donors of spleen cells of as heavily irradiated recipients. When the cells are injected intravenously they lodge in the spleen. If donor and recipient are of the same histocompatibility type there is no enlargement of the spleen, but if they differ there is marked enlargement of the spleen when the mouse is killed five to seven days later. Weight increase in the spleen is used as a measure of the intensity of the graft-versus-host reaction.

of various sorts, T cells seem to have approximately as wide and sensitive a range of specificity for foreign antigens as B cells and antibodies have. It is hardly conceivable that the same species should evolve two such similar types of receptors on two wholly different principles, and most workers would tend to favor the concept of a T-cell receptor that, for the present, can be called an IgT receptor. This accepts the fact that it is immunoglobulin-like in character and has a standard variable-region combining site, but leaves the nature of its heavy chain unspecified. To say that T cells carry an IgT receptor, however, is not to say that the receptor is necessarily synthesized by the cell that carries it. The receptor could just as well be received passively from B cells.

At this point we move to another set of antigens, the alloantigens on the surfaces of cells from an unrelated animal of the same species. As one example we can take the graft-versus-host reactions that are responsible for the pocks on the chorioallantoic membrane on which adult chicken lymphocytes have been dropped. Of almost exactly the same quality is another example—the enlargement of the spleen when lymphocytes from a mouse of type *A* are injected intravenously into a mouse of a different major histocompatibility type *B* that has been immunologically paralyzed by a dose of X-rays. [*See the illustration above.*] In both of these experiments it can be calculated that the reaction is specific for each of the dozen distinct major histocompatibility types that have been tested in each species. But what is disconcerting—or was originally—is that in most T-cell populations as many as 2 to 5 percent of the cells will react against a single allogeneic tissue. That finding is extremely difficult to interpret in terms of a single system of immunoglobulin receptors and a consistent rule that one immunocyte (T or B) reacts effectively only with a single antigenic determinant. In fact one would have to agree that unless some second set of receptors is also available for the work done by the T cell, the result could well be fatal to the whole idea of clonal selection.

A number of immunologists would agree that there must also be a different system present and that it is intimately related to the major histocompatibility antigens that determine whether or not a rapid, decisive rejection of a skin transplant between two individuals will occur. The simplest formulation, which will almost certainly have to be developed into some more elaborate and sophisticated form, is to assume a clonal system in which there are receptors corresponding in complementary fashion to each of the major histocompatibility antigens (MHCA) of the species. [*See the illustration on page 78.*] Each T lymphocyte expresses only one, and when it meets a cell carrying the corresponding MHCA, it can react by proliferation to produce a descendant clone, each cell of which also has the same receptor. The receptor is presumably a protein quite unrelated to an immunoglobulin. It should be noted, however, that though this receptor, which can be called a primitive allogeneic receptor (AR), can react only with the right MHCA, the MHCA can also react with immunoglobulin receptors and antibodies of the right types—in more conventional terms, the MHCA can induce the formation of antibodies. At the present time many immunologists would probably summarize their views on T-cell receptors as follows:

1. Most T-cell immune responses are mediated by an immunoglobulin receptor which is, or closely resembles, IgM in monomeric form (IgM1); many consider it wise to refer to the receptor noncommitally as IgT.

1(a). The IgM1 receptors are received passively from adjacent B cells at an early stage of their response to specific antigenic stimulation; or

1(b). the IgT receptors are synthesized by the T cells themselves but the process develops no further than the IgM1 stage.

2. A primitive allogeneic system of receptors of the type just described is intrinsic to some or all T cells and is quite distinct from the IgT system.

The weight of the evidence favors a passive origin for the IgT receptors, and two sets of experimental data may be cited in support. The first and probably the most impressive was recognized in the course of Warner and Szenberg's work in 1961–1962 but has been largely overlooked. They completely inhibited the development of the bursa by administering 2 mg of testosterone to 12-day embryos and found that after hatching, the chicks, in addition to failing to produce antibody, could not be sensitized to tuberculin or give an accelerated vaccinia reaction. They rejected skin grafts normally and when their lymphocytes were deposited on the chorioallantoic membrane, these T cells were present, but no B cells. On the present hypothesis these T cells would be fully capable of reacting with allogeneic cells, but in the absence of B cells to "arm" them with passive IgT receptors they could not produce delayed hypersensitivity against a foreign antigen. It should be noted that surgical removal of the bursa after hatching, or even at 18 days incubation, does not guarantee that all B cells will be removed from the animal; B lymphocytes will already have begun to develop in and leave the

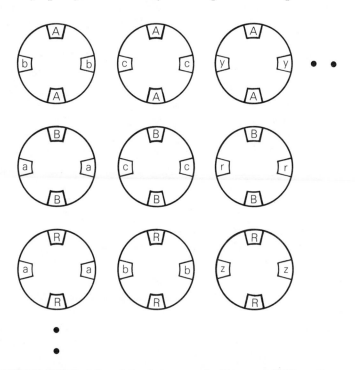

ONE FORMULATION of the relation between major histocompatibility antigens and allogeneic receptors. Each horizontal row represents cells from an individual mouse of a strain having different major histocompatibility antigens (MHCAs) of types A, B, and R, shown as upper case letters. The allogeneic receptors (ARs) are shown lower case, a, b, and so on, to correspond to and react with upper case A, B, and so on, and it is assumed that all except the autologous allogeneic receptor exist among the cells in each individual. Each T lymphocyte expresses one receptor. When it meets a cell carrying the corresponding MHCA, it can react by proliferation to produce a descendant clone, each cell of which also has the same receptor.

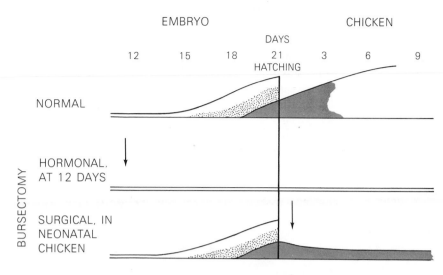

A COMPARISON OF HORMONAL BURSECTOMY at 12 days of incubation (indicated by the arrow at the left side of the middle diagram) and surgical bursectomy at the time of hatching (arrow in the bottom diagram). The white area indicates the development of the bursal epithelium; the dotted areas mark the entry and proliferation of lymphoid cells; gray areas show the relative amounts of differentiated B cells liberated in the circulation; after hatching, only the level of liberated cells is shown. There can be a sharp difference between the result of never allowing the bursa to develop and of removing it after it has developed and liberated even a small proportion of differentiated cells.

bursa. Surgical removal is therefore bound to be less effective than when the whole development of the bursa is inhibited by the administration of testosterone from 12 days of incubation onward. In chicks treated with hormone injections there has been *no* development of lymphocytes in the bursal epithelia. [*See the illustration above.*]

The second set of experiments is due to Morten Simonsen, working with graft-versus-host reactions in mice. His primary interest was to find whether preliminary immunization of the mouse supplying the graft—in these experiments blood lymphocytes—resulted in accentuation of the reaction induced by the graft in the recipient. When the mice used differed in their *major* histocompatibility antigens, it made no difference whether a normal animal was used as cell donor or one that had been immunized with cells of the recipient's type. The normal cells produced a strong reaction, as measured by splenic enlargement in the recipient, and immunization produced no further increase.

Quite contrasting results were obtained when donor and host differed only in respect to one of their *minor* histocompatibility antigens. A recipient injected with normal donor cells responded with only a trivial degree of splenic enlargement. When the donor was immunized with recipient cells or tissues, its cells became capable of producing a much more active graft-versus-host reaction, as much in fact as was shown when host and donor had major histocompatibility differences.

The difference between the two results depends in all probability on the fact that a large proportion (2 to 10 percent) of normal T cells carry an allogeneic receptor against any specific major histocompatibility antigen, and any increase in that proportion as a result of immunization is insignificant. In the second instance, no allogeneic receptors can be involved and the reactions must be mediated through the Ig receptor system. The normal donor has only very small numbers of T cells carrying Ig receptors capable of reaction with a minor histocompatibility antigen, but immunization against the recipient's antigen will allow the effective arming of a large enough proportion of T cells to give a major response in the recipient animals.

There are plenty of difficulties; most of the workers dealing with reactions that involved foreign antigens have implicitly assumed that the receptor they were concerned with was produced by the T cell itself and that on stimulation a specific clone developed, much as a clone of a B-cell plasma cell does. It would need very careful planning to devise a situation in which no clonal proliferation of B cells was going on parallel with the apparent clonal expansion of "armed" T cells. To date there is no evidence that IgM1 is liberated from activated B cells, though IgM1 is known to be abundant in the cytoplasm and most recent writers favor it as the receptor of IgM-secreting B cells. Nor has it been shown that there is any receptor for the crystallizable fragment (Fc) of IgM1 on T cells; the one on B cells is specific for IgG. However, there is no doubt that T cells of both rat and mouse will take up IgM reversibly when placed in an individual of a different allotype, though it remains to be shown that material bound with such relative looseness can act as a specific receptor. The verdict for the present is "not proven."

7

Delayed Hypersensitivity

by Alfred J. Crowle
April 1960

*This type of allergy has been identified as the cause
of rash in poison ivy, pains in rheumatoid arthritis,
lung cavitation in tuberculosis and nerve degeneration
in multiple sclerosis*

For some people poison ivy seems to have no poison. While other campers and gardeners must be wary of the paths that they tread and the leaves that they touch, such a person is able to uproot the plant with his bare hands and to suffer no harmful consequences. But the leaves may be touched once too often, and one day, following a brush with poison ivy, that person finds himself afflicted with the skin rash and blisters that make almost everyone else avoid the plant.

Like hay fever, the reaction to poison ivy is an allergy. Just as most people have a hereditary resistance to developing hay fever, so a few people can handle poison ivy with impunity. In either case, however, this impunity may be overwhelmed by repeated exposure to the allergen that proved so innocuous on first exposure. But the hypersensitive reaction that troubles the sufferer from hay fever follows quickly upon his exposure to ragweed or other irritating pollen. The reaction to poison ivy, in contrast, takes more time to develop. Poison-ivy attacks thus are identified with a little-understood group of allergies characterized as "delayed hypersensitivities."

This simple distinction early divided allergic reactions into two main classes. But the underlying reason for the immediacy of the one reaction and the delay of the other was obscured until recently because it was often difficult to provoke delayed hypersensitivity in experimental animals. Techniques developed for this purpose now have begun to expose the mechanisms of delayed hypersensitivity. This understanding in turn has implicated this type of allergy in a wide range of medical problems aside from straightforward allergic conditions: the cavitation of lung tissue in tuberculosis, the rejection of grafted tissue in surgery, the degeneration of nerves in multiple sclerosis, and the stiffening and swelling of joints in rheumatoid arthritis.

The allergic reaction is itself an expression of the body's biochemical integrity. The body reacts to most foreign materials of an organic nature by manufacturing special substances called antibodies. These combine with the foreign material, or antigen, ordinarily without harmful (and often with helpful) results. By this means, for example, the body generates immunity to infectious disease. In allergic reactions, however, the interaction of antigen and antibody does harm to body tissues. For this reason allergies often have been called immunological mistakes. Indeed, such a "mistake" often attends the development of immunity to disease organisms, though there it turns out to be useful. Skin tests based on the allergic reaction are employed by physicians to diagnose diseases such as tuberculosis and undulant fever or to measure the effectiveness of immunization to tuberculosis and smallpox. Epidemiologists sometimes use these tests to trace the spread of an infection in a human population.

The skin is a sensitive indicator of allergies. In animals hypersensitized to a substance the skin test generally indicates whether the allergy is of the immediate or of the delayed type. The reaction typical of immediate hypersensitivity causes the test area to become hot, red and softly swollen within a few seconds or minutes after the injection. A short while later the skin returns to a normal condition. The skin reaction of delayed hypersensitivity, on the other hand, takes several hours to appear; the affected skin also becomes red and warm, but the swelling this time is firm. The reaction lasts for several days and may kill part of the tissue involved. Of course the differences between immediate and delayed reactions in skin tests are not always clear-cut. For example, a strong immediate hypersensitivity may cause so much local tissue-damage that it appears to be a mixture of immediate and delayed reactions and can be identified only by microscopic examination.

Animal experiments, however, have provided a more significant distinction between the two types of allergy. If blood serum from animals having an allergy of the immediate type is transferred to another animal, the recipient will become temporarily sensitive to the same allergen, and will respond to the skin test with a reaction of the immediate type. This indicates that the antibodies involved in immediate hypersensitivity circulate in the blood serum. In fact, it is possible to isolate these antibodies by precipitating them from the serum in reaction with the antigen that induced their formation. Many of these antibodies have thus been purified and their chemical and physical characteristics described. But the transfer of serum from one animal to another will not carry over delayed hypersensitivity; the antibodies involved in this kind of allergy ordinarily do not circulate in the serum. Delayed hypersensitivity may, however, be passed from an allergic to a normal animal by the injection of cells from the lymphatic system, of related cells from other tissues (reticuloendothelial cells) and of white blood cells. Immediate hypersensitivity is never conveyed passively by such cells.

Thus it has become clear that the two types of allergy depend upon two basically different kinds of antibody. One kind circulates freely in the serum; the other is closely bound to living cells. With few exceptions the antibodies of

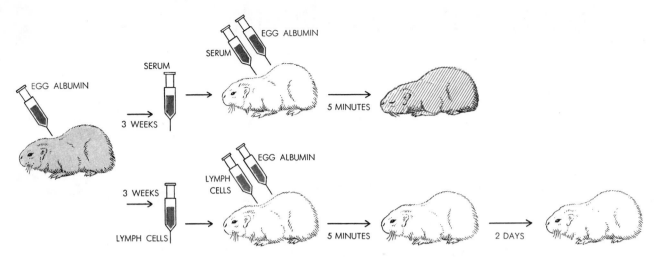

IMMEDIATE HYPERSENSITIVITY is induced by injecting a guinea pig with the antigen egg albumin (*left*). Serum from this animal can transfer the induced allergy to a second animal (*top row at right*), but lymph cells cannot (*bottom row*). After an injection of antigen, guinea pig given serum dies (*hatching*) from an immediate systemic reaction; the one given cells remains well.

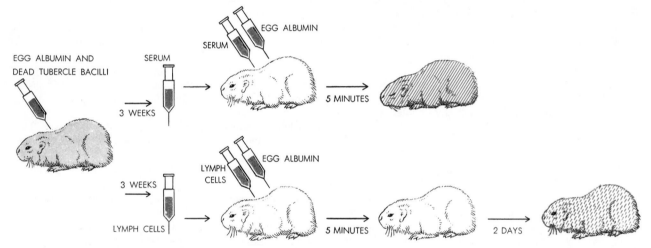

DELAYED HYPERSENSITIVITY to egg albumin is induced along with the immediate type by injecting the antigen and a potentiator, here tubercle bacilli (*left*). Serum from the allergic animal transfers the immediate hypersensitivity to a second animal (*top row at right*); lymph cells transfer the delayed type (*bottom row*). After injection of antigen the animal given serum dies of an immediate systemic reaction; the one given lymph cells later sickens (*broken hatching*) from a delayed type of systemic reaction.

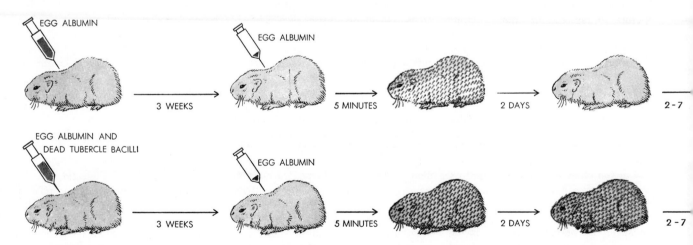

2-7

2-7

DESENSITIZATION is readily accomplished in immediate hypersensitivity but not in the delayed type. A guinea pig with an immediate hypersensitivity (*top*) is given a small dose of antigen; it becomes sick (*broken hatching*) from an immediate systemic reaction but recovers. The animal then does not react to the antigen. A guinea pig having both immediate and delayed hypersensitivity

delayed hypersensitivity lose their activity unless the cells are kept alive and intact. By the same token it has not yet been possible to isolate and identify these antibodies.

For a long time investigators thought that the antigens that induce many kinds of delayed hypersensitivity must be bound equally closely to the living processes of allergenic microorganisms. Infection with certain bacteria will induce both immediate and delayed hypersensitivity in experimental animals. An allergy of the immediate type also can be brought on by extracts of the microorganisms, or indeed by injection of such ordinarily innocuous substances as chicken egg albumin. In early experiments delayed hypersensitivity could be induced only by the living microorganism, so it was often called "infectious allergy." A few years ago, however, various workers found that protein-bearing extracts of killed microorganisms could provoke delayed hypersensitivity if they were injected along with certain lipoidal (fatlike) fractions of these bacteria. Pursuing this lead, they since have succeeded in inducing delayed hypersensitivity to egg albumin and other nonmicrobial proteins by injecting them together with the same type of lipoidal material extracted from bacteria, or simply with the whole killed bacteria.

The role of the lipoidal material is not clear. It may serve to modify the physical nature of the antigen, it may make the responsive cells of the injected animal more reactive to the antigen or it may direct the cells into a new and different response. Some experimenters suggest that lipids in the skin of an affected animal may themselves play the same role in potentiating allergy. It is significant in this connection, incidentally, that the oily poison-ivy allergen, or industrial chemicals that cause the same kind of allergy, hypersensitize an animal only if they are rubbed on the skin.

Since fatty materials are not soluble in water, the antigen and the potentiating agent must be dispersed in an emulsion of water in oil to keep them together in the animal after the injection. Not long ago A. M. Pappenheimer, Jr., of the Harvard Medical School succeeded in inducing delayed hypersensitivity by injecting very minute quantities of protein antigens alone, but the allergy induced seems to differ in some respects from the classic type.

With the means to induce delayed hypersensitivity in experimental animals almost at will, investigators have begun to distinguish its mechanisms more clearly from those of immediate hypersensitivity. One of the most striking characteristics of immediate hypersensitivity is the systemic reaction called anaphylactic shock, which follows rapidly upon injection of a relatively large dose of antigen into the bloodstream. A guinea pig that has been sensitized to egg albumin reacts violently to an amount that would be harmless to the normal animal; it goes into violent convulsions, and moments later it dies of suffocation. The animal also may be readily desensitized to an antigen to which it has immediate hypersensitivity. This is accomplished by injecting a smaller dose of antigen, enough to give the animal a severe but not fatal seizure. Upon recovery it will show no reaction at all to any subsequent injection of egg albumin made during the next few hours or days. An injection of many times the quantity of egg albumin that would have killed the guinea pig before now causes it not the least discomfort.

In an animal in which a delayed hypersensitivity has been provoked the reaction to a heavy injection of the antigen follows a different course. Because the sensitizing technique usually induces immediate as well as delayed hypersensitivity, such an animal may be killed by anaphylactic shock. But if it does recover, it will behave normally for only a few hours. Then its fur begins to ruffle; it breathes uneasily, closes its eyes and crouches apparently senseless to its surroundings. Its body temperature drops and it slowly sinks into a coma to die two or three days later, killed by its delayed hypersensitivity. If the challenging dose of antigen is sufficiently reduced, the animal may recover. But it has not thereby become particularly desensitized to the antigen, for a subsequent injection again will induce the delayed type of systemic reaction, almost as strongly as before.

Although the interpretation of these experimental findings still is controversial, the principal mechanism of delayed hypersensitivity is now discernible. The allergy antibodies are manufactured by some of the body's lymphoid cells when they are confronted with an antigen in a certain form and under specific conditions. These antibodies apparently remain within or on the cells and react specifically with the antigen upon future contact. Probably these antibodies accumulate in large numbers; relatively few lymphoid cells containing them can transfer delayed hypersensitivity from one animal to another. Because delayed hypersensitivity, once actively induced, lasts far longer than the life of any single hypersensitized

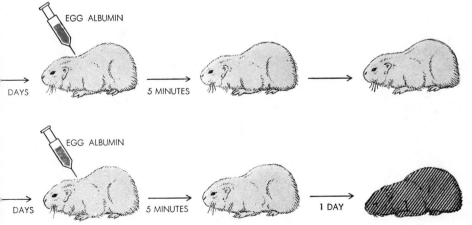

EGG ALBUMIN

DAYS   5 MINUTES

EGG ALBUMIN

DAYS   5 MINUTES   1 DAY

(*bottom row*), on similar treatment, gets nonfatal attacks of both immediate and delayed systemic reactions (*third and fourth steps*). But after the guinea pig recovers, a large dose of the antigen again causes a delayed systemic reaction; the animal then dies (*last step*).

cell, the new cells that replace these either must be freshly sensitized by traces of antigen remaining in the body for a long time, or must inherit the ability to make antibodies through the genetic material of their hypersensitized progenitors. Or the cells may, in some still unknown nonhereditary way, "learn" the art of manufacturing these antibodies from cells already able to do so.

In the delayed allergic reaction the hypersensitive cells seem to be the focus of primary destruction. As the antigen combines with some of the antibodies associated with these cells, it kills the cells. The damaged cells then apparently release uncombined antibodies. The antibodies may be ingested by white blood cells and related phagocytic cells attracted to the site of irritation, and these in turn become hypersensitive and suscep-

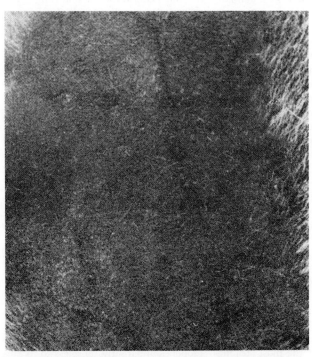

NORMAL MOUSE-SKIN is smooth, and the network of veins is visible through it. In this photograph and the others on this page of mouse-skin tests the areas are enlarged about seven diameters.

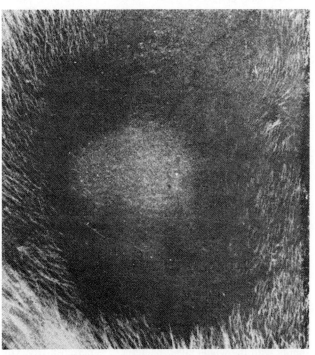

SKIN REACTION in immediate hypersensitivity to bovine serum albumin is shown after one and a half hours. Edema is visible as a blanching of the skin and interruption of the normal vein pattern.

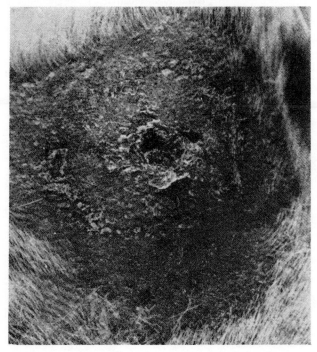

CONTACT DERMITITIS, a form of delayed hypersensitivity, is manifested by a firm swelling (*blanched area*) and central necrosis (*dark scaly area*). This part of a hypersensitive mouse had been exposed to a drop of 2,4–dinitrochlorobenzene 48 hours earlier.

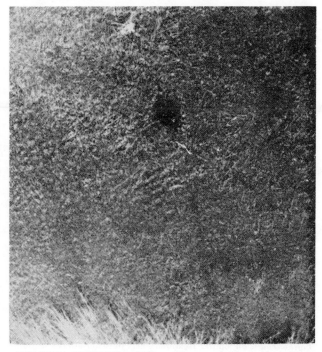

DELAYED SKIN-REACTION persists much longer than the immediate type. Ulceration (*dark spot*) and some swelling are still visible a week after the injection of tuberculoprotein, the antigen to which this mouse had developed a delayed hypersensitivity.

tible to destruction by antigen. This chain reaction evidently continues until antigen or antibody is exhausted. In breaking down, the injured cells release various substances that are toxic to other tissues, thus causing secondary damage that may be more harmful to the body than the primary damage. Secondary effects may account for the death of the skin in a skin test, or for the systemic shock that follows exposure to a large dose of antigen.

The cavities of tuberculosis appear to be formed by delayed-hypersensitivity reactions between protein constituents of the infecting tubercle bacilli and allergic tissue-cells of the lungs, with the secondary toxic products of these reactions causing the destruction of the lung cells. Thus if proteins of tubercle bacilli are injected directly into the lungs of a normal rabbit (in water-oil emulsion to prevent their spread from the site of injection), they cause no cavities to form. But if they are so injected into a rabbit previously hypersensitized by an injection of whole tubercle bacilli elsewhere in the body, they regularly produce cavities. Even a rabbit with delayed hypersensitivity to egg albumin can develop turbercular-like lung cavities if egg albumin is subsequently injected into its lungs.

In many diseases that are chronic enough for delayed hypersensitivity to develop strongly while the body still harbors large or moderate quantities of the infecting agent, it seems likely that gross tissue destruction characteristic of some of them may be traced to the allergic reaction. Recovery from various illnesses caused by bacteria, yeasts, molds and the like thus may depend on how hypersensitive the patient has become to the constituents of the disease germs and on how badly his tissues are injured in allergic reactions with them. Not a little of the itching and sometimes burning irritation of athlete's-foot infection may be due to delayed hypersensitivity to the disease organisms.

Of perhaps less consequence than these manifestations of delayed hypersensitivity is the troublesome and familiar contact dermatitis. This is the itching rash of allergic origin, which can result from repeated exposure of the skin to various nonprotein substances, from the oily constituent of poison-ivy leaves to detergents and industrial chemicals. The substances that cause contact dermatitis seem to have little in common save that they usually combine readily with body proteins; the significance of this tentative finding is not yet completely understood. How readily an individual be-

comes hypersensitive to such substances depends both on his hereditary susceptibility and on the sensitizing potency of the substance. Most people handle the various household detergents with impunity, but the chemical 2,4–dinitrochlorobenzene will sensitize almost anyone upon a single good contact, a fact which makes it a popular experimental chemical for contact-dermatitis experiments in animals. With this chemical, dermatitis can be induced quite easily in an experimental animal simply by dropping a solution of the allergen onto a small area of shaved skin; no lipoidal potentiator is needed. However, if the chemical is injected into the body without touching the skin, it first must be combined with some such potentiator to sensitize the animal. Strangely, the sensitivity associated with contact dermatitis apparently does not make an animal susceptible to the violent systemic reaction that attends the classic form of delayed hypersensitivity to proteins.

An important type of delayed hypersensitivity is that which frustrates surgeons in their age-old ambition to transplant tissues and organs. Unless the donor and recipient are identical twins, tissue transplanted from one to the other almost invariably dies after a few days or weeks. (Grafts of bones or blood vessels only appear to take permanently; actually the foreign tissue is gradually replaced by regeneration of the recipient's own tissues.) A second graft from the same donor is rejected more rapidly than the first. Although immediate hypersensitivity cannot yet be entirely excluded, it appears to have little if any significance in the homograft reaction, as this allergic annihilation of transplanted tissue is called. Often no antibodies appear in the blood serum, and the injection of serum from an animal that has rejected a graft does not cause another animal to reject a graft from the same donor any more speedily. On the other hand, the transfer of lymphoid cells makes the recipient animal reject a graft just as quickly as it would if it were sensitized by prior direct exposure to the donor tissue. Both the animal that has rejected a graft and the animal that has received lymphoid cells will show a skin reaction of the delayed type following intracutaneous injection of cells taken from the donor of the graft. Homograft hypersensitivity differs from classic delayed hypersensitivity, however, in that it can be transferred only with lymphoid tissue cells and not with the white blood cells.

Investigation of the homograft reac-

tion has developed an interesting finding that may have wider implications. Extracts of the material from nuclei of the cells of one animal will provoke the hypersensitivity in another animal as effectively as the intact cells themselves. Yet it is not the nuclear material but material from the cytoplasm (that part of the cell which surrounds the nucleus) that enters into the allergic reaction. This cytoplasmic material, on the other hand, does not induce hypersensitivity. The nuclear substance of animal cells presumably directs their synthesis of cytoplasmic proteins; perhaps when it is transferred to another animal it is ingested by that animal's antibody-making cells, enters their nuclei relatively unchanged and directly induces them to begin making antibodies against the cytoplasmic antigens of cells from which it was originally extracted. Thus the animal would become hypersensitive to cytoplasmic material by having been injected with nuclear material. If this idea is verified, it will have considerable bearing upon our understanding of the fundamental mechanisms of antibody formation.

The homograft reaction reflects the capacity of the body, through its immunological system, to "recognize" its own tissues. This capacity apparently develops shortly before or after birth. Mice of one strain become tolerant to tissues from an unrelated strain if they receive injections of cells of the second type before birth, when their immunological system is still immature. Induction of tolerance in infant human beings by this means is scarcely practical. However, recent experiments with kidney transplants indicate that tolerance can be provoked in adults if the immunological system is depressed by chemical or X-ray treatment before foreign tissue is introduced [see "The Transplantation of the Kidney," by John P. Merrill, beginning on page 187].

Under certain circumstances the body's self-recognition fails. It then develops hypersensitivity to one or another of its own tissues, with consequent injury and destruction to that tissue. Such autosensitization can be of either the immediate or the delayed type. It may be provoked by antigens liberated from the body's own tissue cells. In some instances these antigens may be so well "sheltered," by their usual residence within cells or organs, from the body's antibody-making system that they are genuinely foreign to this system. This seems to be true, for example, of nuclear substances, of physiologically isolated eye substances and of thyroid-gland proteins.

On the other hand the tissues may be damaged in such a way as to alter their normal antigenic character by which the body's immunological system recognizes them. Sensitization may also be provoked by antigens of foreign tissues that are similar to but not identical with those of the tissues subsequently affected by the allergy: mammalian tissues upon which viruses for human vaccination are cultured might be a source of such antigens when they are injected inadvertently along with the virus suspension. Thus antibodies directed against antigens closely similar to normal cellular constituents of the body can cross-react with and injure the normal tissues. It is thought that rheumatoid arthritis develops when streptococci, which have a special affinity for joint tissue, remain in the joints long enough for antibodies against the combination of joint tissue and streptococci to form; these antibodies then cross-react with and damage normal joint tissue.

Some types of induced autosensitivity in experimental animals resemble certain diseases in human beings. One of these experimental diseases seems to be closely related to multiple sclerosis and similar degenerative nerve-tissue afflictions in man. In multiple sclerosis portions of the nervous system are destroyed, rendering useless the muscles controlled by those nerves. This grave disease may rapidly reduce someone in the prime of life to a veritable vegetable.

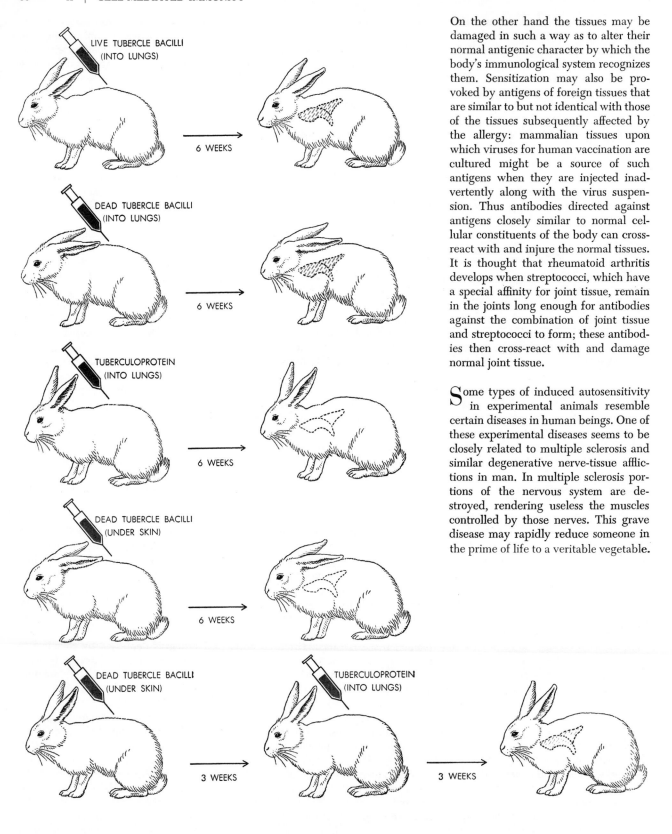

LUNG CAVITIES typical of tuberculosis result from delayed hypersensitivity to the protein fraction of tubercle bacilli. The injection of live tubercle bacilli (*top row*) or of whole killed ones (*second row*) directly into the lungs of a rabbit produces lung cavities (*broken hatching*). Killed bacilli injected under the skin do not induce cavities (*fourth row*) because there is then no protein antigen in the lungs. On the other hand, neither does tuberculoprotein, the actual antigen in this case, produce cavities when injected alone into the lungs (*third row*). If the animal has already developed a delayed hypersensitivity to tuberculoprotein as from the injection of whole bacilli under the skin (*fifth row*), cavities develop in the lungs in the area around the injected antigen.

The nearest experimental counterpart of this disease, called experimental allergic encephalomyelitis, or EAE, is provoked by injecting a guinea pig with a homogenate of another guinea pig's brain or of a portion of its own brain, along with tubercle bacilli (for the potentiating lipid that they contain) in water-in-oil emulsion. Two or three weeks later the animal begins to lose its ability to balance, and before long its hind legs, and sometimes all four of its legs, become useless hanging appendages. Sometimes slowly, sometimes rapidly, the animal wastes away and dies; occasionally it recovers. Other species can be made to develop the disease, but not always with equal facility.

In many instances antibodies to nerve tissue can be detected in the blood serum, but these antibodies (apparently indicative of an immediate hypersensitivity) are not present in all cases and sometimes show up in measurable quantities in animals that never develop the illness. If serum containing the antibodies is transferred from an afflicted animal to a healthy animal, the recipient is not harmed. If the circulatory systems of a normal and a hypersensitized animal are surgically connected, however, the disease is transmitted to the normal animal. This suggests that it is the white blood cells that carry the damaging antibodies, in accord with the established mechanism of delayed hypersensitivity. Moreover, the animal afflicted with EAE gives a delayed type of reaction to a skin test with nerve tissue.

The damage to nerve tissue in EAE is similar to that in multiple sclerosis. It also closely resembles that seen in the type of encephalomyelitis which sometimes follows vaccination with viruses grown in nerve tissue. If some of the animal nerve tissue is inadvertently injected along with the vaccine, the vaccinated person becomes sensitized to it and, as in EAE, his antibodies may then cross-react with and destroy his own nerve tissue. This has been a particular hazard of immunization against rabies, because the virus used in the vaccine is grown in rabbit spinal-cord or brain.

Unfortunately, despite intensive experimentation on EAE and similar diseases in many laboratories, no way has yet been found to help those people who develop delayed hypersensitivity to their own tissues. A tremendous amount of research still is required to achieve an understanding of, and eventually to control, the phenomenon of delayed hypersensitivity, but the rewards should be almost unimaginably great.

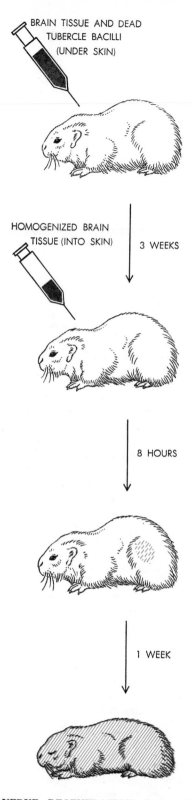

BRAIN TISSUE AND DEAD TUBERCLE BACILLI (UNDER SKIN)

HOMOGENIZED BRAIN TISSUE (INTO SKIN)

3 WEEKS

8 HOURS

1 WEEK

NERVE DEGENERATION disease that mimics multiple sclerosis is produced experimentally by injecting a guinea pig with brain tissue from another guinea pig (*top*). A skin test with the same material (*second from top*) produces an inflammation (*hatched area*) typical of delayed hypersensitivity (*third from top*). The antibodies of the allergy evidently attack the animal's own nerve cells. The animal loses control of its muscles and finally dies (*bottom*).

8   The Thymus Gland

by Sir Macfarlane Burnet
November 1962

*Its function has been poorly understood, largely
because the gland atrophies after childhood. Now
it appears that the thymus founds a line of cells
that is responsible for the production of antibody*

In trying to understand how the body develops immunity to disease, investigators have been finding more and more clues pointing to a crucial role for the thymus gland. Since the thymus of an adult human being is an organ that is barely discernible in the chest, its role in immunity has come as something of a surprise. As the picture has unfolded, however, it is becoming clear that in man and other animals the thymus finishes its task quite early in life. This task is evidently to stock the body with cells of a very special kind called lymphocytes. These cells have the ability to travel freely through the body and are more abundant than any other of the body's wandering cells. It has therefore been a persisting challenge that the function of neither the lymphocyte nor the thymus (except as a producer of lymphocytes) is stated in any textbook of cytology or physiology.

This gap in knowledge is rapidly being filled. It appears, moreover, that the function of the thymus is deeply entwined with the information-carrying role of deoxyribonucleic acid (DNA), the long-chain helical molecule whose genetic role has been so widely discussed of late. There is a certain irony in this emerging view: 20 years ago, when the genetic role of deoxyribonucleic acid was not known, it was called thymonucleic acid because it was found abundantly in calf thymus. This source was also reflected in the name "thymine," which was given to the constituent base now known to be unique to DNA.

There are good reasons why the thymus should be the most convenient source of DNA, the most important component of the cell nucleus. The large majority of the cells in the thymus are lymphocytes, which of all mammalian cells have the greatest ratio of nucleus to cytoplasm. In a young animal the thymus is a big organ; early in the life of a mouse it accounts for .5 to 1 per cent of the total body weight. In such an animal the metabolic activity of the thymus, judged by the turnover of DNA or by the number of cells actually dividing at any given time, is five to 10 times greater than that of the spleen or the lymph nodes, which are the other main reservoirs of lymphocytes in the body.

Today most physiologists would probably agree that the thymus is the primary source of lymphocytes in mammals, and that when these cells are liberated into the circulation, they settle down in organs such as the spleen or a lymph node. There the cells from the thymus, or their descendants, give rise to the cells responsible for some of—perhaps all—the immunological functions of the body. High among these functions is the ability to produce antibodies: substances that help the animal organism to repel invasion by bacteria and viruses. Another major function is to help the body distinguish between "self" and "not self"; that is, between its own tissue proteins, or other large molecules, and those found, for example, in tissue transplanted from another animal.

Without going into detail, one can say that two main theories have been proposed to explain the ability of certain cells to produce antibody. The "instructive" theory holds that the invading protein, or antigen, acts as a template against which an antibody protein somehow molds itself. So molded, the antibody can combine with the antigen and inactivate it. The "selective" theory, of which I have been a strong advocate, proposes that individual cells responsible for immunity are genetically endowed with the ability to "recognize" one kind or perhaps several kinds of antigen, and that collectively these cells can recognize all foreign proteins [see "The Mechanism of Immunity," by Sir Macfarlane Burnet, the article beginning on page 12].

If one accepts the selectivity theory, it seems reasonable to ascribe to the lymphocyte two intimately related functions. First, it must be the primary bearer of information that endows its descendants with immunological activity. Second, it may provide a mobile reserve of chemical building blocks from which new populations of descendant cells can be rapidly produced when and where they are needed.

Anyone with even faintly exotic tastes in food is familiar with calf thymus in the form of sweetbreads. (The term "sweetbread" is also applied to calf pancreas.) In shape and location, but not in size, the thymus of the calf closely resembles that of man or any other of the higher mammals. Some of our Australian marsupials have two thymuses, but the meaning of that is still to be elucidated. In a child the thymus takes the form of two roughly oval lobes that lie in the front of the chest just behind the top of the sternum (breastbone) and in front of the aorta and other great blood vessels in the region where they emerge from the heart. The size of the thymus increases more or less in step with general growth up to the age of eight or 10 years. Thereafter the gland lags behind and slowly begins to atrophy. In an adult the actual substance of the thymus is often hard to distinguish from the fat in which it is normally embedded. The thymus is not easily visualized by X rays and is too close to vital structures to allow the use of biopsy-needle techniques to obtain a small piece of thymic tissue for histological examination. As a

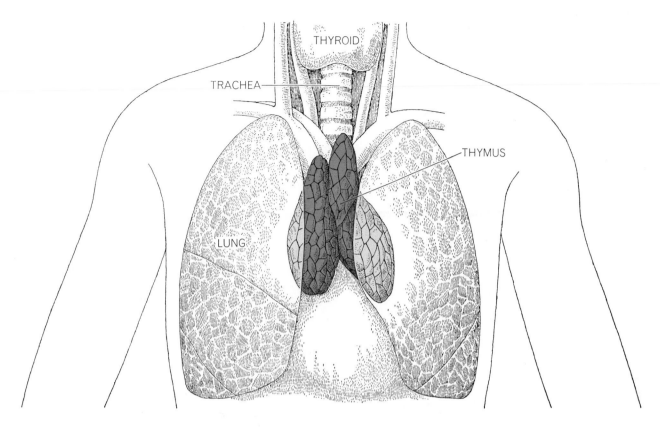

HUMAN THYMUS (*shown here in a child*) is a flat, pinkish-gray, two-lobed organ that lies high in the chest, in front of the aorta and behind the breastbone and partly behind the lungs. The thymus is large in relation to the rest of the body in fetal life and in early childhood; then it grows less quickly, and by the age of puberty it has stopped growing and then begins to atrophy. This course of events suggested that the thymus completes its work early in life, but until recently its exact function was unknown.

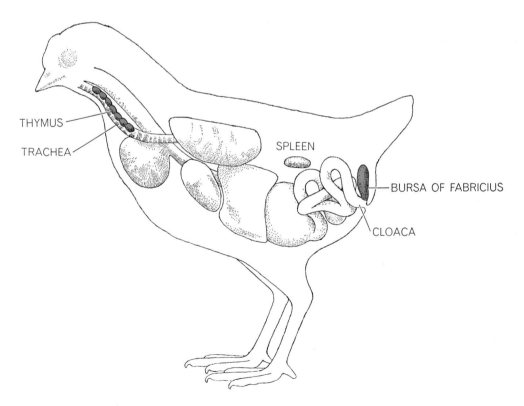

CHICKEN THYMUS (*shown here in a young chicken*) is composed of 14 separate lobes, seven of which are strung out along each side of the bird's neck. The chicken has another organ, called the bursa of Fabricius, which is active in early life and later disappears. The bursa seems to share with the chicken thymus some of the functions performed in the human by the thymus alone.

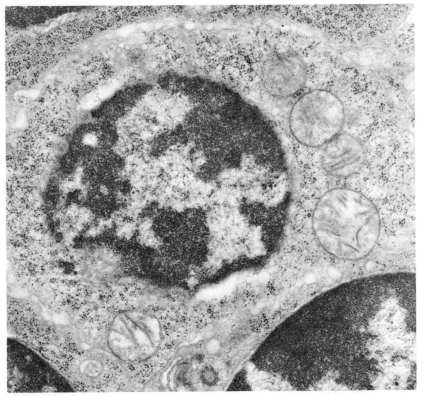

LYMPHOCYTE from rat thymus, enlarged some 29,000 times, fills center of this electron micrograph made by George D. Pappas of the Columbia University College of Physicians and Surgeons. The large nucleus contains a high concentration of DNA, the genetic material. The relatively thin rim of cytoplasm contains energy-supplying mitochondria but no other well-developed organelles; the small, dark grains of ribonucleoprotein are not organized for the task of protein synthesis. Portions of three more nuclei can be seen at the corners.

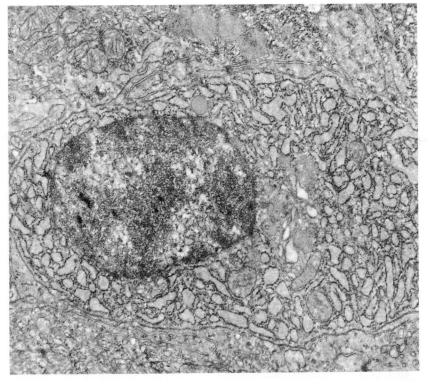

PLASMA CELL from an immunized guinea pig's lymph node is seen, enlarged 24,000 diameters, in an electron micrograph made by Richard A. Rifkind of the College of Physicians and Surgeons. Note the well-organized folds of endoplasmic reticulum filling the cytoplasm. The attached ribonucleoprotein particles, or ribosomes, synthesize protein antibody, which is visible as the amorphous gray material filling the channels of the reticulum.

result most of our knowledge of the human thymus has come from observations made at post-mortem examination.

This limitation gives rise to an interesting difficulty. Of all the organs in the body the thymus is the most responsive to "stress." Acute infection or severe injury, X-irradiation or a large dose of cortisone—any of these will within a day or two destroy millions of lymphocytes in the thymus and shrink its mass to half or less. A child who has died after an illness lasting more than a few days will therefore have a thymus much smaller than that of a healthy child of the same age. Because most children examined post-mortem have died after an illness, the opportunity to see a normal thymus is quite rare. This gave rise to a rather paradoxical situation in the first quarter of this century, when children dying suddenly from no clearly recognizable cause were said to have died from *status thymicolymphaticus*. Such children had a large thymus, and for a long time this was considered the cause of the sudden death. In point of fact the thymus was large because death had been sudden and no stress atrophy had occurred.

Under the microscope a stained section of the thymus has a thick outer cortex of closely packed, deeply stained lymphocytes and an inner medulla with many fewer cells, most of them with nuclei that have taken the stain more lightly. To the microscopist, however, the thymus is a rather uninteresting organ. To the immunologist, on the other hand, the organ is interesting largely because of what is *not* present.

In the body of a mature animal or human being the chief concentrations of lymphocytes are found in the spleen and the lymph nodes. Both are deeply involved in immunity, and there are well-known microscopic changes by which the pathologist can recognize that the organs are responding to an immunological stimulus, such as an infection or an experimental implantation of foreign cells. For example, in a lymph node that is draining an area of skin infection one will find areas of lymphocytic proliferation (germinal centers) often surrounded by accumulations of mature lymphocytes (lymph follicles). Elsewhere in the lymph node one will see accumulations of cells (plasma cells) whose staining qualities depend on the fact that they are actively synthesizing protein; in their case the protein being synthesized is antibody directed against the infecting microorganism. None of these things can be seen in the thymus. There lymphocytes multiply freely but move about in the process and never produce fixed germinal centers, and plasma cells are not formed.

The standard first step toward elucidating the function of an organ is to remove it and analyze the resulting disabilities. In the history of physiology clues have often been obtained from observing what happened in human beings when an organ was destroyed by accident or disease. In more recent times surgical procedures occasionally gave unexpected results that subsequently led to important new understanding of organ function. Removal of large amounts of thyroid gland in cases of goiter, for instance, sometimes caused serious spasms; these were eventually traced to the unintentional removal of the parathyroid glands, resulting in a disturbance of the calcium balance of the body.

The conventional approach of the physiologist is to remove the organ by appropriate surgery in some suitable ex-

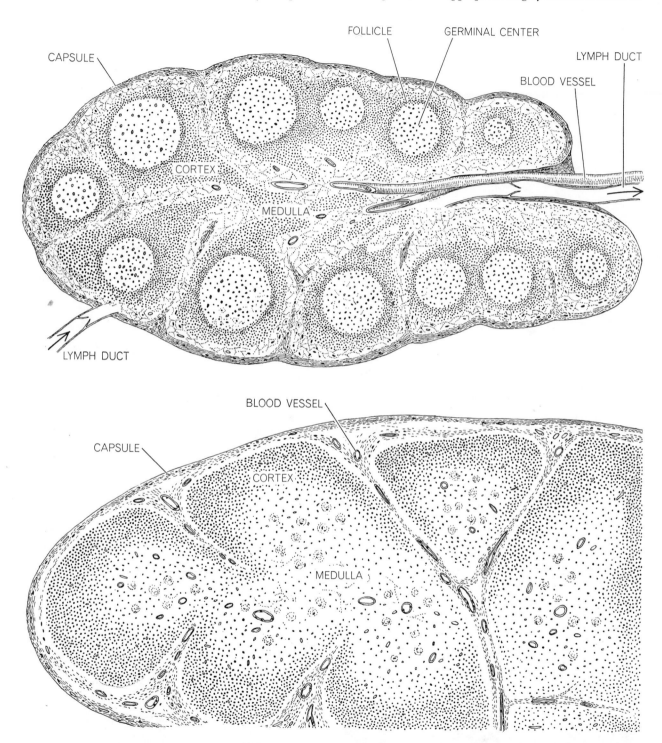

LYMPH NODE AND THYMUS TISSUE are compared in these drawings. The two are somewhat similar, both having a spongy network of structural cells. In the case of lymph node tissue (*top*) lymph filters through this network from the afferent to the efferent ducts. Both tissues have large numbers of lymphocytes. But in the lymph node, and particularly in one that is stimulated immunologically, there are dense round or ovoid concentrations of lymphocytes called follicles, or nodes, surrounding germinal centers in which lymphocytes are proliferating. Elsewhere in the cortex of an active node, plasma cells, which produce antibody, are found. In thymus tissue (*bottom*), on the other hand, lymphocytes do not proliferate in fixed germinal centers and there are no plasma cells.

perimental animal. Until 1961 neither approach had given any clue to the function of the thymus. If one removes the thymus from a mouse a few weeks old, the only significant effect is a minor reduction in the number of lymphocytes in the blood and in the size of the lymph nodes and the spleen. The sole functional effect observed is a beneficial one: a great reduction in the incidence of leukemia in strains of mice genetically predisposed to this disease.

There is a rare human disease, myasthenia gravis, which is just what its Latin name means—a severe weakness of some of or all the muscles. For somewhat obscure reasons it was treated in the 1930's by complete surgical removal of the thymus with rather variable results, but there were enough apparent cures to make this operation a popular method of treating early cases. Most of the patients were young adult women, and evidently complete removal of the thymus did them no harm at all.

Perhaps this is to be expected of an organ that spontaneously atrophies as its owner ages, but a logical study based on that observation was undertaken only last year. Jacques F. A. P. Miller, a young Australian cancer researcher working at the Chester Beatty Research Institute in England, decided to see what would happen if the thymus were removed from mice on the first day of life. It was a tricky operation to suck out the whole of the thymus from an anesthetized newborn mouse without doing other damage, but the results were striking. Most of the mice developed normally for three or four months; then many of them died for reasons that are not yet fully under-

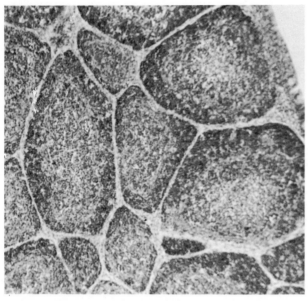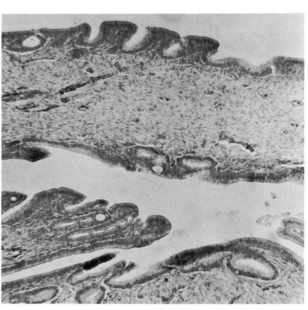

BURSA OF FABRICIUS apparently gives rise to the cells that will produce antibody in the chicken. As shown in the section at the left, a normal bursa has separate follicles packed with lymphocytes. Injection into the chicken embryo of the male sex hormone testo-terone "bursectomizes" the chicken; the bursa (right) atrophies and no lymphoid tissue develops. A chicken so treated produces no antibody. The photomicrographs, in which the sections are enlarged 100 diameters, were made by Noel L. Warner and the author.

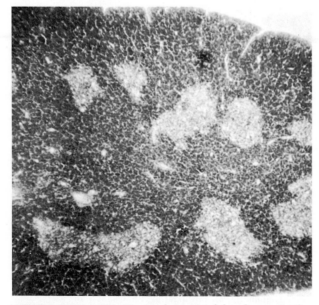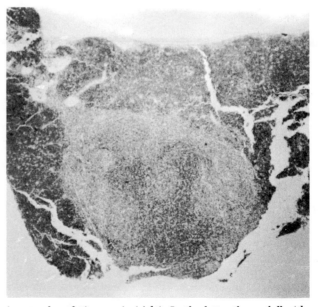

AUTOIMMUNE DISEASE may be initiated by changes in the thymus. Here a section of normal mouse thymus (left) is compared with thymus from a New Zealand Black mouse suffering from auto-immune hemolytic anemia (right). In the latter the medulla (the paler area) is enlarged and lymphocytes proliferate as in a lymph node. The author's photomicrographs enlarge the tissue 40 diameters.

stood. During the period of development, however, the mice showed some important departures from the normal. When the thymus was removed from mice of a particular strain at birth and then, two to four weeks later, skin was transplanted to them, it was found that a majority would retain grafts from any one of several strains of mice and even from rats [*see illustration at right*]. Normal mice reject such grafts in 10 days or less. This work has been confirmed in several laboratories, and extensive investigations are under way to sort out the limitations of the technique and to account for the big differences that seem to exist from one strain of mice to another. Several investigators, including Miller, have also found that a variable proportion of mice, rats and rabbits thymectomized at birth lose most or all of their capacity to produce antibodies.

It seems, then, that the functional activity of the thymus is at its peak in the first few days of life and perhaps also in the last few days of existence *in utero*. Miller's view is that the thymus produces and liberates into the blood the lymphocytes that pass to spleen and lymph nodes and there settle down and mature into the populations of cells that look after the integrity and security of the body.

In studies of the kind just described the mouse yields one great advantage to the chicken. The chicken embryo is easily accessible to experimentation: separated from the mother in the avian egg, it can be treated with drugs or altered surgically. The possibility therefore arises of influencing the immune reactions of the hatched chicken by manipulations of the embryo. In my laboratory in Melbourne, Aleksander Szenberg and Noel L. Warner have developed a method based on one devised by Harold R. Wolfe and his associates at the University of Wisconsin. The method has provided results that have interesting differences from those observed in mice.

The chicken has a thymus whose shape is totally unlike the shape of the thymus in mammals; it takes the form of two strings of seven separate lobes running down each side of the neck. Nevertheless, it has a cellular structure similar to that of the mammalian thymus and evidently its function is similar also. In the chicken, however, there is another organ, somewhat like the thymus in structure, that is situated at the end of the intestinal tract just above the cloaca. This organ is called the bursa of Fabri-

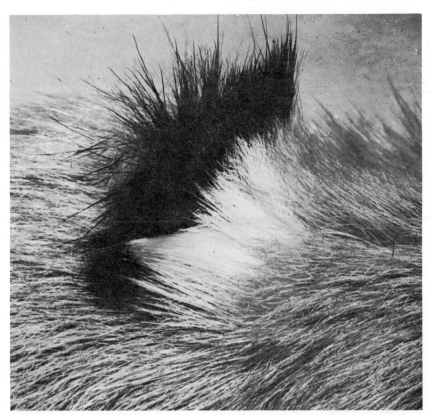

REMOVAL OF THYMUS from mice on the first day after birth leads to their toleration of skin grafts that would be quickly rejected by a normal mouse. This picture made by Jacques F. A. P. Miller of the Chester Beatty Research Institute shows such a mouse carrying two healthy grafts: skin from an unrelated mouse (*black hair*) and from a rat (*white hair*).

cius. Its main microscopic feature, like that of the thymus, is closely packed masses of lymphocytes. Its chief activity is in early life; it vanishes completely at sexual maturity.

This last characteristic may be related to the effect that the male sex hormone testosterone has on the embryo. If two milligrams of testosterone are injected into an embryo 12 days old, the development of the bursa is cut short. It remains a flabby appendage to the bowel and does not produce lymphocytes. The chickens are somewhat unhealthy, but many survive indefinitely and can be used for various immunological studies. The most striking result is that such "hormonally bursectomized" chickens fail completely to produce antibody in response to any of the standard antigenic materials such as serum albumin or bacterial vaccines. Most such birds nonetheless reject skin transplants from other chickens in quite normal fashion.

Szenberg and Warner have found, however, a small proportion of these treated chicks in which both bursa and thymus have failed to develop lymphocytes. In these they have obtained the same kind of result that Miller and others observed in mice thymectomized at birth. Skin grafts from unrelated chick-

ens are *not* rejected for the period that the chicken survives. All such chickens are sickly; the longest survival to date is six weeks from hatching.

There is much more that might be said about the immune responses of chickens, but I can summarize by saying that there are apparently two organs concerned with primary production of lymphocytes. One, the bursa, gives rise to those cells whose descendants are responsible for antibody production; the other, the thymus, seems to produce in chickens, as in mammals, the cells whose descendants are responsible for the rejection of foreign skin grafts. Perhaps the most interesting phase of immunology still to be uncovered is the real function that we recognize by the highly artificial test of transplanting skin.

The results in chickens are almost decisive in showing that the thymus is not involved in antibody production as such, nor in cellular reactions against bacterial components, such as the tuberculin reaction. The cells involved in both of these are derived from the bursa. Perhaps the best suggestion is that the thymus, in both birds and mammals, liberates the cells whose descendants are primarily involved in the surveillance of cellular integrity in the body. When

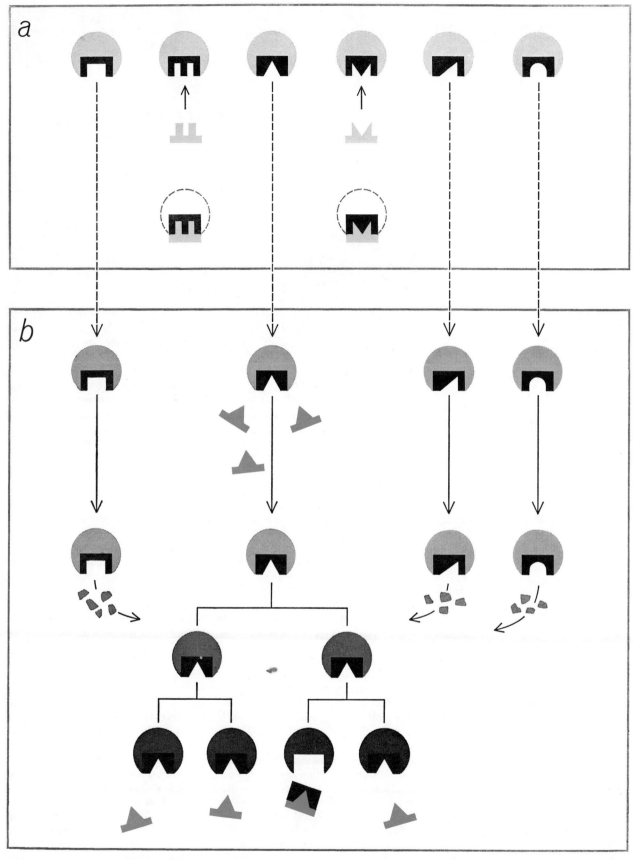

HYPOTHESIS OF THYMUS FUNCTION suggests that lymphocytes are produced in the thymus (a) and give rise to populations of cells (large numbers of which are represented here by only six cells) that have specific antibody potentialities. In the thymus these cells are exposed to "self-components" (*light-colored figures*); any that react are destroyed to guard against autoimmune activity. The descendants of those that remain are concentrated in the spleen and lymph nodes (b). When one of these descendent lymphoblasts is stimulated by an antigen (*dark-colored figures*), it proliferates; its own DNA provides "information" and that of unneeded fellow cells provides raw material. The progressively more mature plasma cells thus formed produce the antibody that neutralizes the antigen.

cell surfaces are changed by toxins or viruses or by simple aging, or, more important, when they are changed as a result of somatic mutation, it is necessary for the survival and proper functioning of the individual that the anomalous cells should be recognized and dealt with. This may be the function of the cell populations that descend from the ancestral lymphocyte cells liberated from the thymus. In mammals it is highly probable that the thymus also carries out the function performed by the bursa of Fabricius in the chicken, which is to feed into the body the cells whose descendants will produce antibody.

Such suggestions represent at present no more than a good working hypothesis to account for the experimental results of removing the thymus and, as we shall now see, for the relation of changes in the thymus to "autoimmune" disease.

Under the heading of autoimmune disease we include a number of conditions in which cells or tissues of the body seem to be attacked by antibodies or immunologically active cells. Rheumatoid arthritis, hemolytic anemia, myasthenia gravis and perhaps multiple sclerosis are examples.

Until recently there were no satisfactory models for the study of these diseases in the laboratory. Now we believe that a strain of mice called New Zealand Black provides a true analogy to one such human disease: acquired hemolytic anemia. This strain of mice was developed at the Cancer Research Laboratory of the University of Otago in New Zealand by Marianne Bielschowsky; she, with her collaborators, first recognized the existence of hemolytic anemia in the mice. The results of breeding experiments indicate that the mice differ from a healthy strain by one or more genetic factors. Their abnormal constitution is manifested by the development, usually at about six months of age, of antibody against their own blood cells. There is also evidence that in some cases there is an attack, either by antibody or perhaps by cells, against one or more components of their other tissues.

My colleague Margaret C. Holmes and I have many lines of study in progress on these mice, but the only finding that is relevant here is the occurrence of immunological activity in the thymus. At approximately the same time as evidence of antibody against their own red cells appears, we find in the medulla of the thymus enlarged areas where lymphocytes are multiplying in germinal centers and producing plasma cells, just as they would be expected to do in a lymph node but never in a normal thymus.

These results find a close and rather exciting parallel in the thymuses of patients with myasthenia gravis. Sections from specimens of thymus removed at operation contain many germinal centers quite similar to those in mice of the New Zealand Black strain. There is a hint here that changes in the thymus may play an essential part in the initiation of autoimmune disease generally, and at the present time there is an urgent need both to determine if other human autoimmune diseases also show the thymic lesions and to locate other strains of animals that will permit comparable laboratory studies.

Obviously there is much more to be learned about the thymus and the lymphocytes it produces. No final interpretation will be possible until we have a better understanding of how cells produce antibodies or exert immunological functions in other ways. The new developments nonetheless seem to be very much in line with selective theories of immunity, although they may demand a more flexible interpretation of how cells can sort themselves out into different clones (descendants of a single cell) in the process of differentiating from unspecialized cells.

All selective theories of immunity and antibody formation are based on the axiom that in the healthy animal or human being no cells should emerge and multiply that can immunologically damage any of the normal components of the body. Autoimmune disease represents a breakdown of the means by which this control is maintained.

The appearance of similar signs of abnormal immunological activity in the thymus of mice with autoimmune anemia and in humans with the autoimmune disease myasthenia gravis strongly suggests that the control process is located predominantly in the thymus. Our present findings fall neatly into place if we look on the thymus as an important source of the lymphocytes involved in what we may call tissue integrity. In the thymus the lymphocytes are produced by proliferation, differentiated into groups with varying immunological potentialities and sorted over to detect any potentiality of reacting with "self-components"; that is, the body's own components. Any reactive cells are inhibited or destroyed, and eventually those that pass the test are liberated into the circulation to help populate the lymphoid tissues elsewhere in the body.

Perhaps we should finish with a look at the lymphocyte—a literal and simpleminded look at an ordinary "small" lymphocyte such as one sees in any stained specimen of blood under a standard optical microscope. (In fact, not much more can be learned by using an electron microscope.) The small lymphocyte has a large, dense nucleus, indicating a rich content of DNA. Surrounding the nucleus one sees little cytoplasm, and the cytoplasm is empty except for a few mitochondria, the granules responsible for supplying energy. Functionally the lymphocyte is a highly mobile cell, able to pass out of the small blood vessels with ease and likely to be found wandering in any tissue or accumulating in areas where there has been mild cellular damage of almost any sort.

There are two ways to look at the cell nucleus that may be particularly important in relation to the lymphocyte. The nucleus is the repository of information that when called into action may determine the conversion of the lymphocyte into a proliferating mother cell from which a clone of functioning cells, plasma cells for example, could develop. At the same time the nucleus is a concentrated source of nucleotides (DNA constituents) and amino acids (protein constituents), which could be drawn off and used as building blocks in the construction of new cells. This may be particularly relevant to the lymphocyte in view of the extreme ease with which it breaks down under stress.

The modern view of lymphocyte function brings us back to our starting point: the high content and rapid synthesis of DNA in the thymus. It is a logical but still unproved hypothesis that the enormous populations of lymphocytes in the body have a double function. Each cell carries a limited range of potentialities for immunological activity and under rare and specific conditions can be stimulated to proliferate by contact with an appropriate antigen. There is much to suggest that active multiplication is only possible when a free supply of the necessary nutrients can be brought into the site of proliferation. For this purpose the DNA of those lymphocytes whose specific activity is not required can readily be made available in the form of nucleotides, or smaller fragments, to allow swift new production of nucleic acid and active proliferation of the cells whose specific qualities are needed to deal with whatever alarm has called them into activity. The best use can thus be made of both qualities of the nucleus and its DNA. The many provide raw material for the construction of new nuclei; the few provide information as to how the new generation of cells should be constructed.

9

The Thymus Hormone

by Raphael H. Levey
July 1964

*The blood cells that manufacture antibodies trace their
origin back to the thymus gland. It has recently been
discovered that the gland also secretes a substance
that enables the cells to make antibodies*

Until a few years ago the function of the thymus gland, a two-lobed structure that lies in the upper chest in front of the aorta, was an enigma to investigators. Removal of the organ from experimental animals or in the course of surgical operations on human patients caused no noticeably harmful effects. In fact, in all animals including man the thymus, although it is prominent at birth, begins to atrophy of its own accord long before the animal reaches maturity. Certain crucial experiments performed only three years ago, however, indicated that the thymus does, after all, play a most important role: it appears to be a principal actor in the body's defenses against infection and similar immunological challenges [see "The Thymus Gland," by Sir Macfarlane Burnet, the article beginning on page 88]. Since then the gland has been the subject of intensive and fruitful investigation in many laboratories. Among other things it has been discovered that the thymus produces a previously unsuspected hormone.

A central figure in this story is the mouse, which has provided most of the information about the activities of the thymus by its responses to various surgical experiments. In a newborn mouse the thymus is about three millimeters long and two millimeters wide. The organ continues to grow until the age of weaning; then it begins to decrease in size in the process known as age involution. If the thymus is surgically removed at that time, the mouse will show no ill effects. A turning point in the investigation of the thymus came in 1961, when Jacques F. A. P. Miller of the Chester Beatty Research Institute in Britain undertook the experiment of thymectomizing mice immediately after birth. These mice grew normally for several weeks or months, but then they became ill and soon died of a wasting disease whose main features were loss of weight, weakness, lethargy and diarrhea. Detailed internal examination showed that the mice had suffered a severe depletion of the white blood corpuscles called lymphocytes.

In the mouse the lymphocytes constitute some 70 percent of all the white blood cells (in the human body they represent only 20 to 25 percent). It has now been established that the thymus is by far the most important source of lymphocytes in the newborn mouse. It serves as the seedbed for these vital cells and sends them forth to the other lymphoid organs: the spleen, the lymph nodes and areas in the small intestine known as Peyer's patches. In these locations the lymphocytes continue to divide. As the primary factory for lymphocytes, the thymus produces them as much as 10 times faster than the other organs do. The cortex, or outer layer, of the thymus is densely packed with these cells in their small, fully developed form. In the other lymphoid organs the production of lymphocytes takes place in nodules that have a "germinal center" where medium-sized lymphocytes can be seen actively dividing. This division becomes particularly active, and the germinal center enlarges, in the nodules of lymph nodes that are responding to an infection or a graft of foreign tissue.

Various experiments have demonstrated clearly that the thymus is essential for the normal development of immunological competence, at least in the mouse. A mouse whose thymus has been removed at birth fails to produce circulating antibodies against foreign substances. In fact, such a mouse will accept a skin graft from an unrelated animal, whereas normal mice invariably reject such foreign grafts. Without much doubt these effects can be attributed to the depletion of small lymphocytes in the mouse that has been thymectomized at birth. Lacking these cells, the animal loses most of its immunological potential. There is considerable evidence that the small lymphocytes from the thymus not only seed the lymph nodes for further lymphocyte pro-

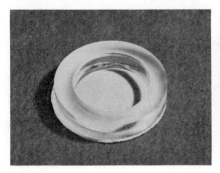 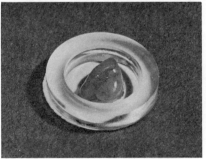

DIFFUSION CHAMBER ensures that no cells from an implanted thymus reach the host animal's bloodstream; any effects of an implant can be ascribed to a humoral factor. The chamber is made by gluing a fine filter to a plastic washer 1/4 inch in inside diameter (*left*). With a newborn-mouse thymus inside (*right*), the capsule is closed with a second filter.

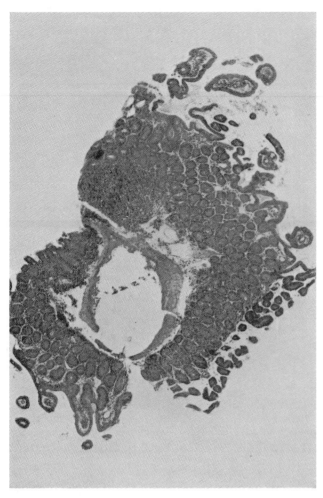

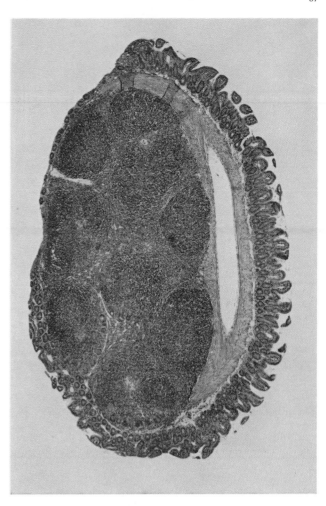

PEYER'S PATCH, an area of lymphoid tissue in the wall of the intestine, atrophies in mice thymectomized at birth (*left*) but remains large and active in thymectomized mice that receive a capsule implant (*right*). In the control animal the patch has been reduced to the small, rounded granular area at the top center; it is here enlarged 55 diameters. In the implanted animal the patch, enlarged 30 diameters, is the oval area at left, occupying most of the photograph. It is filled with "germinal centers" rich in lymphocytes.

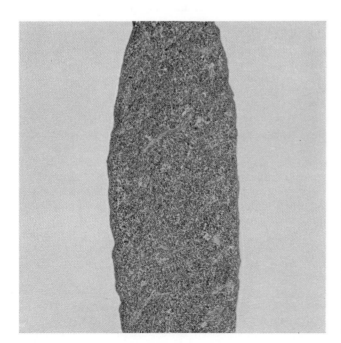

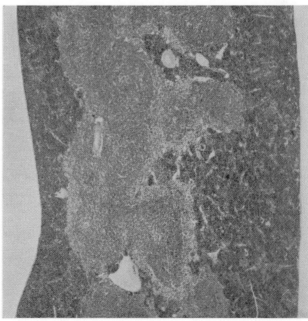

SPLEEN is another lymphoid organ that demonstrates the effect of implantation of a capsule-enclosed thymus. The section of spleen at left, enlarged 50 diameters, came from a mouse thymectomized at birth and is atrophied. The section at right, enlarged 40 diameters, came from a thymectomized mouse that received an implant; it is large and well developed and is filled with lymphocytes.

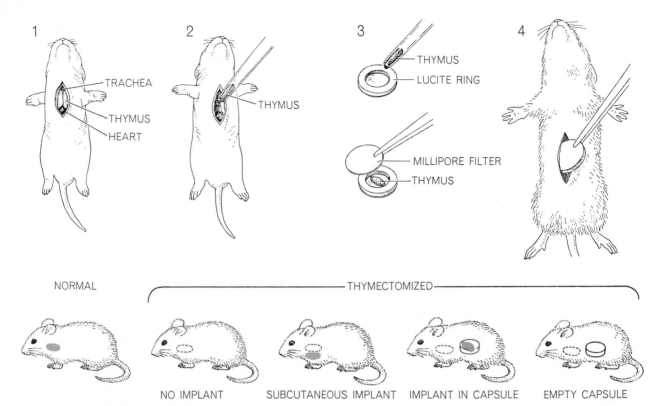

1

TRACHEA

THYMUS

HEART

2

THYMUS

3

THYMUS

LUCITE RING

MILLIPORE FILTER

THYMUS

4

NORMAL — THYMECTOMIZED

NO IMPLANT   SUBCUTANEOUS IMPLANT   IMPLANT IN CAPSULE   EMPTY CAPSULE

EXPERIMENTS BEGIN with a thymectomy performed on a newborn mouse (*1*). The thymus is removed by suction (*2*) and placed in a Millipore diffusion chamber (*3*). The capsule is implanted in a two- or three-week-old mouse (*4*). The bottom row shows the conditions of the animals involved in these experiments: normal mouse with its own thymus intact and thymectomized mice without any implant, with thymus implanted under the skin rather than in a capsule, with thymus inside a capsule and with an empty capsule.

duction but also are precursors of the plasma cells, which synthesize antibodies. (Plasma cells are found in the lymph nodes but not in the thymus.)

The immunological importance of the small lymphocytes shows itself in another and more direct way. Consider a normal newborn mouse. Apart from the lymphocytes in its thymus gland, it has not yet developed any significant immunological defenses of its own. If this mouse is inoculated with foreign lymphoid cells that are capable of growing in its tissues, we should expect the graft to take over and grow at the expense of the mouse's own tissues, a process that is known as the graft-against-host reaction. That is precisely what happens. The mouse's growth slows down; the animal becomes anemic and in general exhibits a stunted development that is called "runt disease." Most important, the mouse is drastically depleted of lymphocytes, which have been sacrificed in an immunological battle against the foreign cells. As the body's sole defense against the graft, the lymphocytes of the thymus, spleen and lymph nodes have been overwhelmed and used up. It is significant that runt disease is similar to the wasting disease that overtakes mice

deprived of the thymus gland, and therefore of lymphocytes, at birth.

All these experimental findings gave a strong indication of the function of the thymus gland, but they were still not direct proof. The classic method of determining the role of a gland is to remove it from an experimental animal, observe the effects closely, then reimplant the same tissue and investigate how and to what extent this restoration counteracts the effects of removal. Until recently this approach had not produced much enlightenment about the thymus, because there was very little effect to investigate when the organ was removed from grown or growing animals. But after Miller's demonstration that striking effects emerged when the thymus was extracted at birth, experimenters promptly began to test the results of reimplanting the thymus in such animals.

The results were both dramatic and in the classic tradition. When mice that had been thymectomized at birth received, within three or four weeks, subcutaneous grafts of thymic tissue from donor mice of the same strain, they did not fall victim to the wasting disease. Their lymphoid organs produced lymphocytes at about the normal

rate, and the animals proved capable of evincing all the normal immunological reactions.

Two of the outcomes of this kind of operation were, however, rather puzzling. In the first place, most of the lymphocytes produced in the thymic graft turned out to be related genetically to the cells of the host mouse, not to the cells of the donor that had supplied the grafted tissue! (The cells could be distinguished because the donor cells were marked by an unusual chromosome.) The same was true of the lymphocytes multiplying in the target lymphoid organs (the spleen and lymph nodes); they too were of the host type rather than the donor type.

This fact suggested that the thymus gland does something more than merely supply lymphocytes as seeds, or parents, to produce new lymphocytes by division. The thymic grafts in these mice were somehow stimulating the hosts to make lymphocytes out of their own cells.

The second curious outcome of the thymus-grafting experiments pointed in the same direction. It was found that when thymic tissue from a newborn mouse was placed under the skin of an older mouse whose thymus was deteriorating, the grafted thymus continued to show its own characteristic rapid rate of production of lymphocytes. This again suggested that the young thymic tissue contained an intrinsic stimulating factor.

I was intrigued by these observations, and my interest was shared by two colleagues in the Laboratory of Biology of the National Cancer Institute: Nathan Trainin and Lloyd W. Law. The thymus has been much on the minds of investigators of leukemia, a cancerous disease marked by the uncontrolled increase of lymphocytes and other white blood cells [see "Leukemia," by Emil Frei III and Emil J. Freireich; SCIENTIFIC AMERICAN, May 1964]. Trainin, Law and I undertook to investigate the stimulating influence of the thymus gland.

One way to explore the problem would be to expose the target organs—the spleen and the lymph nodes—to the substances produced by the thymus but not to the thymic cells themselves. Fortunately a technique for accomplishing this was available. It was based on the use of a plastic capsule with pores so fine that it holds in cells but lets out all the chemical products of the cells. We constructed and tested a suitable capsule for our experiments. It consisted of a Lucite washer, or ring, 6.4 millimeters (about a quarter of an inch) in internal diameter, with Millipore filters of cellulose glued over the top and bottom. This formed a circular diffusion chamber 6.4 millimeters across and 1.6 millimeters deep. The pore size of our filters was less than half a micron —about a fifteenth of the average diameter of the small lymphocytes of a mouse. We evaluated the ability of the capsule to contain cells by filling it with highly malignant lymphoid tumor cells and then implanting it in mice. None of the mice developed tumors; since as few as four viable cells of the tumor are usually capable of producing tumors in a susceptible mouse, this was conclusive verification that the filter was an effective barrier against cells. On the other hand, the pores allowed free passage to fluids and colloids, thus admitting nutrients for the cells into the capsule and letting molecular products pass out.

The standard procedure in the experiments we carried out was as follows. The thymus was removed from the experimental mouse within 12 hours after birth. Three to four weeks later we implanted in the mouse's abdominal cavity a Millipore diffusion chamber

containing a whole thymus taken from a newborn donor mouse of the same strain. Then we watched for the results, comparing them with the simultaneous histories of control groups of mice (some not operated on at all, some thymectomized but not provided with a thymus-containing capsule, some implanted with an empty capsule and some grafted subcutaneously with an unenclosed thymus).

The thymectomized control mice that received no substitute thymus (including those implanted with an empty capsule) all fell victim to the wasting disease. They grew more slowly than normal mice, began to deteriorate at about five weeks of age and died by the seventh or eighth week. All showed a severe loss of small lymphocytes, and their lymphoid organs were stunted and contained no germinal centers.

In contrast, the mice implanted with a substitute thymus, even though it was enclosed in a capsule, grew and survived almost like normal animals. Their body weight increased steadily; they showed no signs of the wasting disease or of any depletion of small lymphocytes in the blood. Their lymphoid organs were normal or even better developed than in nonthymectomized animals. The spleen was sometimes oversized and was filled with many lymphatic nodules containing active germinal centers; the lymph nodes were large and abundant; the walls of the small intestines showed an extraordinary number of large and active Peyer's patches. In short, the lymphoid organs were stimulated to intensely active production of lymphocytes.

When we tested these mice for their immunological potential, they showed

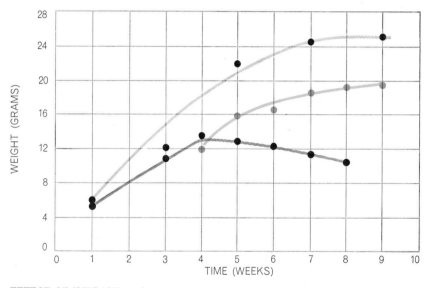

EFFECT OF IMPLANT on body weight is shown. A normal animal gains steadily (*light gray curve*). A thymectomized animal loses weight and dies in about eight weeks (*dark gray*). The implantation of a thymus in a chamber maintains the growth curve (*color*).

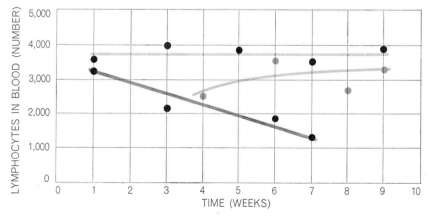

NUMBER OF LYMPHOCYTES in the peripheral blood remains satisfactory in the case of implanted animals (*colored curve*), whereas it falls off sharply in thymectomized mice.

the same remarkably normal reactions. We inoculated the mice with red blood cells from sheep. Normal mice usually produce within one week powerful antibodies, called hemolysins, that destroy these cells. Mice thymectomized at birth, on the other hand, fail to produce any substantial amount of these antibodies. It turned out that an experimental mouse with a capsule-enclosed thymus planted in the peritoneal cavity did produce the antibodies, in an amount approaching that produced in normal animals [*see illustration below*].

Next we subjected such mice to a more elaborate and sensitive test of their immunological behavior. For this experiment we used certain strains of mice that are unusually resistant to the effects of neonatal thymectomy: they do not show symptoms of the wasting disease or any depletion of lymphocytes until they are several months old. They are, however, immunological-

ly defective, as we found in experiments performed in collaboration with Wallace P. Rowe and Paul Black of the National Institute of Allergy and Infectious Diseases. These experiments involved infection of the mice with a highly virulent disease of the central nervous system called lymphocytic choriomeningitis.

When the virus responsible for this disease is injected into the brain of a normal susceptible mouse, the animal invariably dies within eight days. The direct cause of death is presumed to be a dense infiltration of the meninges by small lymphocytes. This produces a hypersensitive reaction similar to the reaction of a tuberculous patient to tuberculin, which also is associated with a rush of lymphocytes to the site of the injection. In both cases the reaction is delayed: for 48 to 72 hours in the case of the tuberculin injection and for seven days in the case of the injection of the meningitic virus into the mouse's brain.

Now we found that mice thymectomized at birth did not succumb to the infection, even when injected with a normally 100 percent fatal dose of the virus. The virus multiplied normally in the mice's tissues, but there was no flood of lymphocytes into the meninges. In other words, thymectomy had prevented the hypersensitive reaction by suppressing the immunological response involving lymphocytes. Would thymectomized mice with a capsule-enclosed thymus show the normal immunological response? We made the test. After implanting the capsule in the mouse at the age of three weeks, we injected into its brain a week later a large amount of the virus: about 200 times the usually lethal dose. Whereas all thymectomized mice not supplied with a substitute thymus survived this dose, 54 percent of our experimental mice with the capsule-enclosed thymus were killed by it. And their meninges showed the characteristic influx of lymphocytes that marked the

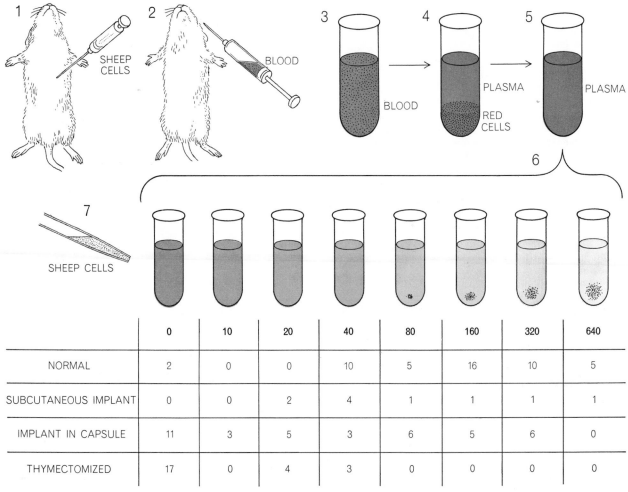

	0	10	20	40	80	160	320	640
NORMAL	2	0	0	10	5	16	10	5
SUBCUTANEOUS IMPLANT	0	0	2	4	1	1	1	1
IMPLANT IN CAPSULE	11	3	5	3	6	5	6	0
THYMECTOMIZED	17	0	4	3	0	0	0	0

IMMUNOLOGICAL TEST measures the ability of mice to form an antibody that destroys foreign red blood cells. Sheep cells are injected into mice (*1*). Seven days later a sample of the mouse's blood is drawn (*2*) and centrifuged (*3, 4*) to remove cells. The remaining plasma (*5*) is serially diluted (*6*) and a measured number of sheep cells are added to each test tube (*7*). The dilution at which most of the sheep cells are destroyed, leaving only a small clump, is the antibody titer of the animal involved; the titer is 80 in the illustration. The table shows that the antibody titer of animals with implants inside capsules compares well with that of normal mice.

reaction of normal mice.

This accumulation of diverse kinds of evidence made quite clear that the thymus in the diffusion chamber, even though it released no cells, nevertheless provided the body of the mouse with agents or services the thymus normally provides. Most impressive was the fact that the thymus implanted in a cell-tight capsule was just about as effective as a subcutaneous graft of a thymus that freely transmitted lymphocytes to the lymphoid organs. The thymecto-mized mouse's protection against the wasting disease and its immunological powers were about the same in both cases.

We must conclude that in normal cir-cumstances the thymus sends some-thing besides lymphocytes to the target organs—the spleen and lymph nodes. It sends a messenger or factor that prompts those organs to produce lym-phocytes themselves from their own cells. It seems safe to surmise that this factor is a hormone; it admirably an-swers the definition of a hormone, name-ly a substance that is secreted by a gland, travels to other organs by way of the bloodstream and produces a specific effect on their activities. This thymic hormone has not yet been given a name, but there is no longer much doubt of its existence.

A capsule-enclosed thymus gland implanted in the body of a mouse ap-parently serves the animal's lifelong needs although the lifetime of the gland in the capsule is not much more than about 60 days. In this respect it mimics the normal situation: the thymus with which an animal is born also has a limited career of activity. The gland tides the animal over a critical period in its early development and then ceases to be indispensable. Once it has acti-vated the other lymphoid organs to pro-duce lymphocytes it subsides to a minor role. Its brief heyday of activity in the first weeks or months of the animal's life has been all-important, however, for the future survival of the animal. The hormone the thymus provides at that time, in an amazingly small amount, directs the development of the system of immunity that will protect the ani-mal for the rest of its life.

Our findings tend to support a modi-fied version of the "selective" theory of immunity that Sir Macfarlane Burnet has described in his article titled "The Mechanism of Immunity" [beginning on page 12 in this volume]. He sug-gested that the body contains a variety of lymphocytes, each of which has a

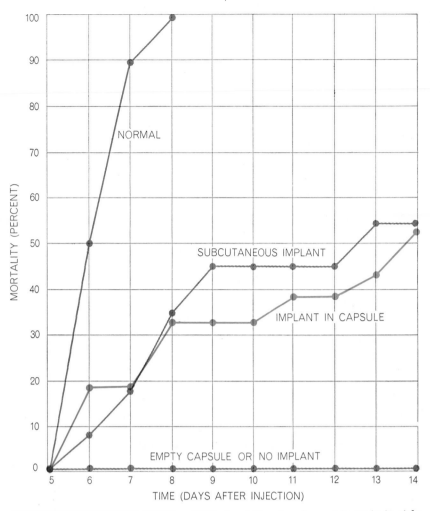

HYPERSENSITIVITY REACTION to LCM virus kills mice of a certain strain in eight days. Thymectomized mice do not succumb to this reaction. The implantation of a thymus under the skin, however, restores the sensitivity, and more than half of such grafted mice die. The implantation of a thymus inside a chamber has just about the same effect.

built-in capacity to produce a specific antibody, or at least to give rise to cells that will produce it. When the right antigen comes along, the particu-lar clone, or group, of cells that is capa-ble of generating production of the specific antibody is stimulated to multi-ply. Recently James L. Gowans of the University of Oxford presented evidence that there may be two classes of lym-phocytes: (1) "committed" ones, which have already reacted with a specific antigen, and (2) "uncommitted" ones, which are free to react to new anti-genic stimuli. In the light of these hypotheses and the available experi-mental evidence, one can outline a general picture of the immunity system in mammals and the role of the thymus in it, as follows:

When an animal is born, the thymus is actively producing lymphocytes. The thymic hormone renders these cells capable of reacting with antigens. They are still uncommitted, but, as Burnet

suggests, each has only a restricted range of response to specific antigens. Shortly after birth the lymphocytes pro-duced by the thymus begin to migrate to the other lymphoid organs. As soon as each competent lymphocyte encoun-ters and reacts with an appropriate anti-gen, it becomes committed and begins to multiply, giving rise to plasma cells that synthesize antibodies to the antigen.

The spleen, lymph nodes and other lymphoid organs contain a small supply of lymphocytes and multipurpose cells called stem cells when the animal is born, but these cells are not able to react with antigens or to multiply until they are activated by the hormone from the thymus. Soon after birth hormonal messengers from the thymus begin ar-riving and render the lymphocytes in these organs capable of proliferating and of becoming "committed." Once a sufficient self-replenishing reservoir of such cells has been established in the spleen and lymph nodes, the main job

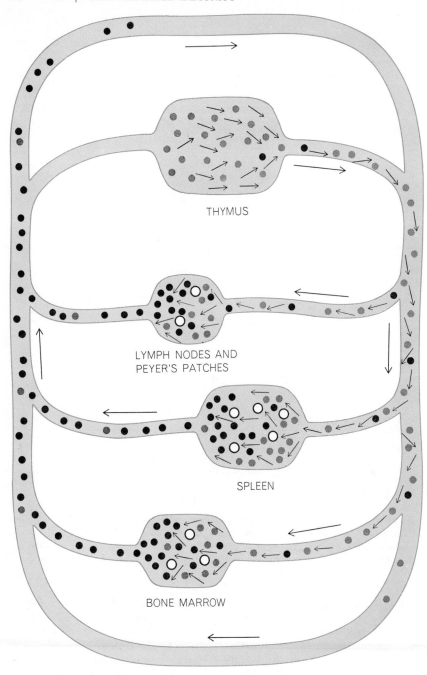

THYMUS

LYMPH NODES AND
PEYER'S PATCHES

SPLEEN

BONE MARROW

of the thymus is done and it can retire.

This kind of scheme can explain the results of our experiments on the immunity reactions of the mouse. Removal of the thymus at birth deprives mice of their source of immunologically competent lymphocytes. In the case of the resistant strains of mice that maintained a high level of lymphocytes in the blood in spite of thymectomy at birth, the explanation of their failure to show an immune response to the virus injection is that their lymphocytes, in the absence of the thymus hormone, were incapable of generating a line of replicating cells that would react against this new antigen.

The next step in the investigation is clear, because the path has been well marked by the classic studies of endocrine glands and their hormones. Now that the specific effects of removing the organ and reimplanting it have been intensively tested, the third step, according to the traditional strategy, is to isolate the hormone—if indeed it is a hormone—and proceed to study its chemical action. When this is accomplished, the chemical basis of resistance to infection and to grafts of foreign tissues may be much clearer.

ROLE OF THYMUS in immunity may be as suggested in this diagram. At birth most lymphocytes are in the thymus; a few are in other lymphoid organs, along with precursor stem cells (*circles*). The lymphocytes are incompetent (*gray dots*), unable to react to antigens, until they are exposed to a humoral factor that originates in the thymus (*black arrows*). The humoral factor travels through the bloodstream to other lymphoid tissues and there produces competent lymphocytes (*black dots*) that can become antibody-producing cells. The factor may also stimulate the stem cells to proliferate and differentiate into lymphocytes.

10

The Human Lymphocyte
as an Experimental Animal

by Richard A. Lerner and Frank J. Dixon
June 1973

*Maintained through many generations in laboratory
cultures, the cells that make antibody lend themselves
to studies of cell differentiation and diseases involving
the immune system, which may include cancer*

Some of the major questions in cellular biology today are these: How does a cell respond to its environment? How does that response alter the expression of the cell's genes? How do cells communicate with one another? How do cells differentiate? How do the specialized functions of a cell (such as secretion) relate to its general functions (such as gene replication)? There is a single class of cells that lends itself to the study of all these major questions. It is the lymphocyte, the cell that stands at the center of the immune response, the process by which an organism responds to its environment. The immune response is not only a defense against disease but also a cause of some diseases. Moreover, it seems increasingly clear that it is implicated in the chain of events that leads to cancer. Lymphocytes can now be cultured, or grown in laboratory glassware. Because of their special properties and the ease with which they can be manipulated, cultured lymphocytes are being exploited in a variety of investigations that are under way in a number of laboratories.

One way of characterizing these investigations is to say that they deal with the specialized functions of cells rather than the general functions (or, as Boris Ephrussi puts it, the luxury functions as opposed to the housekeeping ones). The housekeeping functions are those needed for the cell to stay alive and reproduce itself: energy transfer, the flow of genetic information from DNA through RNA to protein, the formation of cellular· organelles. These functions are common to most cells. The various specialized functions, on the other hand, are peculiar to certain classes of cells and are reflected in the different shapes and duties of, say, brain cells and muscle cells, and the different secretions of, say, pancreatic cells and lymphocytes. When cells are maintained outside the organism in a culture, they can dispense with their specialized functions and still live, grow and divide. Indeed, it has been argued that a cell that can dispense with its luxury functions has a selective advantage over one that cannot, since it can put more of its energy into the housekeeping chores that are necessary for its survival. The differential expression of luxury functions in culture is illustrated by the human melanoma, a tumor that synthesizes the pigment melanin. When melanoma cells maintained in a culture are proliferating rapidly, no pigment is synthesized and the cells appear colorless. When growth ceases, however, the dark pigment granules are synthesized and the cells turn black.

Since about 30 years ago, when biologists began in earnest to remove cells from higher organisms and maintain them in a culture, a great deal has been discovered about what the housekeeping functions of cells are and how they are carried out. For example, we now understand rather well the structure of the genetic material, DNA, how it is transcribed into RNA and how RNA is translated into protein. It is time now to apply the rigorous procedures established over the past 30 years to the study of the luxury functions of cells. That will not be an easy task nor will it soon be accomplished, but it is the route toward a better understanding of the questions we listed at the beginning of this article.

Those questions have in common a relation to one of the central issues in biology: the problem of how events at the surface of a cell alter the expression of the cell's genes. The essential initial step in the immune response is the contact of an antigen—a foreign substance—with receptors on the surfaces of lymphocytes derived from the bone marrow, the so-called *B*-lymphocytes. (This contact may be altered by interaction of the antigen with the white cells called macrophages or with lymphocytes derived from the thymus gland, the so-called *T*-lymphocytes.) The contact alters the expression of the *B*-lymphocyte's genes, setting in motion a series of events during which the cells divide and differentiate [*see illustration on page 106*]. The cell type evolves from one that is

GREEN FLUORESCENT DYE reveals immunoglobulin molecules on the surface of lymphocytes (*see next page*). An antibody against the immunoglobulin molecule is prepared by injecting some immunoglobulin from one species into an experimental animal of a different species. The antibody is coupled to fluorescein, a fluorescent dye, and is allowed to react with the cells. The fluorescein-labeled antibody binds specifically to immunoglobulin molecules on the cell surfaces (which in this case act as antigens). The resulting antigen-antibody complexes are revealed by the yellow-green glow emitted by the fluorescein under ultraviolet radiation. This micrograph and the ones on page 111 were made by Curtis Wilson with a Zeiss dark-field microscope, mercury-arc lighting and special interference and barrier filters, one effect of which is to make unstained cells or parts of cells appear red.

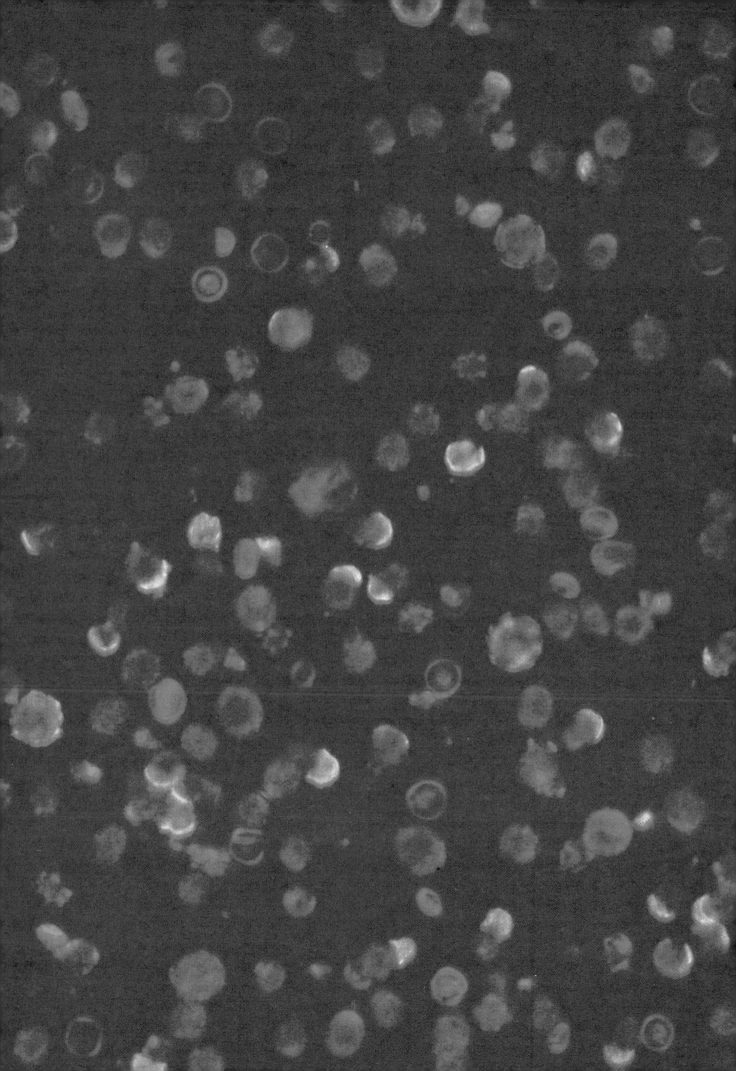

specialized to respond to an event in its environment to one that is uniquely adapted to the synthesis and secretion of antibody molecules. These two cells, the undifferentiated small, or "virgin," lymphocyte and the plasma cell, represent respectively the beginning and the end of the process of lymphocyte differentiation. Just how many times the cells divide in the course of this differentiation is not known, but many of the changes have been documented. There is a progressive decrease in the number of immunoglobulin molecules, or cell-surface receptors, on each cell. The irregular nucleus of the small lymphocyte becomes regular and round, and the nucleus becomes much smaller in relation to the surrounding cytoplasm. In the cytoplasm there is an increase in the number of such organelles as lysosomes, the Golgi apparatus and mitochondria. The organelles called polyribosomes increase in number and become associated with membranes to form an extensive network of endoplasmic reticulum, which is presumably involved in the greatly augmented synthesis and secretion of immunoglobulin molecules.

It would be convenient to be able to induce a culture of lymphocytes to enter the process of differentiation and then observe them as they move through the successive stages. Unfortunately this is not yet possible, but such an experimental system can in effect be simulated. Approximately 100 different lymphocyte clones, or cell lines descended from a single cell, are available. They cover the spectrum of differentiation, since the lymphocytes in any clone appear to be arrested at one point in the process of differentiation. By selecting the proper clone the investigator can therefore work with lymphocytes that represent a particular stage in the process of differentiation.

Lymphocytes in culture have a number of properties that suit them uniquely to the study of the special functions of cells and thus to the process of differentiation. One such property is their exquisite specificity. A single cell is capable of responding to only one antigen or at most to a limited number of antigens with a similar molecular structure. That means the cell-surface receptors for the antigens must be highly specific. What is the nature of the receptors and how many different ones must there be in order to accommodate the different antigens an organism must deal with?

Niels K. Jerne of the Basel Institute for Immunology suggested (in a modification of Paul Ehrlich's original theory

of antibody response) that the remarkable specificity of the immune response could best be accounted for if the receptor for antigen were the antibody molecule itself, in which case the antibody would be both the receptor and the effector. The immunoglobulin, or antibody, molecule is well adapted to serving such a double function [see "The Structure and Function of Antibodies," by Gerald M. Edelman, the article beginning on page 39]. In its simplest form it is a protein composed of two heavy and two light polypeptide chains that are joined by several disulfide bridges. Each chain is divided into two kinds of regions: "constant" regions, in which the sequence of amino acids (the constituent units of the polypeptides) is essentially the same in all antibodies of a given class, and "variable" regions, in which the sequence is different in every antibody [see illustration on page 107]. The variable regions provide the specificity required for the receptor function: the binding of antigen. The constant regions are involved in such effector functions as the binding of complement or fixation to skin (an element in certain inflammation processes).

Studies in several laboratories have indicated that Jerne's hypothesis is correct, at least in its broad outline. At the Scripps Clinic and Research Foundation we have been able to measure the surface receptors in quantitative terms by developing a sensitive radioimmune assay that determines the number of molecules of immunoglobulin exposed on the

surface of cultured lymphocytes [see illustration on page 108]. The number varies between 20,000 and 200,000 in different lines. As lymphocytes proceed along the line of differentiation the number of antibody molecules on the surface decreases; several studies have suggested that most plasma cells have few receptor molecules, if any at all. This is an interesting case of biological modulation. The plasma cell is in effect the end of the line: it is specialized for a high rate of synthesis and secretion of immunoglobulin molecules and has no need for receptor molecules.

Immunoglobulin molecules associated with the cell surface—the presumed receptor molecules—can be visualized by the technique of fluorescence microscopy. Antibody is prepared in one species against the immunoglobulin molecules of the species supplying the lymphocytes to be studied. The antibody is coupled to a fluorescent dye such as fluorescein. When the complex of the antibody and the dye reacts with cells, it binds to the immunoglobulin molecules associated with the cell surface and, when the cells are exposed to ultraviolet radiation, the characteristic green glow of the irradiated fluorescein reveals the location on the cell surface of the immunoglobulin molecules [see illustrations on the opposite page and on page 108]. The surface-associated molecules can be isolated and characterized by a combination of chemical and physical procedures. The exact structure of these molecules is still under study, but the available evidence

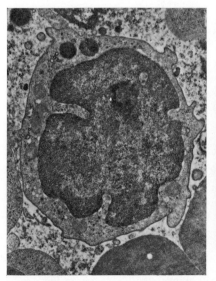 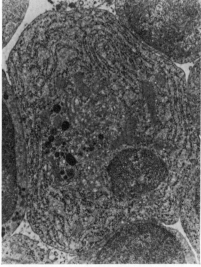

DIFFERENTIATION in the course of the immune response changes a lymphocyte (left) into a plasma cell (right). Noticeable changes include an increase in cell size, a relative decrease in the size of the nucleus and the formation of organelles involved in synthesis and secretion of antibody, including ribosomes (small black dots) arrayed along the membranous endoplasmic reticulum. The electron micrographs were made by Joseph Feldman.

suggests that the surface molecules may differ in some respect from the immunoglobulin that is secreted to become circulating antibody.

One of the characteristics of normal eukaryotic cells (the cells of organisms other than bacteria) is that they synthesize, grow and divide on definite cyclic schedules unless they retire from the cell cycle into a resting phase. Cell biologists conventionally divide the cycle into four phases called G_1, S, G_2 and M; the first three are defined on the basis of the different molecules synthesized in

each of them and the fourth phase is mitosis, or cell division [see illustration on page 109]. The number of temporal segments into which the cycle is thus divided is arbitrary; the degree of detail is limited by incomplete knowledge of the regulation of synthesis in these cells. It is actually likely that cells regulate their activities minute by minute or even second by second, and as we learn more it should be possible to fill in the minutes and seconds on the cell-cycle clock.

Studies in our laboratory and in that of David Pressman at the Roswell Park

Memorial Institute and of Donald N. Buell and John L. Fahey at the University of California at Los Angeles School of Medicine have shown that secretory immunoglobulin is synthesized in lymphocytes during a limited part of the G_1 phase, as is the case for other luxury polypeptides in other cells. In contrast, the surface immunoglobulin receptor molecules appear to turn over throughout the cell cycle with a half-life of about 45 minutes. The reason for this rapid turnover of cell-surface immunoglobulin is not yet clear, but it may well be relat-

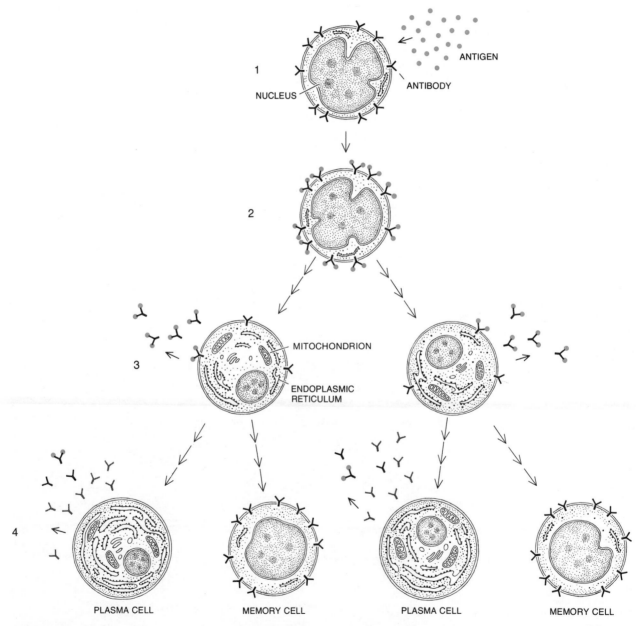

IMMUNE RESPONSE may begin when a small lymphocyte with antibodies (*black Y's*) on its surface encounters antigen molecules (*color*) against which its antibody is specific (*1*). The antigen is bound to the antibody (*2*); this event, together with a second signal involving another kind of lymphocyte, induces the small lympho-

cyte to divide and differentiate (*3*); surface receptor antibodies are lost and replaced by new ones. The lymphocytes differentiate to become plasma cells and memory cells (*4*). Plasma cells synthesize and secrete circulating antibody (*gray Y's*); memory cells, held in reserve, respond sensitively to reappearance of the antigen.

ed to modulation of the immune response, that is, to the requirement that immunoglobulin that has been "hit" by antigen not remain on the surface and that there be enough new receptor immunoglobulin on the surface to respond sensitively to any new hits by new antigen molecules.

Just as there is a temporal order for the synthesis of proteins during the mammalian cell cycle, so there are apparently limited periods during which the synthesis of enzymes can be induced. In liver cells, for example, David W. Martin, Jr., Gordon M. Tomkins and Daryl Granner of the University of California at San Francisco have shown that the enzyme tyrosine aminotransferase can be induced by corticosteroid hormone only during the last two-thirds of G_1 and at any time in S. It seems likely that we shall find a limited period of the lymphocyte cycle during which an antigen can induce cellular proliferation. The role of the antigen would therefore be not directly to trigger the synthesis of immunoglobulin but rather to induce specific resting lymphocytes to enter the cell cycle and so pass through a phase in which such synthesis is obligatory.

David Prescott of the University of Colorado has noted that when nerve cells and striated-muscle cells in living animals retire from the cell cycle, they do so during the G_1 phase; he has suggested that for most cells the control of further proliferation and differentiation is mediated by some event during this phase. An example of such an event occurring in cultured cells was reported by Karlin Nilausen and Howard Green of the Massachusetts Institute of Technology. They found that when certain mouse cells ceased to grow because of contact inhibition (that is, because they had formed a complete single layer in the culture dish), they did so during the G_1 phase. Moreover, some observations made by H. Becker of the Ontario Cancer Institute and his colleagues indicate that there are physiological differences between cells in the resting phase and cells in the G_1 phase. All of this tends to suggest that in the case of lymphocytes contact with antigen molecules may be the inducing event that initiates entry into the G_1 phase and subsequent cellular proliferation.

The rapid increase in antibody formation after an antigenic challenge is hard to explain simply on the basis of an increase in the number of cells that form antibody. Some investigators have proposed that additional cells are "recruited," and that in these cells the genera-

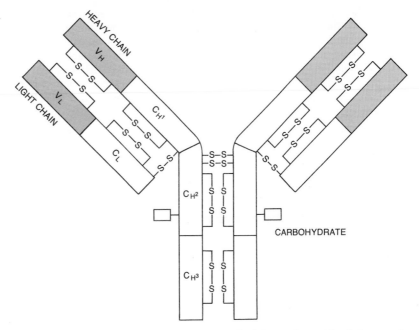

ANTIBODY MOLECULE is a protein composed of four polypeptide chains, two long "heavy" chains and two shorter "light" ones. Each chain has a variable region (*color*), whose amino acid sequence provides the specificity for binding antigen, and one or more constant regions. The four variable regions are homologous (their amino acid sequences match up), as are the eight constant regions. The chains are connected by disulfide bridges.

tion time is shortened, so that the cells divide with particular rapidity. Our data show, however, that as cells proceed through the G_1 phase the synthesis of immunoglobulin can increase as much as fivefold without cell division or even the synthesis of DNA. Recruitment, then, can be explained as the passage of an increasing number of cells to a point in the cell cycle where the rate of antibody synthesis is greatly increased. This contention is supported by the finding that during the induction of an immune response neither DNA synthesis nor mitosis is a necessary predecessor of antibody synthesis.

Like other cells in culture, lymphocytes can be used for studies of mutation and other kinds of variation. In this application lymphocytes have a number of advantages. They apparently have an infinite life-span in culture, during which their phenotypic expression persists, that is, their shape, physiological functions and other characteristics remain constant. They retain the normal diploid (double) set of chromosomes, whereas in most other cultured cells the chromosome complement changes. And they are easily cloned: a single cell with specific properties can be isolated from a culture and its progeny can be grown into a large population.

A number of inherited disorders af-

flicting humans are caused by inborn errors of metabolism such that the patient's cells fail to synthesize a necessary enzyme or some other kind of product. By obtaining and culturing lymphocytes from such patients one can track down the defect, quantify it and perhaps in time find ways to remedy it. Arthur D. Bloom and his colleagues at the University of Michigan Medical School have examined a number of such defects in this way. One was the Lesch-Nyhan syndrome, a serious defect in a metabolic pathway that converts preformed nucleosides (DNA precursors) into DNA. Bloom's group found that lymphocytes from these patients produce only 1.4 percent of the normal amount of HGPRT, a key enzyme in the pathway. Production defects of this kind may someday be corrected by manipulating or replacing the defective cells.

One way of manipulating would be through cell fusion: if two lines of cells are cultured together, some cells may fuse and form hybrid daughter cells that contain chromosomes, and thus genetic information, from both parent cells. It may be possible to remove cells from a patient, fuse them to cells that contain the gene for the missing enzyme and return the "corrected" cells to the patient. Henry Harris of the University of Oxford has shown that (at least in one system) fused cells may incorporate some foreign genetic material without bringing about the synthesis of foreign surface antigens, so that apparently one need not be concerned that the fused cells would be rejected.

Cells that start out with the same genotype, or hereditary constitution, may come in time to have subtly different phenotypes. The immunoglobulins are ideally suited to the study of lymphocyte phenotypes because they are so readily detected, characterized and quantified by sensitive immunoassays. It has long been known that when cells from mouse plasma-cell tumors are cultured, some of the cells spontaneously lose the ability to synthesize the heavy-chain parts of the immunoglobulin molecule. (There is a much smaller tendency to lose the ability to synthesize light chains, presumably because any heavy

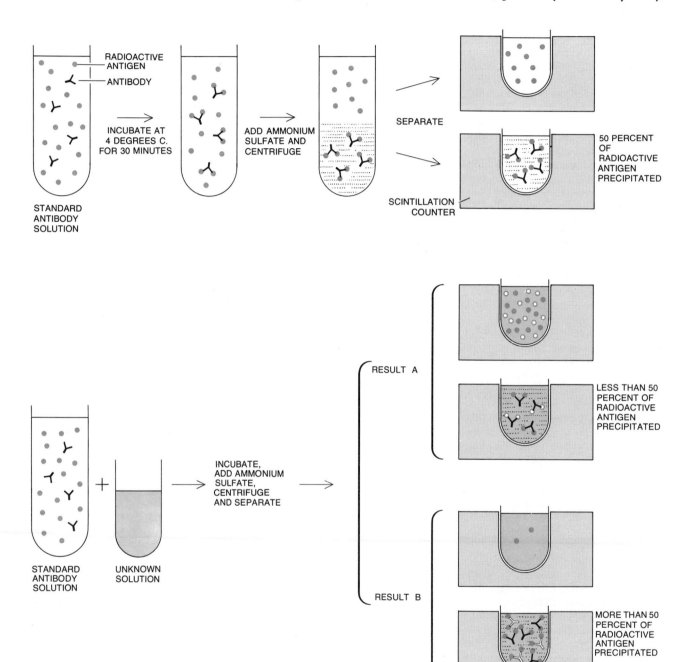

RADIOIMMUNE ASSAY determines the number of antigen or antibody molecules in a solution or on the surface of cells. It utilizes a standard solution (top) of antibody molecules (black Y's) and radioactively labeled antigen molecules (colored dots). The proportions are such that the antibody can bind 50 percent of the antigen. When ammonium sulfate is added and the preparation is centrifuged, the antibody and the bound antigen are precipitated, and measuring the amount of radiation in the precipitate and the remaining solution (right) shows how much of the antigen was bound. If now a solution to be tested is added to the standard solution (bottom) and the procedure is repeated, the assay shows whether there is antigen or antibody in the test solution, and how much. If there is unlabeled antigen (open colored circles) in the test solution (Result A), it will compete for binding sites on the antibody, so that less than 50 percent of the labeled antigen is precipitated (right). If there is antibody (open Y's) in the test solution (Result B), it will provide extra binding sites for antigen, so that more than 50 percent of the labeled antigen is precipitated.

chains without light chains are quite insoluble and are precipitated within the cell and destroy it; the loss of light-chain synthesis may be a lethal mutation and one that is therefore not seen.)

At the Albert Einstein College of Medicine, Matthew D. Scharff and his colleagues have devised an ingenious method of measuring the rate of loss of heavy-chain synthesis in individual mouse plasma cells [*see top illustration on next page*]. They have established that cells lose the ability to synthesize heavy chains at the rate of one loss per 900 cell generations. The event that causes this loss is not yet known, and it will be hard to track down because the appearance of immunoglobulin outside the cell entails the completion of a complex process involving transcription, translation, assembly, transport and secretion of the molecule; an alteration in any molecule or structure that plays a role in this process could cause the failure of secretion that Scharff detects.

The cause may or may not be a simple mutation, in which the substitution of a single amino acid subunit can alter the structure and/or the configuration of a single polypeptide and thus lead to a change in phenotype. Scharff has therefore called the rate of loss he measures a variation frequency rather than a mutation frequency. As a matter of fact many of the phenotypic properties of cells in higher organisms may involve the synthesis and secretion of polypeptides as the result of just such complicated processes. Although variation frequencies may not yield the precise information about the organization of genes that mutation frequencies provide, they may be more to the point in studies of the alteration of certain phenotypes in eukaryotic cells.

In the study of disease, lymphocytes have an important added advantage in that they are part of the system that generates the immune response and may therefore reflect abnormalities peculiar to that system. These include failures of the immune response, certain viral infections, autoimmune disease (in which the organism makes antibodies against components of itself) and perhaps cancer.

In the case of systemic lupus erythematosus (SLE), a serious autoimmune disease, the study of lymphocytes may have yielded important information not only about the disease itself but also about its relation to other conditions. In human SLE (and in a similar disease in the New Zealand strains of mice) the immune

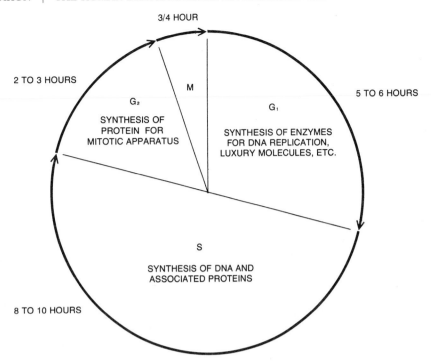

CELL CYCLE is conventionally divided into four phases on the basis of molecules synthesized in each. The times given here are for the HeLa cell, a human tumor cell. The cycle begins with G_1 and ends with M (mitosis), when the cell divides to form two daughter cells.

system synthesizes autoantibodies—often against the victim's own red blood cells and regularly against a variety of specific antigens found in the nuclei of the victim's cells. In many cases the most serious effects of these diseases have been shown to be caused by highly inflammatory antigen-antibody complexes in which at least some of the nuclear antigens are present.

Why, we wondered, do such patients and mice make antibodies almost exclusively to red blood cells and those particular nuclear antigens? What set of events would present those particular antigens to an affected mouse? One clue lay in the fact that many strains of mice harbor C-type RNA tumor viruses. Such viruses have RNA (rather than DNA) as their genetic material, they replicate by transcribing their genetic information into DNA (which can presumably integrate into the host's own genetic material) and they cause tumors in animals they infect [see "RNA-directed DNA Synthesis," by Howard M. Temin; SCIENTIFIC AMERICAN Offprint 1239]. Could the mice be infected by a virus that was replicating and could the intermediates in that replication constitute the antigens in question? When we investigated, we found that the mice were in fact making antibodies that reacted with virtually every polypeptide or nucleic acid intermediate involved in

the replication of the viruses [*see bottom illustration on next page*]. Was it possible that the immune system of the mice had been mobilized against an RNA tumor virus and that in fighting the war against the virus the mice had developed inflammatory antigen-antibody complexes and autoimmune disease?

An answer to that question might shed light not only on the origin of at least one autoimmune disease but also on the possible interrelation of viruses, the immune response and cancer. The connection between viruses and some animal tumors and leukemias has been known for many years. More recently it has come to seem likely that the immune system is somehow implicated in cancer. Since the affected mice had autoimmune disease and made antibodies to viral intermediates, it was obviously important to try to isolate the virus in question. And, for theoretical as well as technical reasons, it seemed to us that the cultured lymphocyte was a better place to find it (perhaps in large amounts) than the very occasional tumors these mice develop.

Let us outline the reasoning. Since a virus is an obligatory parasite that can only survive and multiply in living cells, a tumor is of no advantage to the virus; after all, it may kill the host and the virus as well. Certainly a tumor is of no advantage to the host. Moreover, a tu-

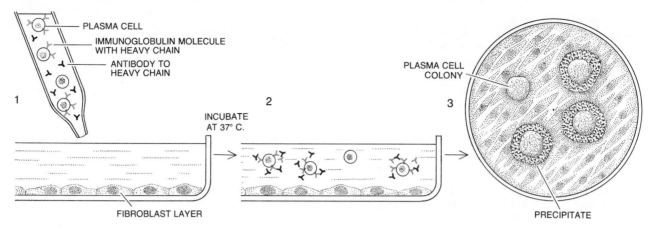

VARIANT CELLS that fail to synthesize the heavy chain of an immunoglobulin molecule are detected and cultured by a technique developed by Matthew D. Scharff of the Albert Einstein College of Medicine. The plasma cells to be tested are pipetted into a culture medium in which a "feeder" layer of fibroblast cells has been established (1). Plasma cells, most of which contain heavy chains, are introduced, along with antibody to heavy chains. The antibody (acting as antigen) becomes bound to the heavy chains, forming antigen-antibody lattices around the cells that contain heavy chains (2). After a few days each plasma cell has proliferated to form a colony of cells (3). The colonies descended from those of the original cells that produced heavy chains are surrounded by an antigen-antibody precipitate; the colony from the cell that did not make the chains has no precipitate. The variant colony is easy to distinguish and its cells can be cultured for further studies. (The third drawing is done at a much smaller scale than the first two.)

mor may not be a valid guide in the search for an oncogenic, or tumor-causing, agent. The reason is that the very formation of the tumor suggests that the host's defenses have been inadequate. The oncogenic agent (perhaps a virus) and the antigens it induces in tumor cells have failed to alert the host's defenses; they may well also evade the investigator.

How might the failure have come about? One possibility is that in a cancer that results from virus infection some process (an immune response?) causes a selection of cells with viral genomes, or gene complements, that are incompletely expressed—genomes in which only a few genes, whose products render the host cells cancerous, are expressed and other genes are not. From the point of view of selective advantage for the tumor this would be an ideal situation, since the unexpressed genes might have coded for more and/or stronger anti-

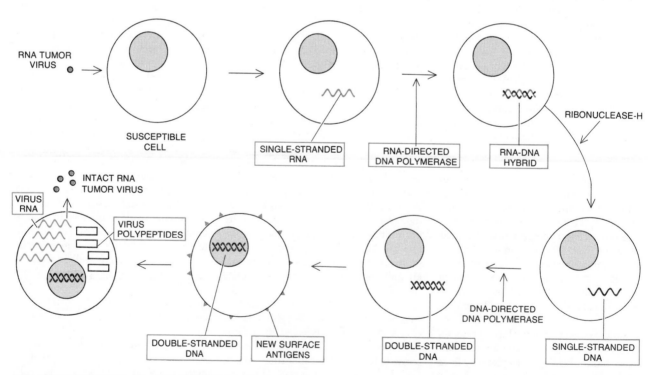

RELATION BETWEEN AN AUTOIMMUNE DISEASE and a tumor-inducing virus was suggested by the fact that human patients suffering from systemic lupus erythematosus (SLE) or mice with a similar disease make antibodies to a variety of antigens, almost all of which are related to similar molecules formed during the replication of an RNA tumor virus. The diagram shows the successive steps in the replication of such a virus, which is unusual in that its genetic information is carried in RNA that is transcribed into DNA in the cell by an RNA-directed DNA polymerase. This significantly broadens the range of foreign nucleic acids that is presented to the host. The molecules against which specific antibodies were found to be made by affected mice are indicated by the colored boxes.

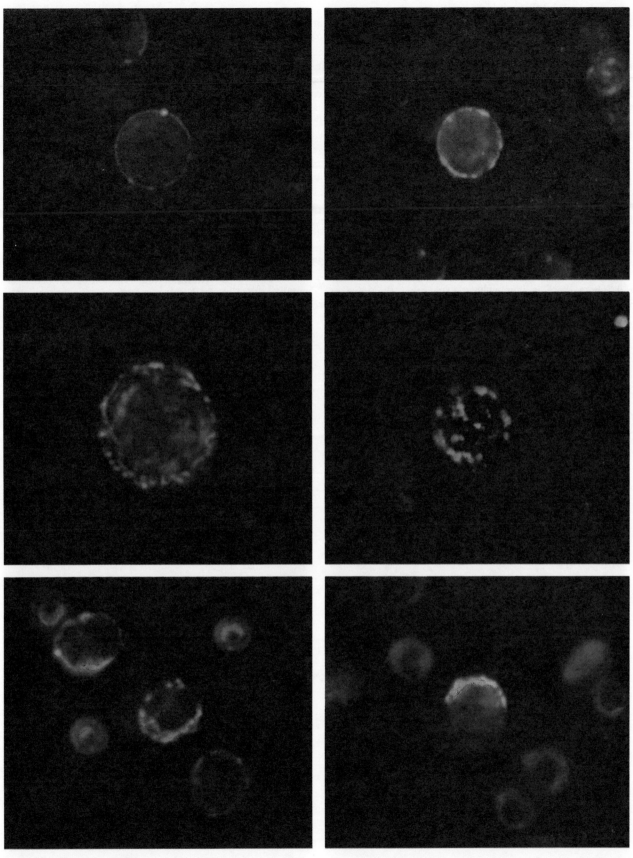

IMMUNOGLOBULIN MOLECULES associated with the cell surface and visualized by fluorescent staining move over the surface of the cell. At first, thinly distributed over the surface, they appear as thin rims at the circumference (*top*). Then they become more concentrated, giving a granular appearance (*middle*). Finally they seem to collect in a restricted area, forming increasingly concentrated "caps" (*bottom*). The movement may represent a sweeping action in which complexes are removed from the surface. The way they move may lend support to the "fluid mosaic" model of the structure of the surface membrane, which sees the membrane as a fluid in which molecules are mobile. If energy supply is blocked (by low temperature, for example), only rim fluorescence is seen.

genic polypeptides that would stimulate the host's defenses.

If this proposed chain of events should be correct, then tumors would not be the most profitable place to look for tumor viruses. It seems reasonable to assume that the growth of a tumor may be the rare and extreme result of the incomplete expression of the viral genome, and that the same virus or similar ones may be present in other disease states or even in apparently well individuals. In cancer, that is, the war has been lost and the virus has gone underground. In other situations the immunologic war may still be being fought against a detectable virus, and a disease (such as SLE) may develop as a result of the battle. We would suggest that the time and place to search for an oncogenic agent is when and where there is immunologic evidence that the host is defending against such an agent.

These concepts are predictive ones and they can be tested. Our prediction is that if a virus is isolated from the New Zealand mice, it should, on being injected into other mice, cause both autoimmunity and cancer. Together with Fred Jensen, we established a number of lines of cultured lymphocytes from New Zealand mice with the autoimmune disease. When we examined those lines, we found that each of them produced a unique RNA tumor virus of the C type. In addition, all cells in each of the lines had a distinctive extra chromosome, and some cells had a deletion—a missing segment—in one of the two X chromosomes. The extra chromosome was also found in eight of 38 cells taken from New Zealand mouse fetuses, indicating that the mice are "mosaics" for this chromosomal marker.

Byron Croker and Bert Del Villano isolated the virus produced by one of these lymphocyte lines and injected it into newborn mice of two New Zealand substrains. Their preliminary results suggest that the concepts we outlined above are correct, but many more mice and different combinations of strains remain to be tested before we can be sure that, through an immunologic reaction, autoimmunity is the price of protection against a tumor. The patient may lose either way, but the concept of such a trade-off is nevertheless significant. The immunologic tracks of autoimmunity may turn out to have the same predictive value for a putative (and hitherto elusive) human tumor virus as classical antigen-antibody tests have had for the identification and isolation of the agents of other diseases.

III

IMMUNE
TOLERANCE

11

Tolerance and Unresponsiveness

by Sir Macfarlane Burnet
An original article
1976

It is biologically necessary that most self-components of the body should not stimulate immune responses. There are several ways by which this necessity may be achieved.

In every discussion of immunity, since Ehrlich first spoke of "horror autotoxicus," the problem of why and how foreign material introduced into an animal provokes antibody production and removal of the foreign material has been balanced by the other problem of why and how the body tolerates its own substance apparently without immune response. For many years I have implied that the basic feature of immunity was the capacity to differentiate between self and not-self.

Any subject within the conventional biomedical field almost automatically divides itself into physiological aspects concerned with normal function and pathological aspects that reflect genetic anomalies, effects secondary to disease elsewhere, or experimental manipulations of exceptional—that is, "unbiological"—activity. In the present context it is convenient to keep the word "tolerance" to mean the natural process by which an animal tolerates or fails to react to its own genetically proper substance, and for some rather strictly limited experimental modifications or applications of that process. For those experiments carried out in adult animals in which, by certain manipulations, the animals fail to respond to some standard antigenic stimulus, the word "unresponsiveness" allows a convenient separation from the first group. It is convenient to consider the two conditions of natural tolerance and experimentally produced unresponsiveness separately.

Natural Immunological Tolerance

At first glance there seems no reason why the ability of a body to veto immune action against its own components should not depend simply on genetically programmed qualities. It is clearly essential that such tolerance should exist, and it came almost as a surprise that tolerance was not laid down genetically but had to be learned.

Although many earlier experimenters were aware of the difficulties of transplanting organs in animals and tended to accept without question that these difficulties did not seem to arise in the experimental work on the embryology of amphibians or chickens, a clear idea of the immunological nature of skin-graft rejection dates only from Peter Medawar's work in the period from 1938 to 1945. Only work done since then need be considered in following the way by which the study of tolerance developed.

Cattle breeders have always been interested in the fact that when a male and female pair of twins was born, the female was always sterile—a freemartin. When veterinarians became interested in bovine blood groups, it was natural enough to include twins in studies of inheritance. In 1945 Ray Owen found that nonidentical bovine twins each had the same complex of blood group reactions but that these corresponded to a mixture of the blood types that would be expected if each calf had been born separately. In most instances the mixture of circulating red blood-cells remained almost constant in composition in each individual for years. Yet if calves of identical genetic character had been born as single births, blood of A injected into B (or B into A) would have provoked an immune response and been eliminated.

An analogous situation in man is provided by the much rarer circumstance when nonidentical twins share a common placental circulation in the uterus. They show blood group reactions indicating that two genetically distinct types of blood cells are present and tolerated. In addition they will accept mutual skin grafts, something that never happens between dissimilar twins from separate placentas, who therefore have wholly independent circulations. [*See the top illustration on page 115.*]

These findings are in themselves sufficient to establish that provided there is a mingling of stem cells and lymphocytes from an early stage of development, genetically foreign cells can be implanted and remain tolerated indefinitely. Tolerance is of genetic origin only in the sense that the genetically controlled cellular mechanisms are installed and ready to react appropriately to whatever potentially antigenic patterns may be encountered. In 1957 I suggested that the simplest mechanism to account for tolerance was to assume that a newly differentiated immunocyte—T and B cells were then unthought of—was destroyed or rendered incapable of multiplication when it recognized and reacted with a corresponding antigenic determinant. Only when it reached a certain maturity would the immunocyte react positively, upon encountering the antigenic determinant, by proliferating and producing antibody.

The recognition of T and B cells, and of the necessity for their cooperation if most antigens are to stimulate production of antibodies, has greatly complicated the picture. It means that our first point of view needs to be restated in more modern terms: an animal is tolerant of a given antigen when there is no effective combination of T and B cells in the body with which the antigen can react to induce antibody formation. This would probably be accepted by a majority of immunologists, though there are others who prefer to think that potentially reactive T and B cells are always present but are actively prevented from reacting against "self" material through the action of suppressor T cells or soluble inhibitors in the blood plasma. Here, as in every other aspect of T-cell function, our uncertainty about T-cell receptors makes it impossible to be definite about the part played by T cells in tolerance. Experimental work on the problem has almost all been concerned with unresponsiveness to foreign antigens and is not directly relevant to natural tolerance.

Tolerance in Tetraparental (Allophenic) Mice

A technique devised by Beatrice Mintz allows the deliberate "construction" of a mouse whose cells are of two genetically distinct types. Very briefly, two immunologically distinct breeds of mice, A and B, are used; A and B females are mated each to a male of her own type, and 24 hours later the fertilized ova are collected in the early stage of cell division. An A ovum is caused to fuse with a B ovum, giving rise to a blastocyst stage composed of an equal number of diploid A and B cells. If the blastocyst is now transferred to the uterus of a physiologically receptive foster mother, it will develop into a physiologically normal mouse whose every organ is a mosaic of A and B cells. [*See illustration at lower right.*] Under ordinary circumstances A and B are incompatible, actively rejecting a skin transplant from the other. However, tetraparental mice accept each type of cell as self and are apparently perfectly adequate in immunological function. It should be emphasized that this synthetic mouse is quite different from an F1 A × B hybrid; it is a chimera of two distinct cell types, in contrast to the hybrid, in which all cells contain A and B chromosomes. If a piece of skin from an AB hybrid is transplanted to an A mouse, each cell is recognized for the foreign B antigen it contains and the whole graft is rejected. If a similar experiment is done with the A + B chimera, the graft is partially rejected, developing a "worm-eaten" appearance, which allows an approximate visualization of the mosaic of A and B cell patches in the skin.

Once again, immunologists have two

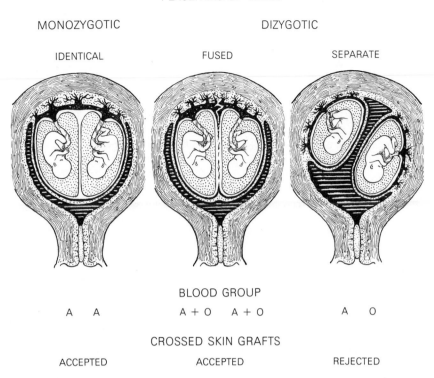

PLACENTAS OF TWINS

MONOZYGOTIC DIZYGOTIC

IDENTICAL FUSED SEPARATE

BLOOD GROUP

A A   A + O   A + O   A O

CROSSED SKIN GRAFTS

ACCEPTED ACCEPTED REJECTED

IMMUNOLOGY OF HUMAN TWINS is shown in this diagram. Monozygotic or identical twins have the same blood group and develop from a single placenta. Dizygotic twins arise from two separately fertilized ova and may have different blood groups. Normally dizygotic twins have separate placentas and after birth reject reciprocal skin transplants. On rare occasions placentas of dizygotic twins fuse to give a common circulation. Under these circumstances the dizygotic twins behave like identical twins in accepting each other's skin grafts.

interpretations of tolerance in tetraparental mice. Mintz and Willys K. Silvers thought it likely that there was complete tolerance in the chimeric mice and an absence of any reactive lymphocytes. Another group—Ingegerd Hellström, Karl E. Hellström, and John J. Trentin—found evidence that there were toxic T cells whose activity was damped by a serum factor. But whatever the mechanism by which the chimeric mice tolerate the skin graft, their tolerance of self is functionally just as complete as it is in any normal mouse.

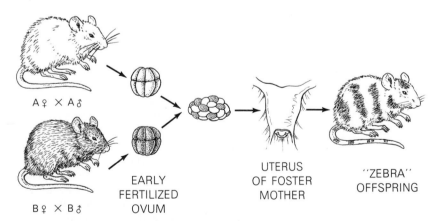

A♀ × A♂

B♀ × B♂

EARLY FERTILIZED OVUM

UTERUS OF FOSTER MOTHER

"ZEBRA" OFFSPRING

WHEN TETRAPARENTAL (ALLOPHENIC) MICE are bred, these accept skin grafts from both parental types. Normally fertilized ova are extracted from pregnant mice at an early stage of segmentation and induced to fuse, forming a chimeric blastocyst. This can be inserted into the uterus of an unrelated foster mother and develops into an anatomically normal mouse. If the original parents were of contrasting colors a "zebra" appearance is seen in a proportion of the tetraparental offspring.

Unresponsiveness

Many serious clinical conditions are due to or associated with immune responses that, in these particular circumstances, seem unwanted and harmful. An autoimmune disease like rheumatoid arthritis or systemic lupus erythematosus is one example, the rejection of a kidney transplant is another, and there are many more. Such occurrences have provided practical justification for attempts over many years to discover ways by which animals, and by implication human patients, can be rendered nonresponsive to one particular antigen or group of antigens without damaging the general capacity of the body's immune system to deal with infections and other everyday responsibilities. In some ways the quest has been successful; there are now at least 20 ways by which this can be accomplished to a significant degree. However, none has provided a really satisfactory method of dealing with immunological disease in man, though the modern method of preventing Rh disease in the newborn promises to be a first-rate example of prophylactic interference with an unwanted immune response [see "The Prevention of 'Rhesus' Babies," by C. A. Clarke, on page 212].

It would be impossible to attempt a comprehensive account of modern work on unresponsiveness. What I shall attempt instead, in this article, is to describe some of the classical studies done before T and B cells were differentiated, then to pay rather special attention to the work of C. R. Parish, which bears on cell-mediated immunity and unresponsiveness, and finally to attempt to outline the simplest statement of the overall results that is broadly consistent with modern experimental findings and the considered opinions of leading contemporary workers in the field.

Classical Experiments Using, as Antigens, Soluble Serum Proteins from a Different Species

In the wake of studies made in the period of World War II on plasma fractionation in relation to blood and plasma transfusions, relatively well-characterized fractions became commercially available, including bovine serum, albumin and gamma globulin, and corresponding fractions from horse and man. These were found very convenient for laboratory studies on the process by which radiolabeled antigens are removed from the circulation, the rate at which antibodies are produced, and the circumstances under which specific unresponsiveness is induced. Out of this work a generally accepted set of results may be outlined in the following, numbered paragraphs based on the work of many authors. In particular, the studies by Frank Dixon, Richard Smith, and William Weigle, all of whom worked with rabbits, and Avrion Mitchison and David Dresser, who used mice, may be mentioned.

1. Relatively large doses of a foreign antigen are needed to induce unresponsiveness in half-grown or adult animals, but unresponsiveness can usually be achieved if large and repeated injections are made. Mitchison's generalization is probably correct that specific tolerance or unresponsiveness to a certain antigen is always developed when circumstances ensure that the antigen is constantly present in the circulation.

2. The earlier in life an antigen is administered, the smaller the dose needed to induce unresponsiveness. In one set of experiments in rabbits that were given a standard dose of bovine serum albumin relative to the body weight of each rabbit, all of those injected during the first week after birth became unresponsive, at three weeks 27 percent, and at four weeks none.

3. Rabbits rendered unresponsive to a single large dose of an antigen early in life slowly and irregularly regain capacity to react in a piecemeal fashion: probably a foreign serum albumin has many distinct antigenic determinants and the reappearance of immunocytes reactive against any one determinant is not related to reappearance of immunocytes reactive against the others. It is rare for an animal to regain its full capacity for brisk and complete response.

4. In adult mice of most strains administration of human or bovine gamma globulin that has been carefully freed of all aggregates is only very slowly eliminated from the body, the mice are unresponsive, and there is no antibody production. If aggregates are present, and particularly if adjuvants are used, antibody is produced. Even after antigen has vanished from the unresponsive mice, immunization with aggregated antigen in adjuvant causes no antibody response.

5. Some mouse strains, notably the "autoimmune strain" of New Zealand Black mice, produce antibody even in the presence of particle-free gamma-globulin antigen.

6. In mice, induced unresponsiveness to injection of serum from another species is not transferable by serum or cells to untreated normal mice. However, by linking a normal untreated mouse in parabiosis with a mouse that has been rendered nonresponsive, a common blood circulation is provided, and if active (i.e., aggregated) antigen is injected into either mouse, both produce antibodies.

Subsequent analysis of these results is consistent with, and generally interpreted as due to, deletion of cells specifically responsible for antibody production, rather than to the appearance of soluble inhibitors or "suppressor cells." This leaves the relative parts played by T and B cells uncertain, but in view of the high and persisting concentration of the antigens used in most experiments it is likely that both kinds of cells are inactivated either by the loss of receptors, by sterile maturation without proliferation, or by directly lethal damage. However, the process by which B and T cells, both reactive to a single antigen, cooperate in the presence of that antigen to produce the corresponding antibody can be analyzed in various ways to throw light on the nature of unresponsiveness. It has been clearly shown that the function of the T cells in this cooperative process can be inhibited more rapidly and by smaller concentrations of antigen than can that of the B cells—in short, T cells are more rapidly "tolerized" than B cells. The evidence therefore points to the absence of specific T cells as being responsible for the later stages of unresponsiveness.

Parish's Work with Chemically Modified Antigen

C. R. Parish, working in G. L. Ada's laboratory in Melbourne and later at Canberra, has introduced a new dimension into research on unresponsiveness by claiming that there is a reciprocal relationship between cell-mediated immunity (the T-cell system) and antibody production (the B-cell system) in that circumstances favoring strong delayed-hypersensitivity reactions are associated with unresponsiveness, as measured by the lack of production of antibodies, and vice versa. There are earlier experiments pointing in the same direction, but Parish's work with chemically treated flagellin represents the only systematic study of a phenomenon that seems to be vitally important for the understanding of immune unresponsiveness.

For historical reasons flagellin, the protein composing the filaments on *Salmonella* bacteria, has for many years been a favorite antigen in the Walter and Eliza Hall Institute. Nossal's early work in establishing an experimental basis for clonal selection theory used antibody from single lymphoid cells to immobilize *Salmonella* microcultures [see "How Cells Make Antibodies," by G. J. V. Nossal, page 22]. That antibody was antiflagellin. Methods of obtaining the predominant protein of the flagella in virtually pure form were subsequently developed and this protein has been extensively used as an experimental antigen in either a monomeric form (FLA) or a polymerized form (POL). When used as POL the protein has the virtue of being composed of a repetitive series of closely spaced antigenic determinants (or what Jerne refers to as "epitopes"). The monomeric form (FLA), which was used in most of Parish's experiments, is actively immunogenic, being capable of producing antibody after administration in very small doses, and it is rapidly eliminated from the body [see upper illustration, this page]. Both these qualities are important in obtaining clear-cut findings.

Parish treated monomeric FLA by acetoacetylation in graded fashion, a process which progressively reduced the capacity of FLA to react *in vitro* with a standard precipitating antiserum. He found, however, that at a stage where only a little of its reactive capacity was lost, its capacity to produce antibody (its immunogenicity) had gone com-

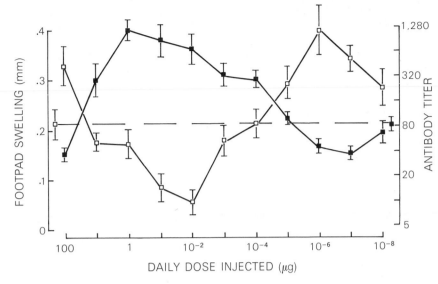

THE PRODUCTION OF TOLERANCE by flagellin (FLA) modified by cyanogen bromide. After a series of daily immunizations with an extreme range of doses of from 100 μg to 10^{-8} μg, rats were challenged with 100 μg of flagellin in saline. Antibody production was measured (as reciprocals of the highest serum dilutions causing agglutination—black squares represent the mean of titers over a four-week period and bars represent standard errors). Twenty-eight days after the first challenge the response of the footpad to a local injection of flagellin was estimated by the degree of swelling (white squares represent the mean of 24-hour swelling). The dashed line represents responses of a control group. The reciprocal relation between the antibody and cellular immunity responses is evident over almost the whole range of doses. Where antibody titers are high, the delayed hypersensitivity responses (footpad swelling) are low. The figure is reproduced from C. R. Parish and F. Y. Liew, *Journal of Experimental Medicine*, 135:298–311 (1972).

pletely. Yet its ability to evoke delayed hypersensitivity to unmodified flagellin had increased and continued to remain high, even when both its *in vitro* reactivity and immunogenicity were zero.

Other experiments showed that in rats previously immunized with flagellin and showing both delayed hypersensitivity and persisting antibody, adequately acetoacetylated flagellin failed to provoke a secondary rise in antibody but sharply increased the effectiveness of

cell-mediated immunity. It was also found that passive administration of antibody to flagellin one hour before injection of a standard immunizing dose could reduce the active antibody response to zero but accentuated the delayed hypersensitivity.

Parish's conclusion, based on a good deal more data than can be included here, may be only partially correct, but it provides an overall way of looking at immune unresponsiveness in terms of

IMMUNOCYTE	RESPONSE OF CELLS MAKING CONTACT WITH ANTIGENIC DETERMINANT (AD)			
	AD OF LOW ACTIVITY		AD OF HIGH ACTIVITY	
	T	B	T	B
T ONLY	ACTIVATION	—	LOSS OF RECEPTORS	—
B ONLY	—	NO EFFECT	—	ONLY A SMALL IgM RESPONSE
T AND B	ACTIVATION	ONLY A SMALL IgM RESPONSE	DEATH	PROLIFIC PRODUCTION OF IgM AND IgG

THE RECIPROCAL RELATION of T-cell and B-cell responses is shown in this table, based in part on the conclusions of C. R. Parish.

By hypothesis, IgM is capable of arming or educating neutral T cells with IgT receptors of the same specificity.

T and B cells that is attractive and at its own level not at variance with the facts. [See *lower figure on page 117.*] First, he finds evidence that T cells that function as (a) helpers in antibody production by B cells and (b) in delayed hypersensitivity to the same antigen are members of the same population, in part, at least. Second, he assumes by implication that T cells have an IgT receptor that is synthesized by the cells themselves. However, it does not seriously embarrass this hypothesis to consider the IgT to be of passive origin, synthesized in the early stage of the specific B-cell stimulation that does not require T-cell cooperation and that produces only IgM. As the work of Simon V. Hunt and Alan F. Williams points strongly toward the conclusion that all IgM on rat T cells is of passive origin, a passive origin of IgT seems preferable. However, once a T cell has its IgT receptor from whatever source, Parish's hypothesis would be unaltered and can be stated as follows.

When an antigenic determinant contacts the T- and B-cell receptors with adequate affinity and the cells are not adjacent, the T cell is stimulated to proliferate and produce functional delayed hypersensitivity and/or "helper" cells, and the B cell is rendered unresponsive. On the other hand, when reactive T and B cells are adjacent in the presence of an antigen with which both can react, the B cells are stimulated to proliferate and produce antibody and the T cells are rendered unresponsive.

IV

NONSPECIFIC ASPECTS
OF IMMUNITY

IV NONSPECIFIC ASPECTS OF IMMUNITY

INTRODUCTION

The mammalian immune system is intimately keyed in with virtually all the other functional systems of the body, some more visibly than others. In many ways it can be regarded as a system for the generation and transfer of information needed to allow cell proliferation, phagocytosis, and vascular adjustments appropriate to various emergency situations. With a little ingenuity one could probably take any anatomical region or functional system of the body and compose an article about its relation to immunity: "Bone marrow and immunity," and "Changes in immunity with age" are just two possible examples.

Three such articles are included in this section. None is primarily concerned with immunity but all deal with matters that are highly relevant to immunology and serve to illustrate the complexity and mutual interactions of the body's mechanisms. It is inevitable that when a scientist writes about his own field he will concentrate on those aspects that have concerned him as an experimenter, and his more general interpretations will be colored correspondingly. Indeed, the knowledge of immunology can be advanced by contributions of this sort. This makes it advisable to offer some introduction to the immunological aspects of the topics taken up in this section: the lymphatic system, lysosomes, and complement.

H. S. Mayerson's article on the lymphatic system deals essentially with its anatomy and its function as the body's drainage system, a system that mops up fluid that has leaked from the blood into the tissues and takes it back to the circulation. Physiologists view the lymphatic system also as a transport system that can handle any molecular or cellular materials in the tissues that need to be moved elsewhere. It is an indication of nature's economy of means to recognize that the lymph drainage system also transports fat from the intestines to the blood and provides the anatomical basis of the immune system. Incidental mention of what happens in the spleen, the lymph nodes, or the thymus—the other important organs of the mammalian immune system—will be found in other articles, but some additional guidance may be useful here in understanding the nature of the lymphatic system.

If foreign material enters the tissues, local inflammation will lead to an increased leakiness of the blood capillaries and the interstitial fluid will include not only some of the offending microorganisms and the liquid lymph filtering from the blood, but also lymphocytes and other cells. Lymphocytes and antigens pass into lymph capillaries and are carried to a regional lymph node which, from the point of view of the hydrodynamics of the lymph circulation, is simply a filter. The part played by the lymph nodes in trapping and making antigens ready to select appropriate T and B lymphocytes for proliferation is described in Nossal's article, "How Cells Make Antibodies," in Section I.

The distribution of the lymphocytes through the body is intensely dynamic. A T lymphocyte newly differentiated in the thymus passes into the blood; it adheres, by some mechanism as yet unclear, to the lining of specialized capillaries in a lymph node, and in a curious fashion it passes *through* the cytoplasm of the endothelial cells [*see the illustration on page 161*]. It comes to rest for a time in a special "thymus-dependent region," either in a lymph node or in an analogous region of one of the lymph follicles of the spleen. Subsequently it will move through a writhing mass of other lymphocytes till it reaches the efferent lymph vessels at the hilus of the node, to be carried by the lymph flow to the next node in the lymphatic system and eventually by the thoracic duct into the blood circulation. B lymphocytes behave in generally similar fashion but arise from the bone marrow, lodge and multiply in the lymph follicles and germinal centers of the lymph nodes, and settle down as plasma cells to secrete antibodies, largely in the medullary cords near the hilus of the node. The foregoing is a much-simplified outline, and under special circumstances various modifications of the standard circulation of lymphocytes will be observed.

Lysosomes, discovered by Christian de Duve and described in his 1963 article, have two main associations with immunity. In phagocytic cells like polymorphonuclear leucocytes and macrophages they play an important part in the ingestion and disposal of microorganisms and fragments of cell debris, the process being greatly facilitated if the material has been coated with antibodies. Lysosomes are normally quite inconspicuous in lymphocytes, but they are probably always present, just as they are in other mammalian cells.

It is generally held that when normal cell necrosis is extensive, as it is in the absorption of the tadpole's tail, which de Duve illustrates in his article, release of the potentially quite destructive mixture of hydrolytic enzymes in the lysosome sac plays the main part in the programmed death and autolysis of the cell. Necrosis in which cell nuclei are pyknotic is characteristic of all regions in which lymphoid cells are actively proliferating. It has been suggested that this may represent the elimination of newly differentiated cells that are reacting lethally to a "self" antigen; it is a reasonable possibility that activation of a T cell to liberate lymphokines and cytotoxic substances could, by involving damage to its own lysosomes, result in the T cell's own death and autolysis.

Complement has a very much closer relationship to classical immune reactions, as is fully discussed in Manfred M. Mayer's article. From many points of view the most important biological lesson about complement is that for decades it was thought of as a single enzyme-like substance, and on that basis the complement fixation tests were used with hundreds of different antigens as the most practically useful of all diagnostic tests for past infection. Subsequent analysis of its numerous components and recognition of the cascade-like character of their interaction has had only minimal influence on clinical serology or pathology, but it has had a salutary effect in establishing that an extraordinarily sophisticated elaboration of checks and counterchecks is needed when macromolecules interact in living substance.

It seems to be a general rule in experimental biology that whenever a conveniently manipulated biological assay is available—and hemolysis is probably the easiest of all of them—the complexity of the control and interaction of macromolecules will reveal itself. Complement is the classical example of this general rule. Blood coagulation and the control of capillary hemorrhage are other examples. In a very different field the genetic analysis of *Escherichia coli*, or bacteriophage T4, has revealed a similar complexity, which allowed decades of illuminating discovery with little indication that final answers were in sight.

Similarly, most of the important aspects of immunological research have reached only crude and tentative conclusions. Even though the chemical structure of several antibody molecules is now known in full detail, a solution of pattern diversification is still far off. Cellular immunology is an almost impossibly difficult experimental field, compared with the ones I just mentioned, and perhaps the real objective we should face is to learn how a sophisticated analysis of this extraordinary biological system can be achieved by considering the system as a whole rather than in terms of its molecules.

The Lymphatic System

by H. S. Mayerson
June 1963

*This second circulation plays an essential role in
maintaining the body's steady state, draining from
the spaces between cells fluid, protein and other
substances that leak out of the blood*

Living tissue is for the most part a collection of cells bathed in a fluid medium. This interstitial fluid constitutes what the French physiologist Claude Bernard named the *milieu intérieur:* the internal environment of the organism that is the true environment of its cells. The interstitial fluid brings nutrients to the cells and carries away waste products; its composition varies in space and time under the control of the co-ordinated physiological processes that maintain homeostasis, the remarkably steady state that characterizes the internal environment of a healthy organism. In the maintenance of the homeostasis of the interstitial fluid the circulation of the blood is obviously of fundamental importance. In the higher vertebrates there is a second circulation that is equally essential: the lymphatic system. Its primary function is to recirculate the interstitial fluid to the bloodstream, thereby helping to create a proper cellular environment and to maintain the constancy of the blood itself. It also serves as a transport system, conducting specialized substances from the cells that make them into the bloodstream. In recent years physiologists, biochemists, physicians and surgeons have been studying the lymphatic system intensively, in health and in disease. Their investigations are providing much new information on how the body functions, explaining some heretofore poorly understood clinical observations and even suggesting new forms of treatment.

The fact that the lymphatic system is an evolutionary newcomer encountered only in the higher vertebrates is significant. In lower animals there is no separation between the internal and external environments; all the cells of a jellyfish, for example, are bathed in sea water. With progression up the evolutionary scale the cells become separated from the external environment, "inside" is no longer identical with "outside" and rudimentary blood circulatory systems make their appearance to conduct the exchange of nutrients and waste products. As the organism becomes more complex the blood system becomes more specialized. The system develops increasing hydrostatic pressure until, in mammals, there is a closed, high-pressure system with conduits of diminishing thickness carrying blood to an extensive, branching bed of tiny capillaries.

At this point in evolution a snag was encountered: the high pressures made the capillaries leaky, with the result that fluid and other substances seeped out of the bloodstream. A drainage system was required and lymphatic vessels evolved (from the veins, judging by embryological evidence) to meet this need.

In man the lymphatic system is an extensive network of distensible vessels resembling the veins. It arises from a fine mesh of small, thin-walled lymph capillaries that branch through most of the soft tissue of the body. Through the walls of these blind-end capillaries the interstitial fluid diffuses to become lymph, a colorless or pale yellow liquid very similar in composition to the interstitial fluid and to plasma, the liquid component of the blood. The lymphatic capillaries converge to form larger vessels that receive tributaries along their length and join to become terminal ducts emptying into large veins in the lower part of the neck. The largest of these great lymphatics, the thoracic duct, drains the lower extremities and all the organs except the heart, the lungs and the upper part of the diaphragm; these are drained by the right lymphatic duct. Smaller cervical ducts collect fluid from each side of the head and neck. All but the largest lymph vessels are fragile and difficult to trace, following different courses in different individuals and even, over a period of time, in the same individual. The larger lymphatics, like large veins, are equipped with valves to prevent backflow.

Along the larger lymphatics are numerous lymph nodes, which are of fundamental importance in protecting the body against disease and the invasion of foreign matter. The lymph nodes serve, first of all, as filtering beds that remove particulate matter from the lymph before it enters the bloodstream; they contain white cells that can ingest and destroy foreign particles, bacteria and dead tissue cells. The nodes are, moreover, centers for the proliferation and storage of lymphocytes and other antibody-manufacturing cells produced in the thymus gland; when bacteria, viruses or antigenic molecules arrive at a lymph node, they stimulate such cells to make antibodies [see "The Thymus Gland," by Sir Macfarlane Burnet, beginning on page 88].

Starling's Hypothesis

The present view of the lymphatic circulation as a partner of the blood system in maintaining the fluid dynamics of the body stems from the investigations early in this century by the British physiologist Ernest H. Starling. "Starling's hypothesis" stated that the exchange of fluid between the capillaries and the interstitial space is governed by the relation between hydrostatic pressure and osmotic pressure. Blood at the arterial end of a capillary is still under a driving pressure equivalent to some 40 millimeters of mercury; this constitutes a "filtration pressure" that tends to make plasma seep out of the capillary. Starling visualized the wall of the capillary as being freely permeable to plasma and all its constituents except the plasma proteins albumin, globulin and fibrinogen, which could leak through only in very small amounts. The proteins remaining in the capillary exert an osmotic pressure that tends to keep fluid in the capillary, countering the filtration pressure. Similar forces are operative in the tissue spaces outside the capillary. At the arterial end of the capillary the resultant of all these forces is ordinarily a positive filtration pressure: water and salts leave the capillary. At the venous end, however, the blood pressure is decreased, energy having been dissipated in pushing the blood through the capillary. Now the osmotic force exerted by the proteins is dominant. The pressure gradient is reversed: fluid, salts and the waste products of cell metabolism flow into the bloodstream [see top illustration on page 127].

It follows, Starling observed, that if the concentration of plasma proteins is decreased (as it would be in starvation), the return of fluid to the bloodstream will be diminished and edema, an excessive accumulation of fluid in the tissue spaces, will result. Similarly, if the capillaries become too permeable to protein, the osmotic pressure of the plasma decreases and that of the tissue fluid increases, again causing edema. Capillary poisons such as snake venoms have this effect. Abnormally high venous pressures also promote edema, by making it difficult for fluid to return to the capillaries; this is often one of the factors operating in congestive heart disease.

A fundamental tenet of Starling's hypothesis was that not much protein leaves the blood capillary. In the 1930's the late Cecil K. Drinker of the Harvard Medical School challenged this idea. Numerous experiments led him to conclude "that the capillaries practically universally leak protein; that this protein does not re-enter the blood vessels unless delivered by the lymphatic system; that the filtrate from the blood capillaries to the tissue spaces contains water, salts and sugars in concentrations found in blood, together with serum globulin, serum albumin and fibrinogen in low concentrations, lower probably than that of tissue fluid or lymph; that water and salts are reabsorbed by blood vessels and protein enters the lymphatics together with water and salts in the concentrations existing in the tissue fluid at the moment of lymphatic entrance." In other words, Drinker believed that protein is continuously filtering out of the blood; the plasma-protein level is maintained only because the lymphatic system picks up protein and returns it to the bloodstream.

Unfortunately Drinker had no definitive method by which to prove that the protein in lymph had leaked out of the blood and was not somehow originating in the cells. Perhaps for this reason his conclusions were not generally accepted. Teachers and the writers of textbooks continued to maintain that "healthy" blood capillaries did not leak protein. It was in an effort to clarify this point that I undertook an investigation of lymph

TWO CIRCULATORY SYSTEMS, the blood and the lymphatic (color), are related in this schematic diagram. Oxygenated blood (light gray) is pumped by the heart through a network of capillaries, bringing oxygen and nutrients to the tissue cells. Venous blood (dark gray) returns to the heart and is oxygenated in the course of the pulmonary (lung) circulation. Fluid and other substances seep out of the blood capillaries into the tissue spaces and are returned to the bloodstream by the lymph capillaries and larger lymphatic vessels.

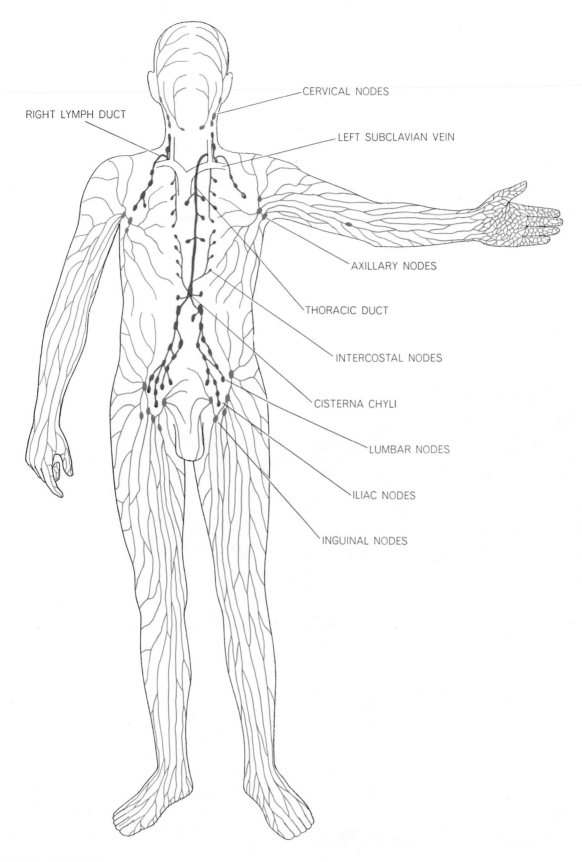

CERVICAL NODES

RIGHT LYMPH DUCT

LEFT SUBCLAVIAN VEIN

AXILLARY NODES

THORACIC DUCT

INTERCOSTAL NODES

CISTERNA CHYLI

LUMBAR NODES

ILIAC NODES

INGUINAL NODES

LYMPHATIC VESSELS drain the entire body, penetrating most of the tissues and carrying back to the bloodstream excess fluid from the intercellular spaces. This diagram shows only some of the larger superficial vessels (*light color*), which run near the surface of the body, and deep vessels (*dark color*), which drain the interior of the body and collect from the superficial vessels. The thoracic duct, which arises at the cisterna chyli in the abdomen, drains most of the body and empties into the left subclavian vein. The right lymph duct drains the heart, lungs, part of the diaphragm, the right upper part of the body and the right side of the head and neck, emptying into the right subclavian vein. Lymph nodes interspersed along the vessels trap foreign matter, including bacteria.

and the lymphatics some 15 years ago. At that time I was working with a clinical group measuring the retention of blood by patients given large infusions. We saw that the patients were retaining the cellular components of the blood quite well but were "losing" the plasma. The loss was clearly into the tissue spaces, not by way of excretion from the kidneys.

If blood capillaries did indeed leak plasma, together with its proteins and other large molecules, then Drinker was correct. If the proteins entered the interstitial fluid, they would stay there, since Starling's measurements and Drinker's findings made it clear that large molecules could not get back into the blood capillaries—unless they were picked up by the lymphatic system. If they leaked from the blood vessels and were in fact returned by the lymphatic vessels, the evolutionary reason for the development of the lymphatic system would be established beyond question. I decided to return to my laboratory at

the Tulane University School of Medicine and investigate the problem.

Over the years I have had the enthusiastic assistance of several colleagues—notably Karlman Wasserman, now at the Stanford University Medical School, and Stephen J. LeBrie—and of many students. Time had provided us with two tools not available to Drinker. One was flexible plastic tubing of small diameter, which we could insert into lymphatic vessels much more effectively than had been possible with the glass tubing available earlier. And we now had radioactive isotopes with which to label proteins and follow their course.

Experiments with Proteins

We injected the blood proteins albumin and globulin, to which we had coupled radioactive iodine atoms, into the femoral veins of anesthetized dogs. The proteins immediately began to leave the bloodstream. By calculating the slope of the disappearance curve in each ex-

periment we could arrive at a number expressing the rate of disappearance [see top illustration on page 128]. The average rate of disappearance of albumin, for example, turned out to be about .001; in other words, a thousandth of the total amount of labeled albumin present at any given time was leaking out of the capillaries each minute. If we infused large amounts of salt solution, plasma or whole blood into our dogs, the disappearance rate increased significantly. The same thing happened in animals subjected to severe hemorrhage. In some experiments we simultaneously collected and analyzed lymph from the thoracic duct [see bottom illustration on page 128]. As before, labeled protein left the blood; within a few minutes after injection it appeared in the lymph, at first in small quantities and then at a faster rate. It leveled off, in equilibrium with the blood's protein, seven to 13 hours after injection.

We were able to calculate from our data that in dogs the thoracic duct alone

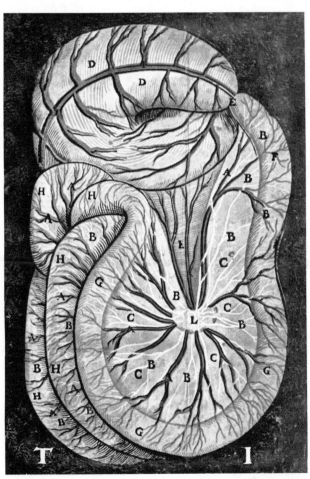

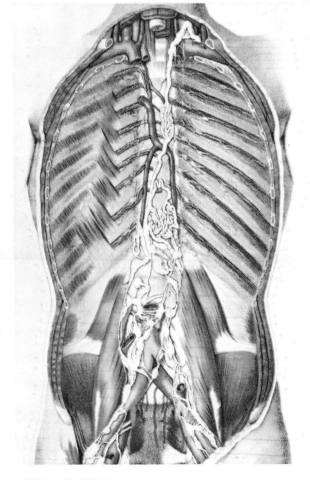

LACTEALS, the lymphatics of the intestine, were first described by the Italian anatomist Gasparo Aselli in 1622. They were pictured in his *De Lactibus*, the first anatomical work with color plates. This plate shows veins (*A*), lacteals (*B*), mesentery (*C*), stomach (*D*), small intestine (*F, G, H*) and a lymph node (*L*).

THORACIC DUCT and the major lymph vessels of the lower extremities and trunk that contribute to it are seen in this plate from a French book of 1847, *Atlas d'Anatomie Descriptive du Corps Humain*. The duct arises from a plexus of abdominal vessels and arches up into the lower neck before entering the subclavian vein.

returned about 65 per cent of the protein that leaked out of the capillaries. Extension of this kind of experiment to man showed similar rates of leakage. In the course of a day 50 per cent or more of the total amount of protein circulating in the blood is lost from the capillaries and is returned to the bloodstream by the lymphatic system.

The importance of lymphatic drainage of protein becomes clear if one considers its role in lung function, which was elucidated by Drinker. The pulmonary circulation, in contrast to the general circulation, is a low-pressure system. The pulmonary capillary pressure is about a quarter as high as the systemic capillary pressure and the filtration pressure in the pulmonary capillaries is therefore considerably below the osmotic pressure of the blood proteins. As a result fluid is retained in the bloodstream and the lung tissue remains properly "dry."

When pulmonary capillary pressure rises significantly, there is increased fluid and protein leakage and therefore increased lymph flow. For a time the lymph drainage is adequate and the lungs remain relatively dry. But when the leakage exceeds the capacity of the lymphatics to drain away excess fluid and protein, the insidious condition pulmonary edema develops. The excessive accumulation of fluid makes it more difficult for the blood to take up oxygen. The lack of oxygen increases the permeability of the pulmonary capillaries, and this leads to greater loss of protein in a vicious circle. Some recent findings by John J. Sampson and his colleagues at the San Francisco Medical Center of the University of California support this concept. They found that a gradual increase in lymphatic drainage occurs in dogs in which high pulmonary blood pressure is produced and maintained experimentally. This suggests that the lymphatic system attempts to cope with the abnormal situation by proliferating, much as blood capillaries do when coronary circulation is impaired.

Leakage from blood capillaries and recirculation by the lymphatic system is, as I indicated earlier, not limited to protein. Any large molecule can leak out of the capillaries, and it cannot get back to the bloodstream except via the lymphatics. All the plasma lipids, or fatty substances, have been identified in thoracic-duct lymph. Even chylomicrons, particles of emulsified fat as large as a micron (a thousandth of a millimeter) in diameter that are found in blood during the digestion of fat, leak out of the bloodstream and are picked

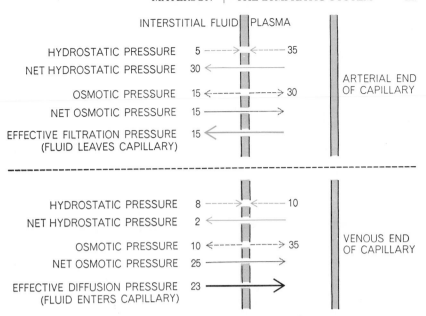

STARLING'S HYPOTHESIS explained the exchange of fluid through the capillary wall. At the arterial end of the capillary the hydrostatic pressure (*given here in centimeters of water*) delivered by the heart is dominant, and fluid leaves the capillary. At the venous end the osmotic pressure of the proteins in the plasma dominates; fluid enters the capillary.

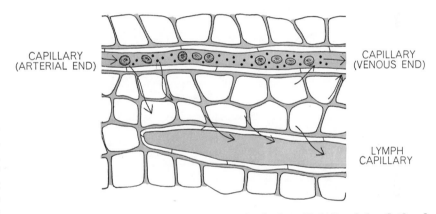

FLUID EXCHANGE is diagramed as postulated by Starling. He believed that fluid and salts (*arrows*) left the blood capillaries, mixed with the interstitial fluid and for the most part were reabsorbed by the capillaries. Excess fluid was drained by the lymph vessels. He took it for granted that most of the protein in the blood stayed inside the blood capillaries.

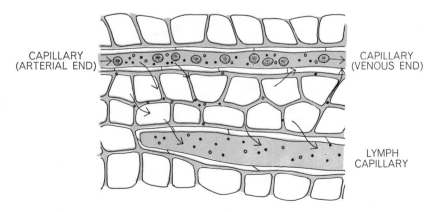

PRESENT VIEW of fluid exchange is diagramed. It appears that such large molecules as proteins (*black dots*) and lipids (*open circles*) leave the blood capillaries along with the fluid and salts. Some of the fluid and salts are reabsorbed; the excess, along with large molecules that cannot re-enter the blood capillaries, is returned via the lymphatic system.

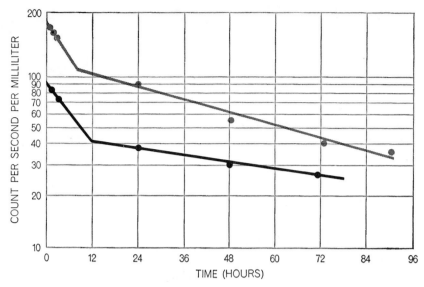

LABELED PROTEINS were injected into dogs' veins. Measuring the radioactivity per milliliter of blood withdrawn from an artery showed how quickly the globulin (*gray*) and albumin (*black*) disappeared. The steep slopes represent disappearance, the shallow slopes subsequent metabolism of the proteins. The radioactivity is plotted on a logarithmic scale.

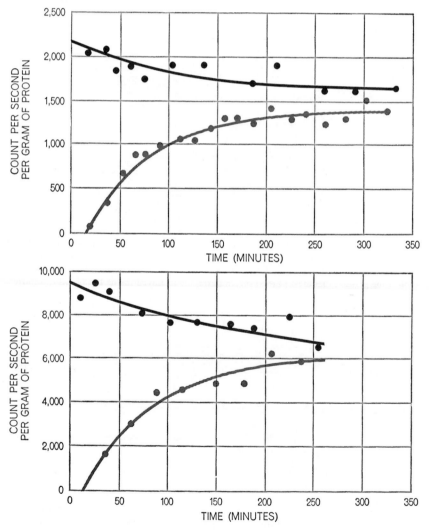

PROTEIN appeared in thoracic-duct lymph (*gray curves*) and increased in the lymph as it disappeared from the blood (*black curves*). The upper graph is for albumin, the lower one for globulin. In time the labeled protein in blood and lymph reached equilibrium.

up and recirculated to the vascular system by the lymphatics. As a matter of fact, there is evidence that they may leak out even faster than proteins. The significance of these findings remains to be explained. Aaron Kellner of the Cornell University Medical College has suggested that atherosclerosis, a form of hardening of the arteries in which there is infiltration of the walls of the arteries by lipids, may have its origin in the fact that under normal conditions there is a constant flow of fluid containing lipids and proteins across the blood-vessel lining into the vessel wall. Ordinarily this fluid is removed by the small blood vessels of the wall itself and by the lymphatics. It is conceivable that something may interfere with the removal of lipids and cause them to accumulate in the blood-vessel wall. It is even conceivable that the high capillary filtration that accompanies hypertension may increase the leakage of lipids from capillaries to a level exceeding their rate of removal from the interstitial fluid, which would then bathe even the outer surfaces of the arteries in lipids.

In addition to demonstrating that the lymph returns large molecules from the tissue spaces to the bloodstream, recent investigation has confirmed the importance of lymphatic drainage of excess fluid filtered out of the capillaries but not reabsorbed. Experiments with heavy water show that blood is unquestionably the chief source of the water of lymph. In dogs the amount of lymph returned to the bloodstream via the thoracic duct alone in 24 hours is roughly equivalent to the volume of the blood plasma. Most of this fluid apparently comes from the blood. In some of our experiments we drained the thoracic-duct lymph outside the dog's body and found that the plasma volume dropped about 20 per cent in eight hours and the plasma-protein level some 16 per cent. Translated to a 24-hour basis, the loss would be equivalent to about 60 per cent of the plasma volume and almost half of the total plasma proteins circulating in the blood. Thus the return of lymph plays an essential role in maintaining the blood volume.

One situation in which this function can be observed is the "lymphagogue" effect: the tendency of large infusions into the vascular system to increase the flow of lymph. As we increased the size of infusions in dogs, lymph flow increased proportionately; with large infusions (2,000 milliliters, about the normal blood volume of a large dog) the thoracic-duct lymph flow reached a peak value about 14 times greater than that

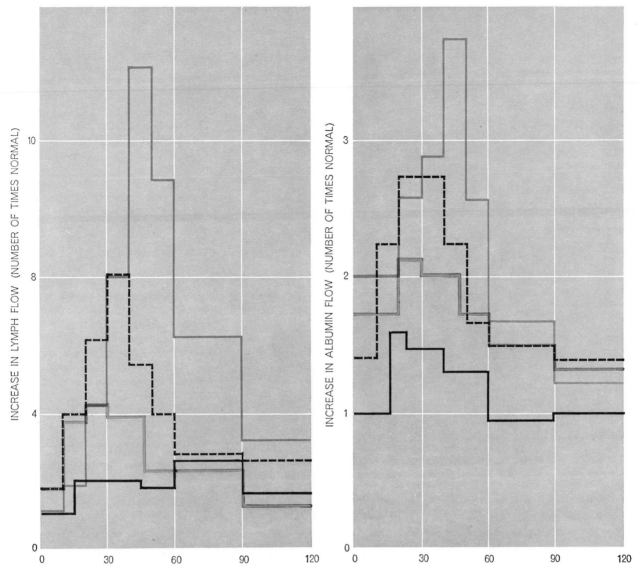

EFFECT OF INFUSIONS on lymph flow (*graph at left*) and on albumin flow in lymph (*graph at right*) in dogs is illustrated. Each curve shows the ratio of the flow after an infusion of a given size to the flow before the infusion. The curves are for infusions of 250 (*solid black*), 500 (*gray*), 1,000 (*broken black*) and 2,000 (*colored*) milliliters. The larger the infusion, the more leakage.

of the preinfusion level [*see illustration above*]. Most of the excess fluid is excreted by the kidneys in increased urine flow. But the displacement of fluid from the blood circulation into the lymph "saves" some of the fluid. In other words, it can be considered as being a fine adjustment of the blood volume so that not all the fluid is irrevocably lost from the body. Large infusions also increase protein leakage, but again the fact that the protein goes to the lymph and slowly returns to the bloodstream minimizes changes in total circulating protein and the loss of its osmotic effect.

The Mechanism of Filtration

The exact processes or sites of the filtration of large molecules through the capillary wall, and through cell membranes in general, are still unclear. As Arthur K. Solomon has pointed out in these pages [see "Pores in the Cell Membrane," by Arthur K. Solomon; SCIENTIFIC AMERICAN Offprint 76], "some materials pass directly through the fabric of the membrane, either by dissolving in the membrane or by interacting chemically with its substance. But it seems equally certain that a large part of the traffic travels via holes in the wall. These are not necessarily fixed canals; as the living membrane responds to changing conditions inside or outside the cell, some pores may open and others may seal up."

This last point appears to explain our results with infusions in dogs. The massive infusions overfill the closed blood system, raise filtration pressure in the capillaries and result in increased leakage through the capillary walls; lymph flow is copious and the lymph contains more large molecules. Small infusions do not do this. The reason, then, that patients did not do as well as expected after receiving large infusions or transfusions was that the plasma and proteins leaked out through stretched capillary pores. A similar effect accounted for the case of animals subjected to severe hemorrhage: there was not enough blood to oxygenate the capillary walls adequately, the walls became more permeable and the protein molecules passed through.

We found that the rate of leakage for any molecule depends on its size. Globulin, which has a molecular weight of

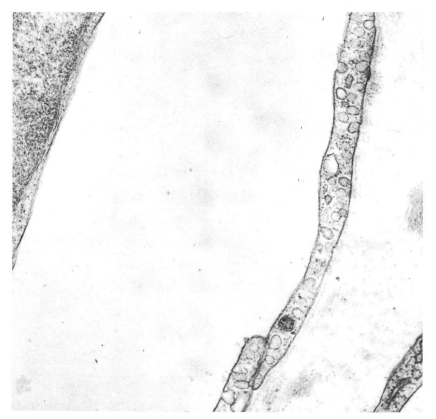

LYMPH CAPILLARY (*lightest area*) of mouse arterial tissue is enlarged 30,000 diameters in this electron micrograph made by Johannes A. G. Rhodin of the New York University School of Medicine. At upper left is part of the nucleus of an endothelial cell of the vessel wall. The thin ends of two other cells overlap near the bottom. The faint shadow in the connective tissue outside the wall is a slight indication of a basement membrane.

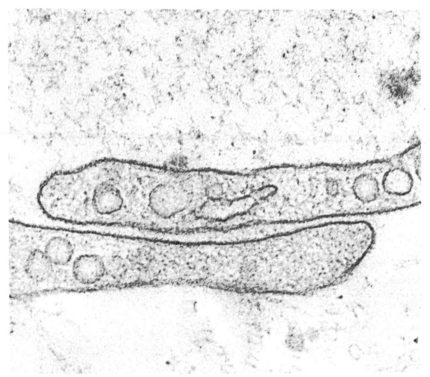

"LOOSE JUNCTION" between the overlapping ends of two endothelial cells of a vessel wall is seen in this electron micrograph, also made by Rhodin, of a lymphatic in mouse intestinal tissue. The lymph vessel is at the top, connective tissue at the bottom. In this case there is no sign of a basement membrane outside the wall. The enlargement is 90,000 diameters.

250,000, leaked more slowly than albumin, which has a weight of 70,000. The third plasma protein, fibrinogen, has a molecular weight of about 450,000 and leaves the blood still more slowly. By introducing into the blood various carbohydrate molecules, which unlike protein molecules do not carry a charge, we were able to demonstrate that it is size and not electrical charge that determines a molecule's rate of movement through the wall.

When, after infusing the carbohydrates, we collected lymph from different parts of the body, we found larger molecules in intestinal lymph than in leg lymph, and still larger molecules in lymph from the liver. This indicated that capillaries in the liver have substantially larger openings than leg capillaries do, and that the vessels of the intestine probably have both large and small openings. There are other indications that liver capillaries are the most permeable of all; for example, apparently both red cells and lymphocytes pass between the blood and the lymph in the liver. Recent studies with the electron microscope confirm the indirect evidence for variations in the size of capillary openings; the structure of the capillaries seems to vary with the organ, and these differences may be related to differences in function.

Transport by the Lymph

When Gasparo Aselli first described lymphatic vessels in 1622, the ones he noted were the lacteals: small vessels that drain the intestinal wall. The dog Aselli was dissecting had eaten recently; the lacteals had absorbed fat from the intestine, which gave them a milky-white appearance and made them far more visible than other lymphatics. The transport of certain fats from the intestine to the bloodstream by way of the thoracic duct is one of the lymphatic system's major functions. Studies in which fatty acids have been labeled with radioactive carbon show that the blood capillaries of the intestine absorb short-chain fatty acid molecules directly, together with most other digested substances, and pass them on to the liver for metabolism. But the lacteal vessels absorb the long-chain fats, such as stearic and palmitic acids, and carry them to the bloodstream via the thoracic duct. The lymphatic system is also the main route by which cholesterol, the principal steroid found in tissues, makes its way into the blood.

Since the lymphatics are interposed between tissue cells and the blood sys-

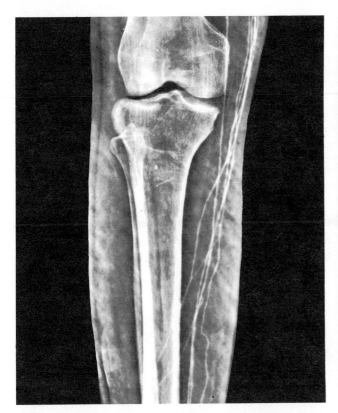 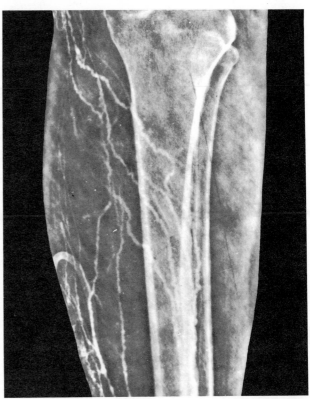

LYMPHANGIOGRAM is an X-ray photograph in which the lymphatic vessels are made visible by injecting into them a radiopaque dye. In the normal leg (*left*) the vessels are straight and well defined. In lymphedema (*right*) there is insufficient drainage of fluid and proteins, in this case because there were too few vessels in the thigh. The extra pressure on the lower-leg vessels increased their number and made them tortuous. These pictures were made by Carl A. Smith of the New York University School of Medicine.

tem it is not surprising to find that they serve as the channel for transport to the bloodstream of substances that originate in tissue cells. The lymph is probably the route by which at least some hormones, many of which are very large molecules, are carried to the blood from the endocrine glands where they are synthesized. Some enzymes, found in lymph in small concentrations, may merely have leaked out of the capillaries. But others are apparently picked up from their cells of origin and carried to the blood by the lymph. Certain enzymes, including histaminase and renin, are present in greater concentrations in lymph than in the blood. The finding on renin, reported by A. F. Lever and W. S. Peart of St. Mary's Hospital Medical School in London, is of particular interest to investigators working on the problem of hypertension. One concept ascribes high blood pressure in some individuals to the production of renin by a kidney suffering from inadequate blood circulation; the renin is thought to combine with a globulin in the plasma to form hypertensin, an enzyme that narrows the arterioles and results in high blood pressure. It has been difficult to establish this concept because no one has been able consistently to demonstrate the presence of renin in the blood of hypertensive patients. Now that it has been discovered in lymph coming from the kidney it is clear that renin is indeed being formed in these patients, although in amounts so small that it usually escapes detection after being diluted in the blood.

Recently Samuel N. Kolmen of the University of Texas Medical Branch in Galveston has provided what may be a confirmation of the renin concept. He produced hypertension in dogs by removing one kidney and partially constricting the artery supplying the other one. When he shunted the thoracic-duct flow into the dog's gullet or allowed it to escape, the hypertension diminished. The implication is that renin was being kept out of the bloodstream. When Kolmen stopped lymph flow in the shunt, presumably inhibiting the diversion of the renin, the hypertension returned.

The Lymphatic Circulation

To the investigators of the 19th century the lymphatic system was "open-mouthed": its capillaries were assumed to be open to the tissue spaces. More recent evidence has shown that the lymphatics form a closed system, that fluid enters not through the open ends of vessels but through their walls. The walls of the terminal lymph capillaries, like those of blood capillaries, consist of a single layer of platelike endothelial cells. This layer continues into the larger vessels as a lining but acquires outer layers of connective tissue, elastic fibers and muscle. Although the capillaries of the blood and lymphatic systems are structurally very similar, recent electron micrographs show differences in detail that may help to explain the ease with which the lymph vessels take up large molecules. Sir Howard Florey of the University of Oxford and J. R. Casley-Smith of the University of Adelaide in Australia believe that the most important difference is the poor development or absence in lymph capillaries of "adhesion plates," structures that hold together the endothelial cells of the blood capillaries. They suggest that as a result there are open junctions between adjacent cells in lymph capillaries that allow large molecules to pass through the walls. Johannes A. G. Rhodin of the New York University School of Medicine puts more emphasis on the apparent absence or poor development in lymph capillaries of the "basement membrane" that surrounds blood capillaries.

Certainly it is clear that very large particles do enter the lymphatic vessels: proteins, chylomicrons, lymphocytes and red cells—the last of which can be as much as nine microns in diameter. Bacteria, plastic spheres, graphite particles and other objects have been shown to penetrate the lymphatics with no apparent difficulty. Yet we have found that when we introduce substances directly into the lymphatic system, anything with a molecular weight greater than 2,000 is retained almost completely within the lymphatics, reaching the blood only by way of the thoracic duct. If large particles can get into the lymphatic vessels, why do substances with a molecular weight of 2,000 not get out by the same channels?

I have spent many hours trying to formulate an answer to this question without arriving at a sophisticated concept, and have had to be content with a simple explanation that is at least consistent with the current evidence. Assume that the smallest terminal lymphatics are freely permeable to small and large molecules and particles moving in either direction through intercellular gaps. Compression of these vessels in any way would tend to force their contents in all directions. At least some of the contents would be forced along into the larger lymph vessels, where the presence of valves would prevent backflow. And once the lymph reaches a larger vessel it can no longer lose its large particles through the thick and relatively impermeable wall of the lymphatic.

One can argue that this seems to be a rather inefficient and even casual way of getting the job done. Indeed it is, and this physiological casualness is a characteristic of the lymphatic system as a whole. There is no heart to push the lymph, and although lymphatic vessels do contract and dilate like veins and arteries this activity does not seem to be an important factor in lymph movement. The flow of lymph depends almost entirely on forces external to the system: rhythmic contraction of the intestines, changes in pressure in the chest in the course of breathing and particularly the mechanical squeezing of the lymphatics by contraction of the muscles through which they course.

Lymphatic Malfunction

In spite of the casualness of the lymphatic system, its development, as I have tried to show, was an absolute necessity for highly organized animals. Its importance is most visibly demonstrated in various forms of lymphedema, a swelling of one or more of the extremities due to the lack of lymphatic vessels or to their malfunction. In some individuals the lymphatic system fails to develop normally at birth, causing gradual swelling of the affected part. Lymphangiographic studies, in which the vessels are injected with radiopaque dyes to make them visible in X-ray photographs, show that the lymphatics are scarce, malformed or dilated. Insufficient drainage causes water and protein to accumulate in the tissues and accounts for the severe and often disabling edema. There is evidence that genetic factors may play a role in this

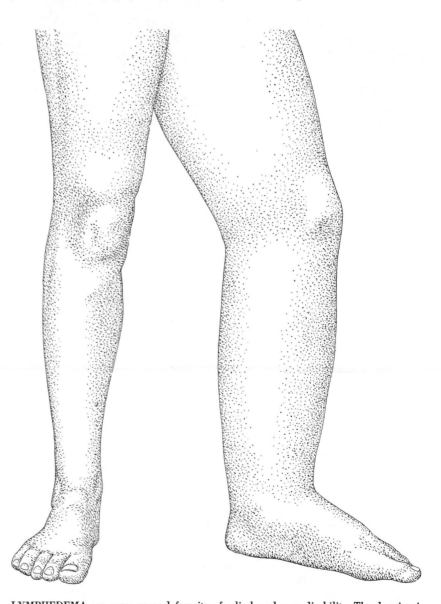

condition. Surgical procedures that destroy lymph vessels may have a similar effect in a local area. Elephantiasis is a specific form of lymphedema resulting from the obstruction of the vessels. It can be caused by infection of the lymphatics or by infestation with a parasitic worm that invades and blocks the vessels.

The lymphedemas have been recognized as such for many years. Recently the view that the lymphatic system is essential to homeostasis—which is to say "good health"—has led to a number of investigations of its role in conditions in which no lymphatic involvement was previously suspected. Our group at Tulane has found that lymphatic drainage of the kidneys is essential in order to maintain the precise osmotic relations

LYMPHEDEMA can cause gross deformity of a limb and even disability. The drawing is based on a photograph of an 11-year-old girl whose leg began to swell at the age of seven, probably because of an insufficiency of lymphatic vessels. The patient's condition was greatly improved by an operation in which the tissue between skin and muscles was removed.

on which proper kidney function depends. This may explain the dilution of the urine observed in some patients after kidney operations: the lymph vessels may have been damaged, decreasing their capacity for draining proteins and interfering with the reabsorption of water by the kidney tubules.

At the New York University School of Medicine, John H. Mulholland and Allan E. Dumont have been investigating the relation between thoracic-duct flow and cirrhosis of the liver. Their results suggest that the cirrhosis may be associated with increased lymph flow in the liver and that the inability of the thoracic duct to handle the flow may bring on the accumulation of fluid, local high blood pressure and venous bleeding that are frequently seen in cirrhosis patients; drainage of the duct outside the body temporarily relieves the symptoms.

These and other clinical observations are consistent with my feeling that the lymphatic system does a capable job when all is going well but that its capacity for dealing with disturbances is limited. As a phylogenetic late-comer it may simply not have evolved to the point of being able to cope with abnormal stresses and strains. The role of the second circulation in disease states is currently under intensive investigation. As more and more is learned about its primary functions and its reactions to stress, the new knowledge should be helpful in diagnosis and perhaps eventually in the treatment of patients.

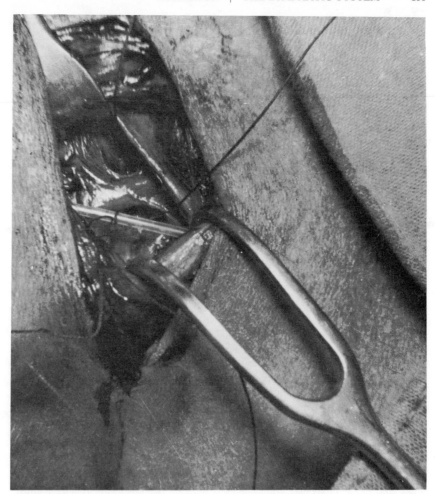

DILATED THORACIC DUCT of a patient with cirrhosis is seen in this photograph made by Allan E. Dumont and John H. Mulholland of the New York University School of Medicine and reprinted from *Annals of Surgery*. The plastic tube just below the duct is a tenth of an inch in diameter. A normal duct would be smaller than the tube.

13

The Lysosome

by Christian de Duve
May 1963

*This small particle acts as the digestive tract of the
living cell. Its enzymes dissolve the substances ingested
by the cell and under certain circumstances can
dissolve the cell itself*

The study of the living cell has in recent years established an increasingly complete catalogue of its working parts and identified these with their functions. The new understanding has come from a collaborative effort of, on the one hand, the cell anatomist, whose electron micrographs portray the internal structures of the cell in almost molecular detail, and, on the other, the biochemist, who disrupts and fractionates the cell so that he can observe the activity of the cellular organelles and their molecular components in isolation from one another. This concurrent study of structure and function has shown, for example, that the organelles called mitochondria conduct the primary energy transformations of the cell and that the smaller organelles called ribosomes are the centers of enzyme manufacture. The latest addition to the list of organelles is the lysosomes. They serve a function more comprehensible in terms of the grosser life processes of multicelled organisms. The lysosomes are tiny bags filled with a droplet of a powerful digestive juice capable of breaking down most of the constituents of living matter, much as these constituents are fragmented in the gastrointestinal tract of higher animals. In point of fact, the lysosomes function in many ways as the digestive system of the cell.

First identified in rat liver cells in 1955, lysosomes are now known to occur in many—possibly in all—animal cells. (It remains to be shown if they are present in plant cells.) It is significant that they are particularly large and abundant in cells, such as the macrophages and the white blood cells, that are called on to perform especially important digestive tasks. Lysosome function and malfunction appear to be in-

volved in such vital processes as the fertilization of the egg and the aging of cells and tissues and in certain diseases. Challenging questions are presented by the properties of the membrane of the lysosome, which enable the organelle to contain enzymes that, on liberation, are capable of digesting the entire cell. Indeed, the death and dissolution of the cell following rupture of the membrane may play a part in the developmental processes of some animals and in a number of degenerative phenomena. This suggests the possibility that cell "autolysis" might be deliberately promoted or retarded for therapeutic purposes by the use of substances affecting the stability of the lysosome membrane.

Although lysosomes are frequently above the lower limit of visibility in the light microscope and are well within the range of the electron microscope, they were not discovered by optical methods. They were undoubtedly seen many times, but their nature and function were not recognized until they had been characterized chemically. The first clue was provided by a chance observation in our laboratory at the Catholic University of Louvain in 1949.

We had just begun to use the then newly developed technique of centrifugal fractionation, in which cells are disrupted in a homogenizer and then spun in a centrifuge at successively higher speeds to yield a number of fractions containing organelles of different types. When isolated in this manner, the organelles still maintain many of their functional properties, which can then be explored by means of biochemical methods. Our object was to localize in such fractions certain enzymes involved in the metabolism of carbohydrates in the liver of the rat and thereby to determine

with which cellular structures these enzymes are associated. The standard procedure in this work is first to assay the homogenate of the disrupted cells for the presence of a given enzyme and then to look for the activity of the enzyme in the fractions. Among the enzymes included in our routines was the enzyme called acid phosphatase. This enzyme, which splits off inorganic phosphate from a variety of phosphate esters, is not directly connected with carbohydrate metabolism. We included it largely for control purposes.

To our surprise the acid-phosphatase activity in the homogenate was only about a tenth of what we had come to expect from previous assays of preparations that had been subjected to the more drastic homogenizing action of a Waring Blendor. The total of the activities found in the fractions, about twice that observed in the homogenate, was still only a fifth of the expected value. When the assays were repeated five days later on the same fractions (they had been kept in the icebox), the enzyme activity was much greater in all the particulate fractions, especially in the fraction containing mitochondria. The total activity was now within the expected range.

Fortunately we resisted the temptation to discard the first series of results as being due to some technical error, and a few additional experiments quickly gave us the clue to the mystery. In living cells the enzyme is largely or entirely confined within little baglike particles; the surface membrane of these particles is able not only to retain the enzyme inside the particle but also to resist the penetration of the small molecules of phosphate esters used in the assay. What we measured in our assays was only the amount of enzyme that

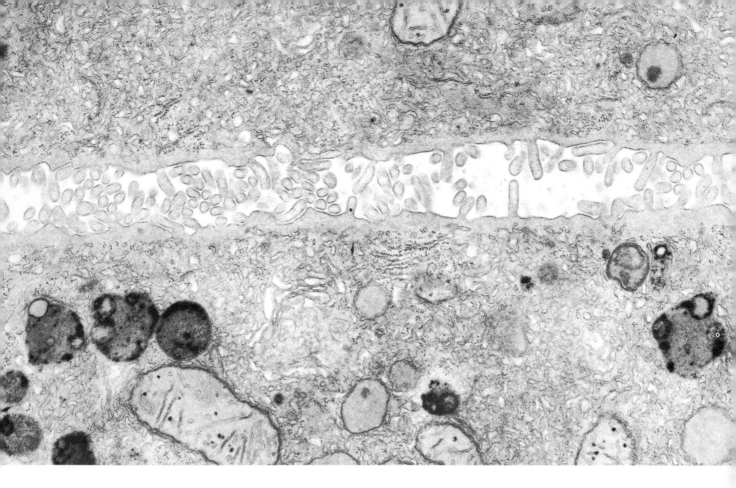

LYSOSOMES appear as relatively large dark objects in the electron micrograph above, which shows parts of two rat liver cells separated by a bile canaliculus. The canaliculus is the light strip running horizontally through the micrograph; the protuberances in the canaliculus are microvilli. The oblong body near the six lysosomes at bottom left is a mitochondrion. The micrograph was made at the Rockefeller Institute by Henri Beaufay of the Catholic University of Louvain. The magnification is 26,000 diameters.

TWO TYPES OF LYSOSOMES in a nephrotic rat kidney cell are magnified 60,000 diameters in the electron micrograph below: the kidney-shaped "digestive vacuole" at upper right and the two round "residual bodies" near the center and at lower left. Layered structures in the latter are "myelin figures," probably consisting of undigested fats. Minute black areas in the lysosomes are lead phosphate precipitated in staining. The micrograph was made by Alex B. Novikoff of the Albert Einstein School of Medicine.

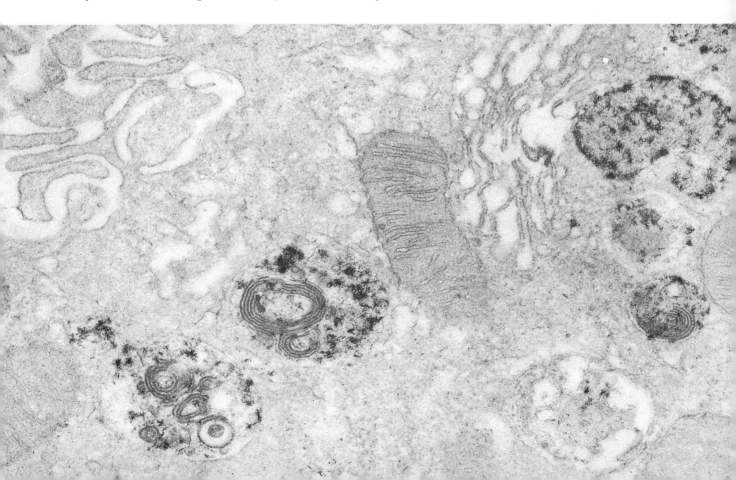

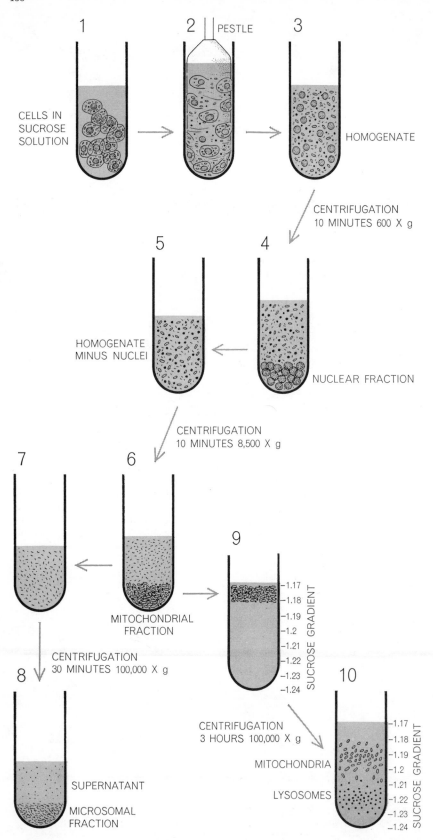

1 CELLS IN SUCROSE SOLUTION

2 PESTLE

3 HOMOGENATE

CENTRIFUGATION 10 MINUTES 600 X g

5 HOMOGENATE MINUS NUCLEI

4 NUCLEAR FRACTION

CENTRIFUGATION 10 MINUTES 8,500 X g

7

6 MITOCHONDRIAL FRACTION

9

−1.17 −1.18 −1.19 −1.2 −1.21 −1.22 −1.23 −1.24 SUCROSE GRADIENT

CENTRIFUGATION 30 MINUTES 100,000 X g

8 SUPERNATANT MICROSOMAL FRACTION

CENTRIFUGATION 3 HOURS 100,000 X g

10

MITOCHONDRIA

LYSOSOMES

−1.17 −1.18 −1.19 −1.2 −1.21 −1.22 −1.23 −1.24 SUCROSE GRADIENT

CENTRIFUGAL FRACTIONATION separates cells into fractions containing various cell components. Rapid mechanical rotation of the pestle ruptures the cells, setting the intracellular particles free in the medium. Successive centrifugations of the resulting homogenate produce fractions in which certain cell particles predominate. Steps *1* through *8* represent a method developed by W. C. Schneider of the National Institutes of Health. Steps *9* and *10* show a modification developed by the author and his co-workers; the mitochondrial fraction (*Step 6*) is sedimented by centrifugation for 10 minutes at 25,000 times gravity. Numbers associated with the sucrose gradient give density in grams per cubic centimeter.

either was free in the cell or had escaped from particles injured by our manipulations. Whereas the Waring Blendor disrupts essentially all the particles, the gentler homogenizing procedure we had been using in our fractionation work ruptured only about 10 per cent of the particles, thus accounting for the low result obtained in the original homogenate. Further fractionation released an additional 10 per cent of the total activity from the fractions; the remainder came out as a result of the aging of the particles for five days in the refrigerator.

When these observations were transposed to the living cell, they suggested an interesting means of control of the enzyme activity. Living cells contain numerous phosphate esters of great importance to cellular function. Most of these phosphate compounds can be broken down by acid phosphatase, and investigators had often wondered why this breakdown does not occur in cells where the enzyme is present in large amounts. It now appeared from our results that the protective agent preventing the enzyme from acting indiscriminately on all the compounds might be simply the particle membrane that segregated the enzyme from the rest of the cell. This possibility, opened up by chance, was so interesting that we decided to make it the primary objective of our work.

At first it was believed that the particles containing acid phosphatase were the mitochondria, but later experiments indicated that they formed a distinct group, different from both the mitochondria and the microsomes on which most biochemists had been working. It took several years to establish the identity of the new particles as a separate group. In the meantime the list of enzymes contained within them began to grow. The number now stands at more than a dozen. In common with acid phosphatase, each new enzyme has demonstrated its ability to split important biological compounds in a slightly acid medium. Ultimately all the major classes of biologically active compounds, including proteins, nucleic acids and polysaccharides, were shown to be susceptible to action by the enzymes contained in these particles. As the spectrum of activity broadened, we became the more impressed with the significance of the new particles and of their surrounding membrane. Considered as a group, the enzymes present in the particles could have but one function: a lytic, or digestive, one. Hence the name "lysosome" (meaning lytic body) that

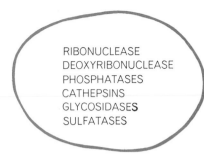
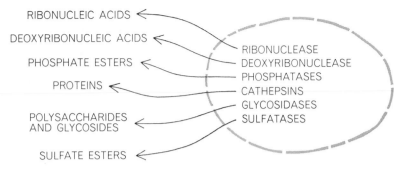

RIBONUCLEASE
DEOXYRIBONUCLEASE
PHOSPHATASES
CATHEPSINS
GLYCOSIDAS**E**S
SULFATASES

RIBONUCLEIC ACIDS

DEOXYRIBONUCLEIC ACIDS

PHOSPHATE ESTERS

PROTEINS

POLYSACCHARIDES
AND GLYCOSIDES

SULFATE ESTERS

RIBONUCLEASE
DEOXYRIBONUCLEASE
PHOSPHATASES
CATHEPSINS
GLYCOSIDASES
SULFATASES

LYSOSOME

INJURED LYSOSOME

LYSOSOME CONCEPT developed by the author is that of a minute "bag" filled with powerful digestive enzymes. So long as the lysosome membrane remains intact, digestion of the substrates on which these enzymes act is confined within the lysosome. But when the membrane is ruptured, the enzymes leak out and digestion takes place externally, often resulting in digestion of the cell.

we gave to the particles. As for the membrane, it must act as a shield between this powerful digestive juice and the rest of the cell. The digestive processes, we deduced, must be confined within the limits of the membrane, and the substances to be digested must somehow be taken up in the particles. Conversely, we were alerted to look for those pathological or normal conditions that might lead to the release of the enzymes inside the cell and the dissolution of the cell.

It was not until 1955 that the electron microscope made its contribution to the identification of the lysosomes. Working in collaboration with Alex B. Novikoff of the Albert Einstein College of Medicine in New York, we obtained our first electron micrographs of cell fractions containing partially purified lysosomes. In addition to known particles, mostly mitochondria, the pictures showed large numbers of characteristic bodies that had occasionally been observed in intact liver cells and that had been named "pericanalicular dense bodies." Their function was quite unknown; their name signified only their preferential location in cells along the bile canaliculi—the smaller bile ducts—and their high electron density, or opacity to the beam of the electron microscope. The identification of the lysosome activity with the dense bodies, made provisionally at that time, has since been confirmed by a variety of techniques.

We hoped that the identification of the liver lysosomes would lead quickly to the recognition of the lysosomes in other cells—much as the characteristic structure of the mitochondrion makes it

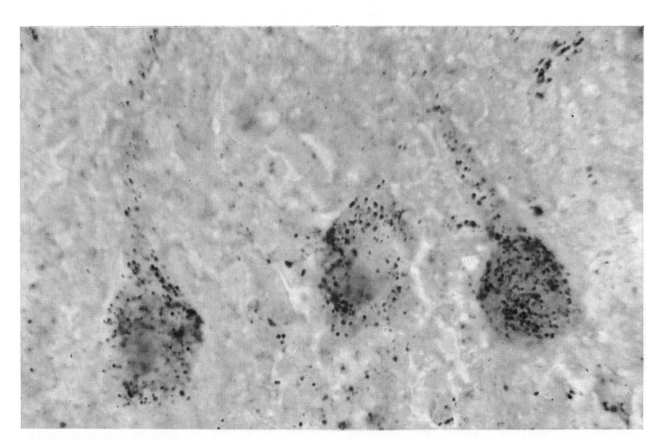

PURKINJE CELLS in the cerebellum of the pigeon contain lysosomes, which appear as tiny dark brown dots. Most of the lysosomes are located in the body of the three cells seen here. Single dendritic processes extending upward from the neurons at left and right also contain a few lysosomes. The magnification of this micrograph, which was made by Novikoff, is 1,600 diameters.

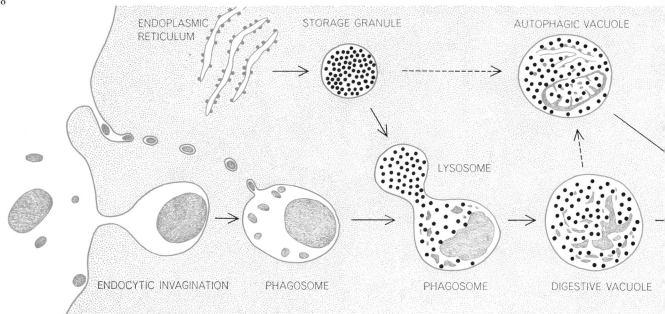

ENDOPLASMIC RETICULUM   STORAGE GRANULE   AUTOPHAGIC VACUOLE

LYSOSOME

ENDOCYTIC INVAGINATION   PHAGOSOME   PHAGOSOME   DIGESTIVE VACUOLE

INTRACELLULAR DIGESTION involves lysosomes in various ways. It is necessary to distinguish four kinds of lysosomes: "storage granules," digestive vacuoles, residual bodies and "autophagic vacuoles." The first three are directly involved in the main digestive process. The storage granule is the original form of the lysosome; enzymes in the granule presumably are produced by the ribosomes (*small colored dots*) associated with the endoplasmic reticulum, but the origin of the lysosome membrane is unknown. When the cell ingests substances by endocytic invagination, a phagosome, or food vacuole, is formed. Several phagosomes may fuse together, forming a single vacuole. A storage granule or other lysosome fuses with the phagosome to form a digestive vacuole. Digestion products diffuse through the membrane into the cell. The digestive vacuole can continue its digestive activity, gradually

readily distinguishable in any type of cell. In this we were disappointed. The lysosomes come in a bewildering assortment of shapes and sizes, even in a single type of cell; they cannot be identified solely on the basis of their appearance. In the continuing study of lyso-

somes, therefore, the cell physiologist or biochemist has had to continue to provide the leads for the cell anatomist and the electron microscopist.

This polymorphism of the lysosomes is now perfectly understandable: their digestive activity causes them to be

filled with a variety of substances and objects in an advanced state of disintegration, and it is their contents that determine their shape, size, density and so on. Nonetheless, the lack of any reliable visual criteria has tended to slow the progress of work in this field. The

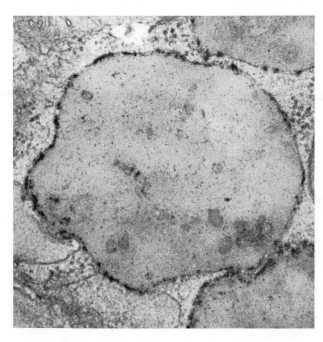

LYSOSOME is magnified 63,000 diameters. Gomori staining precipitated lead phosphate along lysosome membrane. The micrographs on these two pages, all of mouse kidney cells, were made at the Rockefeller Institute by Fritz Miller of the University of Munich.

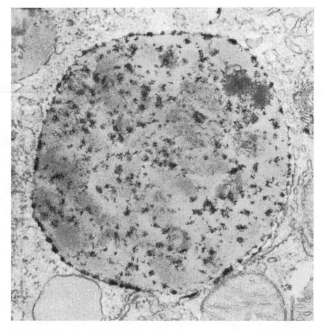

DIGESTIVE VACUOLE from kidney cell of mouse injected four hours earlier with hemoglobin is magnified 41,000 diameters. Lead phosphate appears along the membrane and in the interior. Dark gray patches are hemoglobin in the process of being digested.

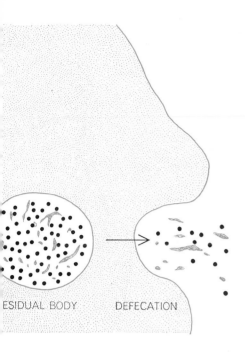

ESIDUAL BODY   DEFECATION

accumulating indigestible material until it becomes a residual body, which may then be eliminated by fusion with the cell membrane. **The distinguishing feature of the autophagic vacuole is the material digested: parts of the cell itself, such as mitochondria and portions of the endoplasmic reticulum.**

approach used on liver cells has been followed successfully in several other tissues, but it is a laborious one, usually requiring a great deal of repetitive work before one obtains fractions sufficiently pure for electron-microscope studies.

Fortunately one of the lysosomal enzymes—the same acid phosphatase that led to the discovery of the lysosomes —lends itself to visual identification. It can be stained by a method first developed by the late George Gomori of the University of Chicago. A slice of tissue is incubated with a compound susceptible to the action of the enzyme and with lead ions present in solution; at the sites where inorganic phosphate is set free by the action of the phosphatase, the phosphate precipitates in the form of an insoluble lead compound. Because lead has a high electron density the compound plainly shows up in electron micrographs; for visualization in the light microscope the compound is converted to black lead sulfide. Thus the enzyme can be localized inside the cell by means of a precipitated product of its activity. This technique, particularly in the hands of Novikoff, has greatly facilitated the study of lysosomes and their function in numerous tissues in both normal and pathological states.

Not all the substances that nurture a cell require digestion by lysosomes. In higher animals tissue cells receive most of their nutrients from the bloodstream in the form of small molecules absorbed through the cell membrane and requiring no digestion in the cell. Some materials, however, are too bulky for direct absorption and too complex chemically for immediate utilization. Objects of this kind must first be "eaten" and digested. Cells are able to engulf large molecules and even bodies as big as bacteria or other cells by a process now generally referred to as "endocytosis." A portion of the cell membrane first attaches itself to the "prey" and then appears to be sucked inward to form a small internal pocket containing the prey. The pocket pinches free from the cell membrane and drifts off into the cell interior, now forming a phagosome, as such bodies have been called by Werner Straus of the University of North Carolina.

The details of the next step vary from one type of cell to another, but they appear in all cases to involve the same fundamental mechanism. The phagosome containing the material to be digested and a lysosome containing the digestive enzymes approach each other; upon contact their membranes fuse to form a single larger vacuole. Digestion then proceeds within the membrane and the products of digestion diffuse into the cytoplasm, leaving behind only such remnants as have proved refractory to attack by the enzymes. Now that the outlines of the process are understood, lysosomes can be recognized in various cells at various stages in the performance of their function, from storage granules for newly synthesized enzymes to digestive vacuoles formed by fusion with a phagosome and finally to bodies containing the residue of previous digestive events.

In some cells, such as the amoeba and other protozoa, the residual bodies are

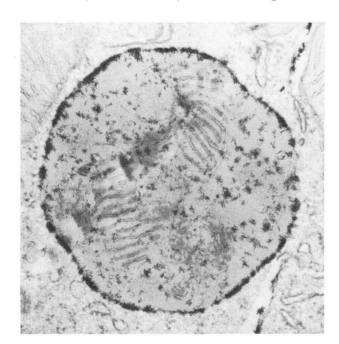

AUTOPHAGIC VACUOLE contains remnants of mitochondria from its host cell. The remnants appear as pairs of lines. "Needles" of lead phosphate were precipitated by the action of acid phosphatase, a lysosomal enzyme. The magnification is 55,000 diameters.

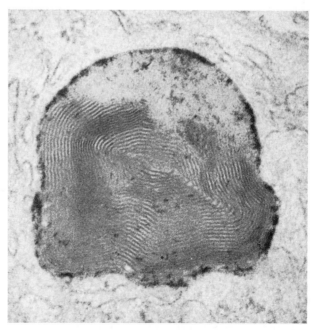

RESIDUAL BODY containing a layered collection of undigested material is enlarged 76,000 diameters. Lead phosphate is deposited mainly at membrane. The first, third and fourth micrographs on these two pages are published by permission of Academic Press.

eliminated by a kind of endocytosis in reverse, called defecation. In other cells, such as liver cells, defecation is slower or absent; the same digestive vacuoles are engaged repeatedly or continuously in digestive activity. After a time they seem to become charged with increasing amounts of residues, and this accumulation is believed to play a part in the aging of such cells.

As James G. Hirsch and Zanvil A. Cohn of the Rockefeller Institute have brought out, the cellular eating and digestive processes assume their most dramatic form in the white blood cells. These cells seem to spend most of their short life preparing for a single big burst of this activity. It has long been known that at the time the white blood cell enters the bloodstream it is filled with large granules; Hirsch and Cohn have shown that the granules are packages of digestive enzymes fitting the specifications of lysosomes. When the

white cell engulfs a particle such as a bacterium, the granules can be seen to disappear one after the other, discharging their contents into the vacuole containing the ingested particle. Eventually the cells lose all their granules and are filled instead with one or more digestive pockets within which foreign particles are in process of dissolution. The cells seem not to recover from this process and eventually die.

This cycle of events in the cell matches at each point—ingestion, digestion and defecation—the process by which higher animals gain their nutrition. Digestion in both cases takes place behind a resistant envelope that protects the rest of the organism from attack by the digestive juices. In higher animals the resistant envelope forms a canal open at both ends; in most cells it surrounds a number of individual pockets. These are able to mix their con-

tents and also to exchange matter with their environment by processes of coalescence reminiscent of the fusion of soap bubbles. Smaller pockets are also seen to pinch off from bigger ones, but the envelope always remains impermeably sealed around each pocket. One can easily imagine how a more permanent and continuous tract might, under some circumstances, evolve from such a flexible and relatively haphazard system. A primitive alimentary canal is indeed found in some single-celled organisms.

There is evidence that some cells may discharge lysosomal enzymes externally and use them to destroy surrounding structures or to open access for themselves. It is possible that the osteoclasts—bone-destroying cells that, along with bone-building osteoblasts, are responsible for the continuous remodeling of bone tissue—gnaw their way into the bone by a mechanism of this sort. They then complete their destructive action by engulfing bone fragments and digesting them in their lysosomes. It has also been suggested that in the process of fertilization spermatozoa may depend on the release of lysosomal enzymes to dissolve some of the structures that surround the egg cell. Subsequent changes in the egg seem in turn to involve the release of enzymes from the cortical granules that cover the outer surface of the cell. As a result the outer layers of the cell are broken down; a new membrane resistant to such attack is built up underneath, and the metabolism of the egg is geared toward division and development. According to Jean Brachet of the Free University of Brussels the cortical granules may belong to the lysosome family. They can also be ruptured by injury such as the prick of a needle; hence the digestive action of these bodies may have something to do with parthenogenesis: fertilization in which no sperm enters the egg.

The death of cells, even when it occurs on a large scale, is not necessarily a disastrous event in the life of a complex organism. Many of the component cells of the animal body are short-lived; they die and are replaced by newly formed cells. This is particularly true of the blood cells and of those cells that form the outer layers of the skin and of the mucous-membrane surfaces of the body. Cell death even plays a role in the early molding of the embryo and in the developmental cycle of some animals. As first shown by Rudolph Weber of the University of Berne and recently confirmed and elaborated by Yves Eeckhout in our laboratory at Louvain, when

REGRESSION OF TADPOLE TAIL, in metamorphosis of the South African frog *Xenopus laevis* into an adult, is accomplished by lysosomal digestion of cells. As metamorphosis proceeds the enzyme concentration increases (the absolute amount of enzyme remaining constant). Eventually the stub contains almost nothing but lysosomal enzymes, and it falls off. Data shown here were obtained by Rudolph Weber of the University of Berne.

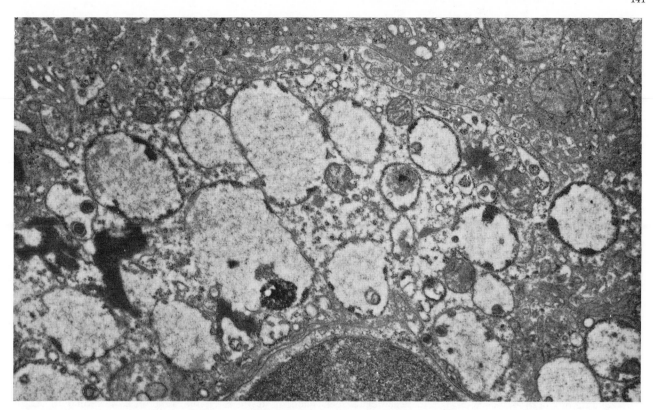

FORCED FEEDING of Kupffer cells from rat liver was achieved by injecting rats with Triton WR-1339, a detergent. The lysosomes become engorged with the detergent because they cannot digest it. Triton WR-1339 is transparent to electrons; hence the lysosomes, magnified 19,600 diameters, appear as light gray amorphous areas bounded by single membranes. The dark gray area at bottom center is a cell nucleus. The micrograph was made by Pierre Baudhuin and Robert Wattiaux of the Catholic University of Louvain.

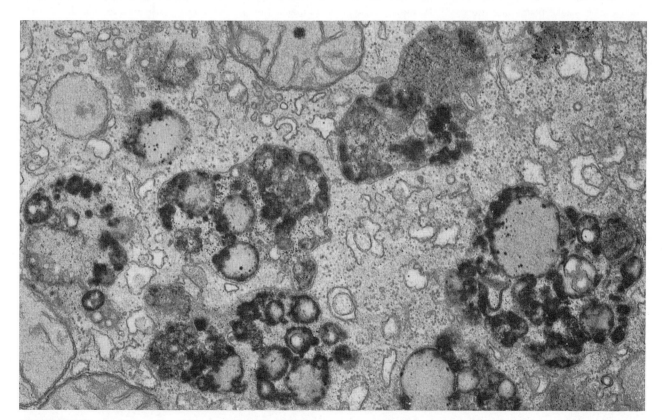

STARVATION caused a number of lysosomes in this cell from a rat liver to become autophagic vacuoles. That is, parts of the host cell (e.g., mitochondria) have found their way into the lysosomes. The mechanism that thus enables the cell to feed on its own substance without damaging itself irreparably is not known. The lysosomes are not stained; they appear as amorphous collections of objects of varying sizes, shapes and shades. The magnification of this micrograph, which was made by Beaufay, is about 38,000 diameters.

a tadpole tail has been reduced to an almost invisible stub, it still contains practically all its original complement of lysosomal enzymes and little else.

Lysosomal enzymes play their role in these processes in three different modes. In the first, white cells and other scavenger cells invariably invade the areas where cell destruction occurs: the lysosomes are there engaged through their normal digestive function inside the cell. A second mode, which has been discovered only recently, can be called cellular "autophagy": portions of a cell somehow find their way inside the cell's own lysosomes and are broken down. How the self-engulfment of the cell fragments takes place is not known. During starvation this process apparently enables the cell to use part of its own substance for fuel and for the renewal of essential constituents without doing itself irreparable damage. As in normal endocytosis, autophagy is kept localized by the limiting membrane.

The third mode of action involves the actual rupture of the lysosome membrane inside the cell and the digestion of the latter as a whole by the released enzymes. It can be described as a perforation of the cellular digestive tract. Such ruptures take place fairly quickly in dead cells, in a manner that recalls the rapid post-mortem putrefaction of the digestive mucosae in higher animals. It is obvious that once repair mechanisms are interrupted the areas most sensitive to dissolution will be those immediately adjacent to destructive enzymes. In the normal life processes of multicellular organisms lysosome rupture following

death of a cell may have some value as a built-in mechanism for the self-removal of dead cells.

Of considerably greater interest is the possibility that the autodissolution of cells may occur as a pathological process. Present evidence indicates that the lysosome membranes may rupture in cells suddenly deprived of oxygen or exposed to cell poisons of certain kinds. As the enzymes are released they attack the cell itself, and they may also diffuse into the surrounding medium, damaging extracellular structures. Honor B. Fell and her co-workers at the University of Cambridge have shown that this is what happens in the cartilage and bones of animals receiving excess vitamin A. Damage by lysosomal enzymes released from the cells apparently explains the spontaneous fractures and other lesions that attend vitamin A intoxication.

Lysosomes can be involved in cell pathology in still other ways. Cells that are forced to engulf large amounts of foreign substances for the digestion of which they are not equipped will tend to accumulate such material in their lysosomes, possibly to the detriment of their general health. Plasma substitutes, such as dextran or polyvinyl pyrrolidone, have been known to cause this condition. It could also be involved in silicosis, the disease that results from the inhalation of silica dust; the particles of silica may accumulate in the lysosomes. Normal substances might accumulate in the same way if a key digestive enzyme is lacking in the lysosomes as a result, let us say, of a genetic abnormality. H. G. Hers of our department at Louvain recently discovered such a deficiency in the tissues

of children who had died of a particularly severe form of glycogen-storage disease; he found that a lysosomal enzyme that attacks glycogen was missing.

If lysosomes can indeed act as "suicide bags"—and we now have good reason to believe that they can and sometimes do act in that way—the question arises as to whether or not their rupture can be influenced by means of drugs. Two possibilities come to mind. Agents acting as stabilizers of the lysosome membrane could be used to protect cells in a critical condition. Or substances that weaken the membrane could be employed to get rid of undesirable cells (for example cancer cells) if their action were sufficiently selective and specific.

So far no conscious attempt has been made to influence lysosomes in either way. But substances of both kinds are already known and some were used therapeutically before their effects on lysosomes were discovered. Vitamin A, in excess, has already been mentioned; although it is not highly specific, it appears to act preferentially on connective-tissue structures. According to recent studies performed by Lewis Thomas and Gerald Weissmann of the New York University School of Medicine, working in collaboration with the Fell group at Cambridge, cortisone and hydrocortisone appear to have a stabilizing influence on the lysosome membrane. This property may account, at least partly, for the well-known anti-inflammatory effects of these drugs. It would seem that in the individual cell, as in the multicellular organism, the digestive system occupies a pivotal position both in physiology and in pathology.

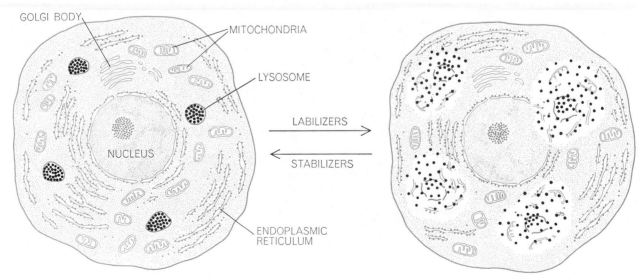

"SUICIDE BAG" is the term coined by the author to describe a lysosome that releases its complement of enzymes within a normal cell. The result is autolysis, or cell death by dissolution. It has been found that some substances affect the stability of the lysosome membrane adversely, thereby increasing the occurrence of autolysis. Other substances are known to have a stabilizing effect.

The Complement System

by Manfred M. Mayer
November 1973

A foreign cell in the body is identified by antibody,
but the cell is destroyed by other agents. Among them
is "complement," an intricately linked set of enzymes

Immunology is the study of the physiological mechanisms by which men and other animals defend themselves against microscopic invaders such as bacteria, viruses and fungi. The immunological defenses also operate against the malignant transformations of cells that result in cancer and against transplanted foreign tissues or organs. Some immunological phenomena are cellular, in that they involve lymphocytes (cells that mediate immunological reactions) and phagocytes (cells that ingest foreign particles and microorganisms or other cells). Other immunological reactions are humoral, in that they involve substances dissolved in the body fluids, such as antibodies and enzymes. Cellular and humoral phenomena can influence each other. For example, the engulfing of foreign particles by phagocytes is promoted by antibodies.

The role of antibodies is well known [see "The Structure of Antibodies," by R. R. Porter, the article beginning on page 31, and "The Structure and Function of Antibodies," by Gerald M. Edelman, the article beginning on page 39]. Less well known is another important feature of the immune system: attack by complement. The term "complement" refers to a complex group of enzymes in normal blood serum that, working together with antibodies or other factors, plays an important role as a mediator of both immune and allergic reactions. The reactions in which complement participates take place in blood serum or in other body fluids and hence are considered to be humoral reactions.

The discovery of complement came between 1880 and 1890 from studies of the capacity of blood serum to kill certain microorganisms. Antibodies had been discovered a short time earlier, but it was found that their capacity to kill bacteria depended on the collaboration of another constituent of serum: "alexin," or complement. The names were intended to indicate that the agent helps antibody to perform its defensive function. As knowledge of complement has unfolded in the intervening 85 years, it has become evident that the relation between antibody and complement is actually the reverse of what it was originally thought to be. It is now recognized that the invading cells are attacked by complement and that the function of antibody is to identify the invading cell as a foreign organism and activate the complement attack.

Antibody and Complement

The relation between antibody and complement resembles the relation between the ignition key of an automobile and the engine. An antibody molecule has sites that combine with a specific pattern on the surface of a foreign cell or with another molecule: an antigen. The fit between the antigen molecule and the antibody molecule is the fit between the ignition key and the ignition lock. The antibody molecule serves to start the complement system, which, like the automobile engine, does the actual work. The analogy can be carried further: Whereas antibody molecules and keys are relatively simple structures, the complement system and the automobile engine are complex assemblies of many different parts.

When complement is activated by antibody, it presents a serious threat not only to invading microorganisms but also to the host's own cells. This self-destructive activity is minimized by the fact that antibody fixes complement on the surface of the invading cell. Thus antibody has three specific functions with respect to complement: (1) recognition of the foreign invader, (2) activation of the complement system and (3) fixation of complement on the invading cell's surface.

The complement system also must fulfill three requirements. It must have a recognition unit of its own so that it can respond to the antibody molecules that have detected a foreign invader. It must have receptor sites that will enable it to combine with the surface of the foreign cell when it is activated. And in order to minimize damage to the host's own cells its activity must be limited in time. This limitation is accomplished partly by the spontaneous decay of activated complement and partly by interference from inhibitors and destructive enzymes. The control of complement, however, is not perfect, and there are times when damage is done to the host's cells. Immunity is therefore a double-edged sword. When an immune system acts against a foreign microorganism, the result is protection; when it acts against the host's own cells, the result is the disruption of body systems. Such disruptions are what are known as allergic or hypersensitive reactions.

The Complement Proteins

There are 11 proteins in the complement system. The complement proteins are designated by the letter C and by number: C1, C2, C3 and so on up to C9. The complement protein C1 is actually an assembly of subunits designated C1q, C1r and C1s. From the studies of Irwin H. Lepow of the University of Connecticut Health Center it is known that the subunits are held together by bonds other than the usual covalent ones, and that the calcium ion Ca^{++} is needed to keep the assembly intact. If the calcium ion is removed by chelating agents, the subunits disassemble. The entire assembly is believed to consist of one molecule of subunit C1q, two molecules of C1r and four molecules of C1s.

The numbers assigned to the complement proteins reflect the sequence in which they become active, with the exception of complement protein C4, which reacts after C1 and before C2. (The numerical assignments were made before the reaction sequence was fully understood.) The recognition of each of the 11 proteins has been achieved through the intensive efforts of many investigators, notably Robert A. Nelson, Jr., of the Lady Davis Institute for Medical Research in Montreal, Kusuya Nishioka of the National Cancer Center Research Institute in Tokyo and William Dean Linscott of the University of California San Francisco Medical Center.

The complement proteins have been isolated in purified form. The concentration of each in human blood serum, along with its molecular weight and electrophoretic mobility, has been determined, largely through the efforts of Hans Müller-Eberhard and his colleagues at the Scripps Clinic and Research Foundation in La Jolla, Calif. [*see illustration below*]. So far little work has been done on the chemical structure of the complement proteins except for the studies of C1q undertaken by Robert M. Stroud of the University of Alabama Medical School and by Müller-Eberhard. These studies reveal that the C1q molecule contains the unusual amino acids hydroxyl lysine and hydroxyl proline. It also contains a large amount of glycine and substantial quantities of carbohydrate (mostly galactose and glucose),

which suggests that it is similar in chemical composition to collagen, the principal protein of connective tissue. In explaining the respective functions of the 11 proteins in the complement system, it is convenient to divide the discussion into three parts: recognition, enzymatic activation and the attack by complement factors that results in destruction of the cell.

Recognition

The recognition unit of the complement system is the C1q molecule. It has the capacity to combine with a segment of the immunoglobulin antibody molecules that bind to antigen molecules. This binding of complement to antibody is the basis of the complement-

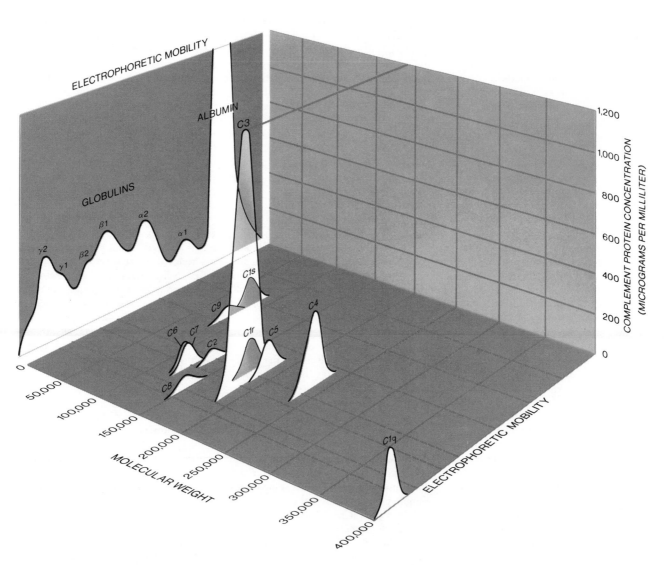

HUMAN COMPLEMENT PROTEINS are characterized by their molecular weight, their electrophoretic mobility (at pH 8.6) and their concentration in blood serum. The C3 protein, which has a molecular weight of about 180,000, is the commonest complement protein; its concentration is about 1,200 micrograms per milliliter. The concentrations of the other complement proteins are much lower. For the purpose of comparison the electrophoretic pattern of globulins (gamma, beta and alpha) and albumin in blood plasma are shown. This illustration is adapted from one prepared by Hans Müller-Eberhard of the Scripps Clinic and Research Foundation.

fixation test that has long been used for medical diagnosis (for example in the diagnosis of syphilis).

Only immunoglobulin M (IgM) and several subclasses of immunoglobulin G (IgG) are able to bind the complement factor C1. IgM is a gamma globulin of high molecular weight that appears in the early stages of infection or immunological challenge; IgG has a lower molecular weight but accounts for about 70 percent of the immunoglobulin in normal human blood serum. Other gamma globulins (for example IgA, which is found in saliva and external secretions, and IgE, which is largely responsible for allergic reactions) do not fix C1. Tibor Borsos and Herbert J. Rapp of the National Cancer Institute have shown that in the case of IgM a single molecule of antibody on the surface of a cell is able to bind C1, but that in the case of IgG two adjacent molecules are required for such binding. Since antibodies are scattered more or less at random over the cell surface, the probability of two IgG molecules occupying adjacent sites is quite small, and the frequency with which IgG binds C1 is low. For example, it has been estimated that with the red blood cells of the sheep as many as 800 IgG molecules per cell are needed to create one receptor site for the complement factor C1. On the other hand, only one molecule of IgM per cell is needed.

Antibody molecules change in shape when they combine with antigen, and this event may be responsible for the conversion of the complement factor C1 from an inactive enzyme into an active one. The active site of the enzyme is on the C$\overline{1s}$ subunit (the bar designates activation). It has been suggested that the C1r subunit plays the role of an intermediate agent between C1q and C1s in the activation process. The recognition by Louis Pillemer and Lepow, and by Elmer L. Becker and Lawrence Levine, that C$\overline{1s}$ is an enzyme, and my own subsequent discovery that its enzymatic action cleaves the complement factor C2, opened the way to an understanding of the enzymatic reactions responsible for complement's attack on cells.

Enzymatic Activation

The second stage involves the complement factors C4, C2 and C3. Their activation is initiated by the enzyme C$\overline{1s}$, and eventually they combine to form another enzyme. The assembly of this enzyme begins with the cleavage of C4 by C$\overline{1s}$ into a large fragment, C4b, and a small fragment, C4a. The C4b

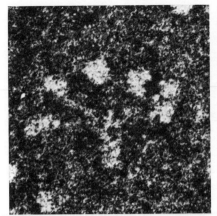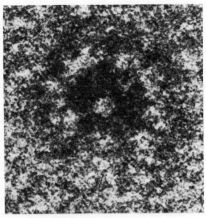

MOLECULE OF COMPLEMENT SUBUNIT C1q is enlarged some 1.2 million diameters in these two electron micrographs, which were provided by Emma Shelton of the National Cancer Institute. The molecule of the subunit consists of three distinct parts: a central part, connecting strands and terminal units. The strands (which are possibly single polypeptides, that is, chains of amino acid units) that join the six terminal units to the central stalk can be seen in the "side" view of the molecule (*micrograph at left*). The "top" view (*micrograph at right*) shows the radial arrangement of the terminal units around the central part.

fragment has an active site that can combine with a receptor on the surface of the cell's membrane, but this binding site has a short life, and only a small proportion of the C4b fragments that are formed become bound. The unbound C4b fragments quickly become inactive and remain in the blood serum. Many molecules of C4 are cleaved by a single C$\overline{1s}$ enzyme, producing a shower of C4b fragments. Only those fragments that become bound to the cell, however, participate in the subsequent reactions. Little is known about the C4a fragment and its fate or about the receptors on the cell that bind the C4b fragment.

The next step, which has been intensively studied in my laboratory at the Johns Hopkins University School of Medicine, involves the adsorption of the complement protein C2 to the cell-bound C4b. This adsorption is promoted by magnesium salts. Following adsorption the C2 molecule is cleaved by a neighboring C$\overline{1s}$ enzyme into two large fragments, one of which, C2a, becomes bound to C4b. Müller-Eberhard has demonstrated that the C$\overline{4b,2a}$ complex is an enzyme. Nothing is known as yet about the receptor on the C4b fragment that binds C2a.

The complement protein C3 is a natural substrate for the C$\overline{4b,2a}$ enzyme. When they combine, the enzyme splits C3 into two fragments. One fragment, C3a, with a molecular weight of about 10,000, is released into the fluid phase and plays a role as a mediator of inflammation; the other, C3b, with a molecular weight of about 175,000, becomes bound to a receptor on the cell's surface. Since the C$\overline{4b,2a}$ complex combination

is an enzyme, it can react more than once and produce a shower of C3b fragments. Only the C3b fragments that become bound adjacent to the C$\overline{4b,2a}$ enzyme, however, are believed to participate in the next reaction, in which the complement protein C5 is cleaved. The C3b fragments that become bound to other sites on the cell surface play an important role as promoters of phagocytosis.

As Hyun S. Shin of Johns Hopkins has shown, the binding of a C3b fragment in the immediate vicinity of the C$\overline{4b,2a}$ enzyme creates a new enzyme that has the capacity to cleave C5. At this point it should be made clear that as the complement proteins are enzymatically cleaved a binding site on the activated complement component is exposed. Because the binding sites have a short life, however, reactivity is soon lost and the complement component disappears as a functional unit. Another matter of importance concerns the instability of the intermediate enzymatic complexes. For example, it has been shown in my laboratory that the C$\overline{4b,2a}$ enzyme is quite stable at zero degrees Celsius, its half-life being about 10 hours. At 37 degrees C. its half-life is only about eight minutes. It loses its activity because the C2a fragment, which contributes the active enzymatic site, migrates into the fluid phase and becomes inactive. The C2a fragment is also released from the C$\overline{4b,2a,3b}$ enzyme. These decay processes may be regarded as one of the factors that limit the ability of the complement system to attack the host's cells.

In the first step of the attack on a cell the complement factor C5 is activated through cleavage by the C$\overline{4b,2a,3b}$ enzyme. The C5a fragment, with a molecular weight of about 15,000, drifts off into the fluid phase, and eventually plays a role as a mediator of inflammation. The larger fragment, C5b, with a molecular weight of about 170,000, may remain on the C$\overline{4b,2a,3b}$ enzyme as it combines with the complement proteins C6 and C7, or it may form a complex only with C6 before it dissociates from the enzyme and combines with C7 in the fluid phase. After the C$\overline{5b,6,7}$ complex is formed, it binds to the cell membrane.

It is believed that the C$\overline{4b,2a,3b}$ enzyme is freed after the dissociation of the C5b,6,7 complex, and that it may then activate another molecule of C5. Direct experimental evidence demonstrating this capacity, however, has not yet emerged. Moreover, although it is be-

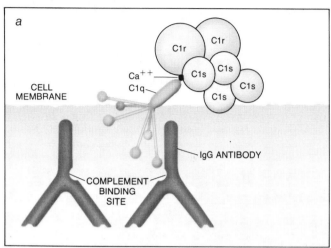

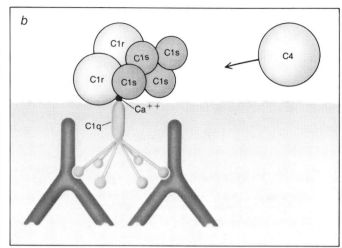

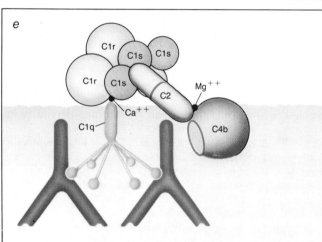

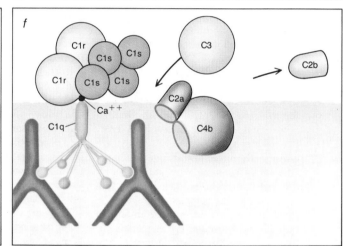

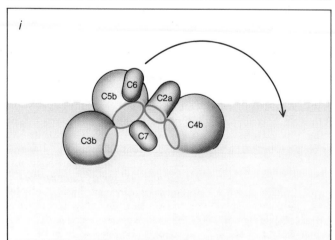

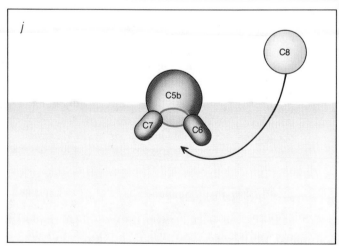

CLASSICAL PATHWAY of complement attack on the cell membrane is depicted. Foreign cells are recognized by antibodies, which bind to antigenic sites on the cell's surface. When two immunoglobulin G (IgG) antibodies are bound to adjacent sites, they can activate complement factor C1, which is inactive until it binds to the antibodies. C1 consists of three subunits, C1q, C1s and C1r, held together by a calcium ion. The C1q subunit is able to bind to the complement binding sites on antibodies (a). When it is bound, the C1 complex becomes enzymatically active and will activate complement protein C4 that comes in contact with a C$\overline{1s}$ subunit (b and c). C4 breaks into two parts, C4a and C4b, and the latter binds to the cell surface nearby (d). When C2 comes in

lieved the C5b,6,7 complex becomes bound to a site distinctly different from the site on the generating enzyme, there is no direct evidence that this happens. There is some evidence that the C5b,6,7 complex transfers to a different site: the C5b,6,7 complex can be transferred from cells with the C4b,2a,3b enzyme to other cells without the enzyme.

Cell Attack

The cell-attack sequence is initiated with the cleavage of protein C5. What role does the protein C6 play? Increasing the temperature or the ionic strength of the fluid phase causes C5b to break away from the C4b,2a,3b enzyme. Once the C5b fragment leaves the activating enzyme, its ability to combine with C6 and C7 is lost. When C6 is combined

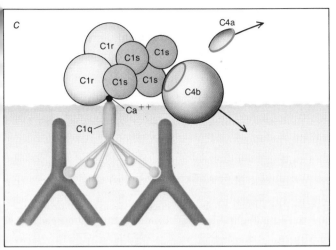

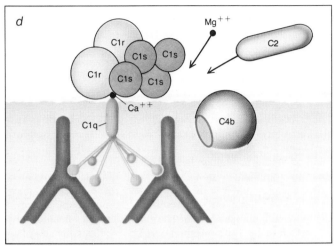

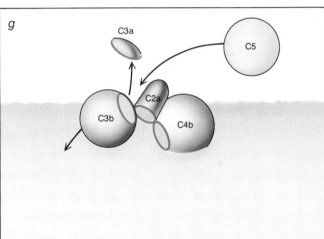

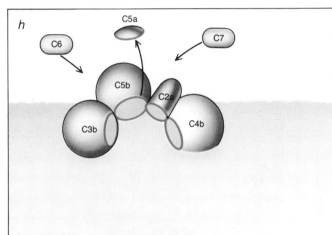

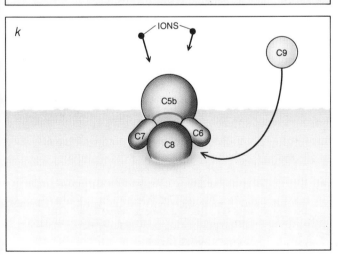

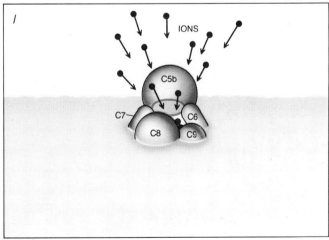

contact with the activated C1s (e), it too is split. The C2a fragment combines with C4b to form an enzyme, which splits C3 (f). The C3b fragment binds to the surface (g). If it is near enough to the C4b,2a enzyme, together they bind C5 (h). C6 and C7 bind to C5b (i). The C5b,6,7 complex then binds to the cell surface at a new site (j). C8 joins the C5b,6,7 complex.

The components assemble themselves in such a way that a small hole is formed in the membrane through which a few ions can pass (k). The addition of C9 greatly enlarges the hole and speeds up the flow of water and ions into the cell (l), causing it to swell and burst. The C3a and C5a fragments produced also play a role in immune and allergic reactions; they cause the release of histamine from cells.

with the C5b fragment, a fair degree of stability is achieved. The C5b,6 complex can be isolated and kept in the fluid phase for extended periods without much loss of its reactivity in subsequent steps. Hence it appears that the C6 complement factor serves as a stabilizer of the activated C5b fragment. It has been shown that C6 itself is not cleaved when it combines with the C5b fragment. It can be recovered in its complete form simply by dissociating the C5b,6 complex.

The complement factor C7 has not been extensively studied. Müller-Eberhard has shown that it binds to the C5b,6 complex. Robert Thompson of the University of Birmingham and Peter Lachmann of the Royal Postgraduate Medical School in London have shown that the combination of C7 with the C5b,6 complex, either in the fluid phase or on the generating enzyme, results in the formation of a new binding site that can attach to the cell's membrane. It is possible that C7 activates a binding site on the C5b,6 complex, or that the C7 molecule itself develops a binding site. The active binding site is short-lived, and the C5b,6,7 complexes that do not couple with the cell's membrane promptly lose their activity and remain in the fluid phase.

The reactions involving the complement factors C8 and C9 are not yet well understood. It is known that both bind by reactions other than covalent ones. C8 combines first with the C5b subunit of the C5b,6,7 complex and then C9 combines with C8. It is believed these reactions take place after the C5b,6,7 complex is bound to the cell's membrane, but interaction in the fluid phase is certainly possible. Cells subjected to the entire complement sequence up to and including C8 dissolve very slowly. The addition of the complement factor C9 greatly accelerates the destructive process.

It should be evident from the many qualifications and uncertainties in this description of the complement sequence that far less is known about the late-acting complement components than about the early-acting ones. The late-acting components present fascinating problems in immunology that are being investigated in many laboratories.

The Properdin Pathway

The activation of C3 by way of antibody, C1, C4 and C2 is designated as the classical pathway. An alternate pathway called the properdin pathway was discovered by Pillemer in the 1950's, and it is currently under intensive investigation. Some believe that it does not require antibody to initiate it and that hence it may be a more "natural" or "nonspecific" mechanism of immune defense. Such a mechanism might obviously be of great importance in infections and possibly in other diseases as well.

The term properdin refers to a system in blood serum that, acting together with complement, participates in several immunological processes, notably the promotion of the engulfing of cells and foreign particles by phagocytes and the production of inflammatory reactions. The incubation of normal blood serum with microbial cells or with certain polysaccharides derived from microbial cells (such as zymosan, a carbohydrate of the yeast cell membrane) gives rise to enzymes that activate the complement factors C3 and C5. Gram-positive bacteria (such as the pneumococcus) and toxic lipid polysaccharides from gram-negative bacteria (such as the colon bacillus *Escherichia coli*) also activate the properdin pathway. Once activated, the properdin system enzymes assemble on the surface of the bacterial cell and activate the complement attack sequence, beginning with production of the C3b fragment [*see illustration on page 150*]. Furthermore, the biologically active fragments C3a, C3b and C5a are also produced. These products mediate inflammatory reactions involved in immune defense and in allergic processes.

It is thought that there are two distinct enzymes in the properdin system: one that activates C3 and another that activates C5. Both enzymes are multiunit complexes and correspond in function to the $C\overline{4b,2a}$ and $C\overline{4b,2a,3b}$ complexes of the classical pathway. A key to understanding the mechanism of the properdin system comes from recent studies in my laboratory by Shin and Volker Brade elucidating the differences, as well as the similarities, between the properdin enzymes and their classical counterparts. Three of the subunits have been recognized, and each is found in each of the properdin enzymes. One of the subunits, called Factor B, can be regarded as the counterpart of the C2a unit in the corresponding complement enzymes. Factor B is also referred to as C3PA (for C3 proactivator) or as GBG (for gycine-rich beta glucoprotein). The other, Factor D, serves to activate Factor B. The complement fragment C3b is also present and plays a role in initiating the properdin system, but its precise function is not yet clear. One of the questions currently under study concerns the sources of the C3b fragment. A related

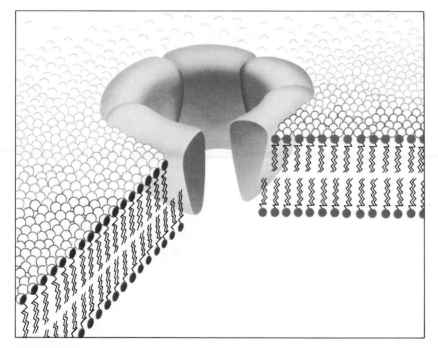

STRUCTURE OF COMPLEMENT LESION postulated by the author is depicted in schematic form. The structure is believed to consist of the five late-acting complement components C5b, C6, C7, C8 and C9. These components are thought to attach themselves to the lipid bilayer of the cell membrane. The bilayer consists of lipid molecules stacked side by side with their polar heads pointing outward and their nonpolar fatty-acid tails pointing inward. The complement components, which are proteins, are believed to assemble themselves into a doughnut or a funnel shape that penetrates the bilayer. The hollow core of the structure could form the lesion through which water and ions flow into cell until it bursts.

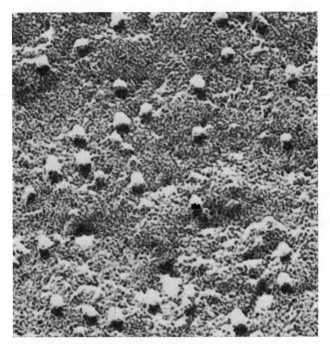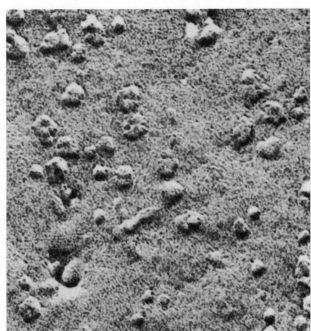

FREEZE-FRACTURED MEMBRANE of sheep red blood cells appears in these electron micrographs. The fracture takes place between the two lipid layers of the membrane, so that the membrane's interior is visible. In cell membrane treated only with antibody the protein globules that penetrate the membrane are normal in size, shape and distribution (*micrograph at left*). Membrane treated with antibody and complement, however, contains large doughnut-shaped aggregates of globules that penetrate to the interior of the cell membrane (*micrograph at right*). There are several doughnut-shaped aggregates in this micrograph; for example, one can be seen in the lower left-hand corner and two other doughnut shapes can be seen to the left of center. Both electron micrographs, which enlarged the structures some 420,000 diameters, were prepared by Bernhard Cinader and his colleagues at the University of Toronto.

study deals with the role of KAF, a regulatory enzyme discovered by Lachmann that destroys the C3b fragment.

Even though the properdin pathway and the classical pathway are initiated differently, various complement components exert an influence on the properdin-system enzymes. The complement factor C4 has been found to accelerate the assembly of the properdin enzymes, and it seems likely that C1 and C2 are also involved in the acceleration, although this has not yet been demonstrated directly. The accelerating effect is probably due to the generation of nascent C3b fragments by the complement enzyme C4b,2a.

One important question about the properdin system is whether or not any antibody is required to initiate it. Since normal blood serum contains at least some antibodies capable of reacting with virtually any bacterial surface, it is possible that in the properdin system the foreign invader is recognized by antibody, just as it is in the classical pathway. Whether or not it turns out that antibody is required, it is already abundantly clear that the classical pathway can be activated only by antibodies of the immunoglobulin-M and immunoglobulin-G classes, and that large quantities of the IgG antibodies are required.

The properdin pathway can be activated by aggregates of immunoglobulins that do not activate complement in the classical way. This has been demonstrated by Abraham G. Osler of the Public Health Research Institute of the City of New York and by Ann L. Sandberg of the National Institute of Dental Research. Although the full implications of these observations are not yet clear, the properdin pathway may represent a mechanism for the activation of immune defenses when sufficient quantities of specific antibody are not available for activation of the classical pathway.

The Donnan Effect

The general nature of complement attack on the cell has been understood for some time. As Burton D. Goldberg of the New York University School of Medicine and Howard Green of the Massachusetts Institute of Technology have shown, when cells are attacked by complement, they swell until the cell membrane is explosively ruptured and the contents of the cell spill out.

The cause of the swelling is a physicochemical phenomenon known as the Donnan effect. It occurs with semipermeable membranes whose pores pass common salts (such as sodium chloride) and water but do not pass large molecules (such as proteins). When such a membrane is set up with a solution of protein, salt and water on one side and a solution of salt and water on the other side, there is a flow of salt and water through the membrane toward the side with the protein.

Since living cells contain protein, they would be subject to the Donnan effect if the cell membrane behaved like a semipermeable membrane. The fact is that the cell membrane does not behave in this way. It has transport mechanisms that actively move various substances through it. When a cell membrane is damaged by complement, however, it does behave like a semipermeable membrane. Then salt and water, and other small molecules, readily flow into it.

There are various ways in which complement might possibly damage the cell membrane. The simplest would be that the complement system makes holes in the membrane. If numerous holes are required for the destruction of the cell, the process would exhibit the characteristic pattern of a multi-hit reaction, and it would have a threshold. If a single hole is sufficient, the system would have the characteristics of a one-hit reaction, in which the number of cells destroyed would be directly proportional to the quantity of complement. In order to determine whether the reaction is multi-hit or one-hit, I undertook experiments to determine how the degree of destruction in a cell population varies with the quantity of complement. The results support the one-hit hypothesis [*see the illustration on page 152*]. I have also examined the question in terms of the kinetics of the reaction, a mode of analysis that involves the measurement of reaction velocity and that has played a major role in the efforts of our group. The results again seem to support the one-hit hypothesis. In this approach, however, the speed of the reaction may be so great that it is not possible to differentiate experimentally between a multi-hit and a one-hit reaction.

Since the complement system has multiple components, it is not possible to study whether the reaction is multi-hit or one-hit in terms of the overall process. Instead it is necessary to investigate the individual reaction steps. It has been found that for C1, C4 and C2 the attack is a one-hit process. It would be tempting to jump to the conclusion that this means that a single hole is sufficient for the destruction of a cell. Indeed, this was the view that was widely accepted until it was learned that several of the complement fragments are enzymes that can produce a shower of the next component. Such a process would result in a cluster of active sites. Particularly for the $C\overline{4b,2a,3b}$ enzyme we must consider the likelihood that it produces a cluster of C5b,6,7 complexes on the membrane surface. When these complexes reacted with C8 and C9, numerous holes would be produced, all of which could be attributed to a single $C\overline{4b,2a,3b}$ site. For this reason studies indicating that reactions involving C1, C4 or C5 are one-hit processes do not really tell us whether one hole is sufficient for the destruction of the cell.

The story is different for C9. Since it is the last component in the reaction series, it should be possible to determine if it is involved in a multi-hit or a one-hit reaction. We have found that adding C9 to cells carrying all the other complement components induces the destruction of cells in a manner indicative of a one-hit process. The efficiency of the C9 reaction is so high that fewer than five molecules, probably as few as one or two, are sufficient for the destruction of a single cell. These results indicate that even if there is a cluster of C5b,6,7,8 complexes, the reaction of only one of them with C9 may be sufficient to produce a hole capable of destroying the cell.

The holes made by complement can be seen in electron micrographs. In micrographs of the surface of a membrane with holes in it the lesion is seen as a light ring with a dark central portion [*see illustration on preceding page*]. The ring appears to be a raised surface and the dark center is thought to be a depression in the membrane. Alternatively, it has been suggested that the light ring is a hydrophobic (water-hating) region and the dark center is a hydrophilic (water-loving) one. John H. Humphrey of the National Institute for Medical Research in London and Robert R. Dourmashkin of the Clinical Research Centre at Harrow in England have studied the relation between the number of lesions

PROPERDIN PATHWAY is an alternate way of activating complement attack. The term properdin refers to a system of factors in blood serum that act together with complement in several immunological processes. The properdin pathway is activated by microbial cells or by bacteria. Little is known about the properdin enzymes, but three subunits—Factor B, Factor D and the complement fragment C3b—have been identified (*top panel*). Other subunits have been indicated in studies but have not yet been implicated definitively. Factor D activates Factor B by cleavage (*middle panel*) and the activated fragment is designated $\overline{B}$. The other B fragment goes into the fluid phase. C3b also plays a role, but its precise function is not known. Possible sources of the C3b that helps initiate the properdin system are the complement enzyme $C\overline{4b,2a}$, or plasmin, trypsin or thrombin in blood serum. Factor $\dot{B}$, Factor D and C3b become assembled on the surface of a microbial cell into a properdin system enzyme that corresponds in function to the complement enzyme $C\overline{4b,2a}$, that is, they split C3 into C3a and C3b (*bottom panel*). C5 also is cleaved (*not shown*), but there are indications that the properdin system enzyme that is involved differs slightly from the enzyme that cleaves C3, possibly with respect to an unidentified subunit. The C3b that is generated may bind to the microbial cell surface, where it promotes phagocytosis (the engulfing of the cell by white cells). Or the C3b may join and yield another properdin enzyme complex, thus setting up a positive feedback process. Reactions after cleavage of C3 and C5 may follow the same sequence as found in the classical pathway, but details are not known.

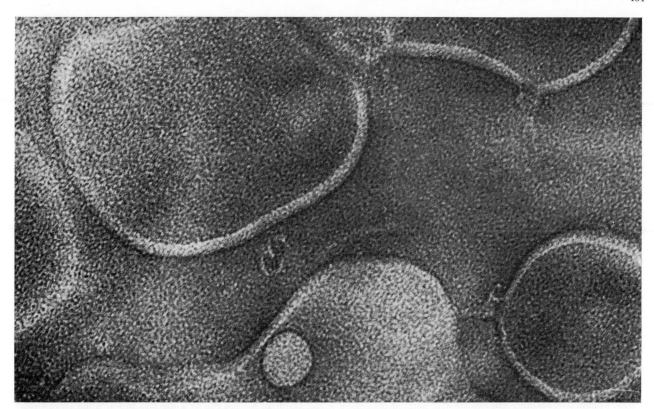

LESIONS MADE BY COMPLEMENT in artificial structures called liposomes provide a simple model for studying the mechanism of complement attack. The liposomes (*large circular shapes*) in this electron micrograph were prepared from the lipids sphingomyelin and cholesterol. The lipids form concentric bilayers that enclose water and ions. When the complement proteins C5b, C6, C7, C8 and C9 from human blood serum are added to the liposomes, lesions are formed in the bilayer (*upper right and lower right in micrograph*). There are also two detached lesions (*left of center*), which suggests that once the lesions are formed they are relatively stable. It is believed that the walls of the lesion consist of complement components, possibly in combination with lipids of the bilayer.

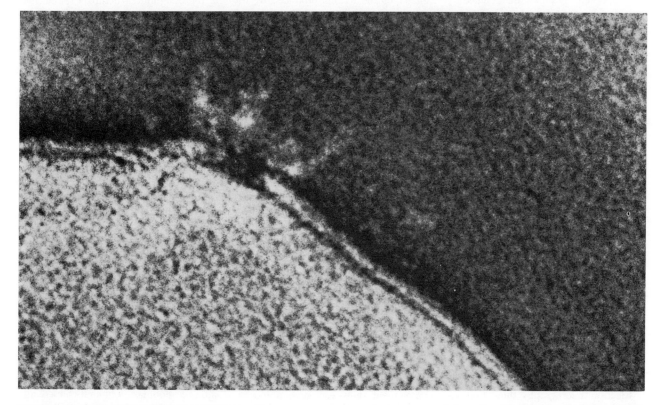

FUNNEL-SHAPED COMPLEMENT LESION in a liposome prepared from the lipid lecithin is about 10 or 11 nanometers thick and has a hollow core that must be hydrophilic (water-loving) because it is penetrated by stain. Magnification is some 880,000 diameters. Both electron micrographs are by E. A. Munn and his colleagues at the Institute of Animal Physiology in Cambridge.

on the cell surface, as seen by electron microscopy, and the number predicted by the one-hit theory. In some instances a one-to-one ratio was found, which supports the one-hit hypothesis; in others the number of lesions exceeded what had been predicted. It may be that in the latter case clusters of lesions were formed as the result of enzymatic showers.

The Doughnut Hypothesis

The fundamental structure of a cell membrane is a double layer of phospholipid, in which the hydrophilic heads of the phospholipid molecules point outward and the hydrophobic tails point inward. Embedded in the phospholipid bilayer are various proteins. Compounds soluble in lipid, such as sterols, may also float in the bilayer. A crucial element in this model of membrane is that the basic structure is a viscous fluid. Under these circumstances at least some of the embedded proteins could move laterally through the membrane.

Significant information about the mode of action of complement has come from studies of the artificial lipid bilayers called liposomes. They consist of a series of concentric lipid bilayers with alternating compartments for water. During their formation ions or small molecules may be trapped in the water compartments. When liposomes are attacked by complement, the trapped ions leak out.

Liposomes are not destroyed by complement in the same way as living cells. The Donnan effect does not come into play. Instead the lipid bilayer is somehow opened and ions from the water compartments flow out. The fact that complement can damage liposomes that consist entirely of lipid and glycolipid, that is, that are totally lacking in protein, strongly indicates that the attack of complement is directed against the lipid bilayer of the cell membrane and not against the proteins embedded in it.

How does complement attack the lipid bilayer? One hypothesis, which has been under consideration since the turn of the century, is that complement induces enzymatic action that gives rise to a leaky patch in the membrane. The crucial element in the leaky-patch hypothesis is that there is a small disrupted patch in the lipid bilayer. Since the bilayer is relatively fluid, the leaky patch must be regarded as a hole lacking rigid structure. Such patches would change in size over a period of time.

Electron micrographs show that lesions on cell membranes attacked by complement are quite uniform in size. Furthermore, lesions produced in red

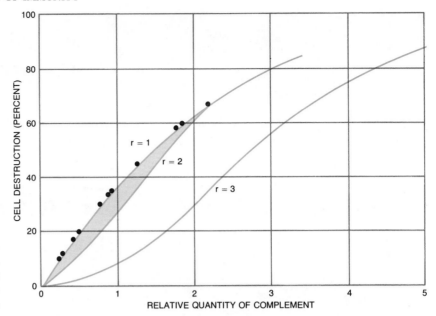

ONE-HIT THEORY states that complement needs only to produce one lesion in the cell membrane in order to destroy the cell. The multi-hit theory states that two or more lesions are required. Theoretical curves were calculated from the binomial probability distribution for threshold values of r = 1, r = 2 and r = 3 (*colored curves*). Measurements were then made in the author's laboratory of the number of cells destroyed by complement reaction in which the amount of complement protein C1, C2 or C4 was varied. The results (*black dots*) fit the one-hit curve. The light colored region is the area in which the experimental measurements make it possible to discriminate between a one-hit model and a two-hit one.

blood cells by guinea-pig complement differ in size from those produced by human complement. The internal diameter of the lesions produced by the guinea-pig complement is between 8.5 and 9.5 nanometers; the internal diameter of the lesions produced by the human complement is between 10 and 11 nanometers. Therefore it appears that the complement from each species can produce lesions of a characteristic size.

The major weakness of the leaky-patch concept is that any lesions that were produced in this way would tend to disappear rather quickly. In my own studies of the stability of membrane lesions I found that they persisted for at least 30 minutes. Now, the leaky patch could be stabilized if it were surrounded by a wall of protein. This concept led me to formulate the doughnut hypothesis: a stable hole is produced by the assembly of a rigid, doughnut-shaped structure in the lipid bilayer of the cell membrane. The hole forms a channel connecting the inside of the cell with the extracellular fluid.

Such a structure could conceivably be assembled from proteins already in the membrane. In view of the fact that liposomes without protein are attacked by complement, however, such a mechanism seems improbable. A second candidate for the structure might be sterols in the lipid, but they too can be rejected

because liposomes without sterols are also attacked. This leaves the complement proteins themselves as the source of the doughnut structure. I see no reason why several of the late-acting complement components could not be arranged to form a doughnut [*see illustration on page 148*]. The outside of the doughnut could be composed of nonpolar polypeptides, that is, protein chains that were hydrophobic; the interior would need polar peptides so that it could be hydrophilic. The structure of the doughnut would be similar to that of the antibiotic Valinomycin, the molecule of which has a hollow core. Another analogous structure is that of glutamine synthetase, which has been shown by electron microscopy to have a hollow core.

Soon after I had formulated the doughnut hypothesis Bernhard Cinader and his colleagues at the University of Toronto produced some electron microscope photographs of lesions that lend support to the concept. Cinader used a freeze-fracture technique, in which a frozen membrane is cleaved along the plane of its bilayer, exposing the membrane's interior. Sheep red blood cells treated with antibody and complement showed globular doughnut-shaped aggregates not found in similar cells treated only with antibody [*see illustration on page 149*]. The aggregates seem to be made up of several units. What is of cardinal importance, however, and what was first demonstrated in these micrographs, is that the complement lesions actually penetrate into the interior of the lipid bilayer.

Electron micrographs of lesions on liposomes, also published after the hypothesis had been formulated, show that the structure of the lesions is like a ring, and that a funnel-like lesion penetrates the lipid bilayer. These micrographs, made by Lachmann, D. G. Bowyer, P. Nicol, R. M. C. Dawson and E. A. Munn of the Royal Postgraduate Medical School in London and the Institute of Animal Physiology at Cambridge in England, show the lesions in top view and in side view [see illustrations on page 151]. Of particular interest is the fact that some of the rings are observed in a free state, that is, not on the liposome's surface. In the light of the procedures followed in the study, it appears likely that the rings were formed out of or derived from C5, C6, C7, C8 and C9. Direct proof of this interpretation calls for electron-microscopic identification of each of the complement components.

Other Activities

Among the activities of complement apart from cell attack are the release of histamine, chemotaxis and immune ad-herence. These activities are an important part of the inflammatory response, which plays a central role in immune and allergic reactions.

The C3a and C5a fragments cause the release of histamine from the cells that store this substance (leukocytes, mast cells and platelets). The histamine increases the permeability of the blood capillaries, which enables leukocytes (white blood cells) to penetrate into tissues where an infectious or allergic process is under way. Both C5a and C5b,6,7 complex are chemotactic for certain leukocytes, that is, they cause the leukocytes to migrate toward the site from which the chemotactic agents are diffusing. This phenomenon promotes the accumulation of leukocytes at tissue sites where immune reactions are proceeding.

The property of immune adherence is bestowed on cells by the C3b fragment. Cells carrying the C3b tend to adhere to leukocytes and other cells. Immune adherence thus promotes phagocytosis (the engulfing of cells by other cells). It is important to note that blood serum contains enzymes that degrade C3a, C3b and C5a, and that these inflammatory factors have a relatively short lifetime. The action of the degradative enzymes is still another device to limit the action of complement.

Many bacteria, notably some of those classified as Gram-negative, are killed by complement, and some are disintegrated in the process. Because bacteria have a cell wall outside their cell membrane, the bactericidal reaction is more complicated than the attack on other kinds of cells. Blood serum contains the enzyme lysozyme, which attacks the glycopeptide responsible for the rigidity of the bacterial cell wall. The attack dissolves the rigid layer of the wall. Tsunehisa Amano and Kozo Inoue of the University of Osaka have shown that lysozyme and complement act synergistically in the attack on bacterial cells. The bactericidal action of complement, however, is overshadowed by the phagocytosis of bacterial cells.

Phagocytosis is a prime mechanism of defense against bacterial infections. It has been known since the 1930's that antibody and complement render bacteria susceptible to phagocytosis, a process called opsonization. Pathogenic bacteria are often resistant to phagocytosis unless they are treated with antibody or complement.

The manner in which complement mediates opsonization was not known until the 1950's, when it was shown by Nelson that the binding of C3b on cell surfaces produced immune adherence. In addition the movement of phagocytic cells toward the infectious agents is facilitated by the histamine-releasing ac-

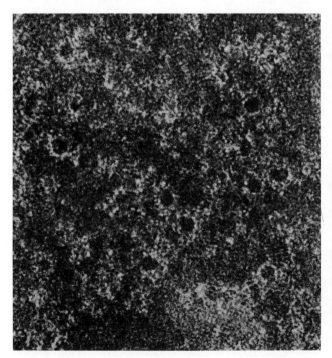 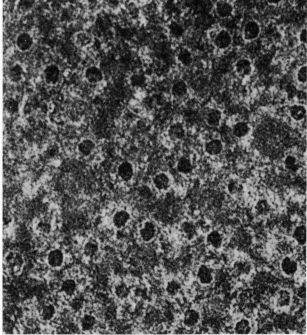

HOLES PRODUCED BY COMPLEMENT appear to be of a uniform and characteristic size for each species. Sheep red-cell membrane treated with anti-Forssman antibody and complement from guinea pig develops holes with an internal diameter of between 8.5 and 9.5 nanometers (micrograph at left). Red-cell membrane from a human patient treated with anti-I antibody and human complement develops uniform holes with a diameter of between 10 and 11 nanometers (right). These electron micrographs, in which the enlargement is some 400,000 diameters, were provided by Robert R. Dourmashkin of the Clinical Research Centre at Harrow in England.

tivity of the C3a and C5a fragments. A directional element is provided by the chemotactic action of the C5a fragment and the C5b,6,7 complex.

The role of complement in phagocytosis is most prominent during the first week of a bacterial infection when an adequate antibody response has not yet developed. The late W. Barry Wood, Jr., Jerry A. Winkelstein and Shin of Johns Hopkins showed that during the preantibody phase the invading bacteria activate the properdin system, which in turn activates the complement system. Patients with certain defects related to C3 exhibit a pronounced susceptibility to pus-producing bacterial infections. Chester Alper and Fred Rosen of the Harvard Medical School have studied a number of patients with such a defect. Their investigations have contributed substantially to the understanding of the role of the properdin system and complement in the immune defense against bacterial infections.

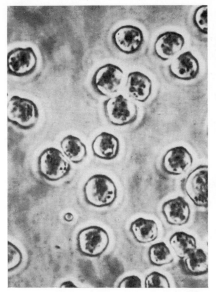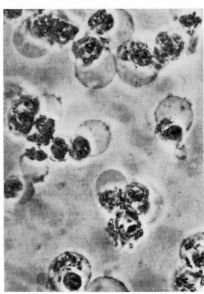

TUMOR CELLS before and after treatment with antibody and complement are shown in these phase-contrast light micrographs provided by Burton D. Goldberg of the New York University School of Medicine. The micrograph at left shows untreated Krebs ascites tumor cells, magnified about 700 diameters. After treatment the cells swell and burst (right).

Anaphylaxis

The processes that protect the body against foreign cells or toxic substances can also produce undesirable effects, which are collectively termed allergy or hypersensitivity. One such phenomenon is anaphylaxis, an untoward reaction to foreign antigen, which may occur following repeated exposure to the antigenic substance. Anaphylaxis due to the sting of bees or wasps is not uncommon. The injection of certain drugs, particularly penicillin, can also cause anaphylaxis. Some people suffer anaphylactic reactions following the inhalation of allergens such as ragweed pollen or after the ingestion of certain foods. Anaphylaxis, which can be severe enough to cause death, is due to an antigen-antibody reaction that brings about the release of massive amounts of histamine and other substances.

It has been suspected for a long time that complement might be involved in anaphylaxis. This view is derived from the discovery more than 60 years ago that the treatment of blood serum with certain bacterial polysaccharides results in the formation of toxic substances, which were named anaphylatoxins. When serum containing such substances is injected into an experimental animal, the symptoms of anaphylaxis are produced. We now know that these bacterial polysaccharides are similar to the polysaccharides that activate the properdin system. Efforts to elucidate this phenomenon were stimulated by the work of Osler. They came to fruition

with the discovery that the properdin system cleaved C3 and C5, and that the resulting C3a and C5a fragments induced the release of histamine.

The role of anaphylatoxins in anaphylactic reactions is quite uncertain. It is known that some reactions such as hay fever are produced by a different mechanism involving antibodies belonging to the IgE class of immunoglobulins. The production of local anaphylaxis with antibody from a different animal species has been extensively investigated, notably by Otto Bier of the Instituto Butantan in São Paulo, Brazil. Although the experiments with heterologous antibodies are not directly relevant to anaphylaxis induced by an animal's own antibody, they nevertheless demonstrate that activation of the complement system by immune complexes, with the consequent production of the complement subunits C3a and C5a, can produce local anaphylactic events.

In general, when immune complexes form in an organ or a tissue, the complement system will be activated at that site, through the classical pathway, the properdin pathway or both. The biologically active complement fragments and complexes can become involved in reactions that damage the host's cells, and these pathogenic reactions can result in the development of immune-complex diseases. For example, in some forms of nephritis complement damages the basal membrane of the kidney, resulting in the escape of protein from the blood into the urine. The disease disseminated

lupus erythematosus also belongs in this category; its symptoms include nephritis, visceral lesions and skin eruptions. The treatment of diphtheria or tetanus with the injection of large amounts of antitoxin sometimes results in serum sickness, an immune-complex disease. Rheumatoid arthritis also involves immune complexes. Like disseminated lupus erythematosus, it is an autoimmune disease, in which the disease symptoms are caused by pathological effects of the immune system in the host's tissues.

How is complement involved in such diseases? As we have seen, the histamine released by the C3a and C5a fragments changes the permeability of the blood vessels near the site of complement activity. The chemotactic property of the C5a fragment and the C5a,6,7 complex, which has been studied extensively by Shin, Peter Ward and Ralph B. Snyderman, results in the migration of leukocytes into the area. Furthermore, the C3b fragment binds to immune complexes, and this action promotes the ingestion of the complexes by phagocytes. Phagocytosis, in turn, is followed by release of lysosomal enzymes that damage the surrounding cells and tissues. The cell-destructive capacity of the complement system may contribute to damage of cell membranes in the immediate vicinity. Activation of the complement system also accelerates blood clotting. This action comes about by way of the complement-mediated release of a clotting factor from platelets.

A genetic deficiency of complement

protein C2 has been found and investigated in some humans, but the most extensive studies of genetic complement deficiencies have been done with guinea pigs, mice and rabbits. Guinea pigs lacking C4 appear to be in good health, presumably because of protection provided through the properdin pathway. Michael Frank of the National Institute of Allergy and Infectious Diseases has shown, however, that under certain experimental conditions the complement-deficient guinea pigs exhibit abnormalities. For example, the ingestion of antibody-coated foreign cells by phagocytes does not always proceed properly. The antibody response to protein antigens is also defective.

Mice deficient in C5 also appear to be healthy, although in appropriately designed experiments their resistance to pneumococcal infection is shown to be impaired. The mice are also less resistant to a pathogen related to the bacillus that causes diphtheria in man.

The rejection of skin and organ transplants is caused by poorly understood mechanisms collectively termed cellular immunity. The participation of complement in the rejection process has been suggested by some investigations. For example, when the mechanism of cellular immunity is interfered with by the injection of an antilymphocyte serum, mice deficient in C5 reject skin grafts more slowly than their normal counterparts do. This result suggests that complement is involved in the rejection of grafts by the normal mice. Slower skin-graft rejection has also been noted by Klaus and Ursula Rother of the University of Heidelberg in studies of rabbits lacking C6.

Future Studies

At the present time we are able only to sketch the general outlines of the complement system. Although some steps of the reactions have been worked out, much remains to be done, particularly with the late-acting complements. It should also be stressed that genuinely effective studies of the biological activities of complement (other than its cell-destroying action) have only begun, and that the information now available should be regarded as no more than the result of initial surveys. A fuller elucidation of the role of complement in the body's immune defense system will undoubtedly open the way to new and better means of controlling infections, allergic disorders and autoimmune diseases.

V

A SUMMARY VIEW OF PART ONE: A Homeostatic and Self-monitoring Immune System

15

A Homeostatic and Self-monitoring Immune System

by Sir Macfarlane Burnet
An original article
1976

The immune system is an intricately controlled mechanism of great versatility and flexibility, capable of dealing with many emergencies.

Immunology, like the rest of the biomedical sciences, has been constructed out of the recording and comparison of countless experiments. The continuing accumulation of data and the integration of each investigator's experience with contemporary results from other laboratories and current theoretical ideas is a process that will always remain the dominant and most worthwhile approach to our subject. But sometimes one must stand back from the detail and try to sense the direction in which the broad functional pattern of the immune system as a whole seems to be developing. The objective of this article is to present that pattern as it appeared to one immunologist during the years of 1974 and 1975.

The picture that seems to emerge is of a homeostatic and self-monitoring system whose function is to maintain the genetically defined integrity of body substance, which end it achieves by transient interchanges of information from random contact between fully mobile units. That condensed version is, I believe, not inconsistent with any of the facts in this collection of *Scientific American* articles and is in a form that would probably be acceptable to most present-day immunologists. To be applicable to actual problems, however, it will need considerable expansion and will undoubtedly become more controversial.

Let us start first with the unique quality of the system that is expressed in its ability to maintain a functioning mechanism for the effective handling of information, virtually without any morphological structure. Niels Jerne has spoken of the resemblance of the immune system to the nervous system but has not stressed the extraordinary difference between the labyrinthine network of neural circuitry and switchgear, most of which is set up to last for life, and the momentary contact of mobile immune cells swirling through the blood- and lymph-circulatory systems. Nor does the immune system have analogies with any manmade technological device, despite the miraculous factory that Nossal used as an analogy in his article [see "How Cells Make Antibodies," by G. J. V. Nossal, page 22]. Instead, the immune system is an intensely biological invention. Any analogies must be sought in another set of biological systems for informational transfer, systems that may be exemplified by the incessant traffic in an ant nest or in any other community of the social Hymenoptera, in which the exchange of information made at each contact between hurrying individuals has a superficially similar counterpart in the immune system. [*See the illustrations on pages 160 and 161.*] It is not too far-fetched even to extend the analogy to the interactions between people in any large human community, and provided one maintains a sense of humor there may well be help occasionally in understanding immunopathology by thinking of analogous situations in human social pathology. Both are intensely biological phenomena.

The immune system is second only to the nervous system in the intricacy of its functioning, and in the genetically sound individual it is equal to that system in maintaining the homeostasis that is virtually a synonym for health. In the process, the system must be kept on perpetual alert to deal with both foreign intrusions and "disloyalty" from within. I might even press the political metaphor further and indicate that one of the chief preoccupations of the system is to maintain a series of checks and counterchecks against inappropriate action by its own agents. The complexity of the system depends on the difficulty—again with political parallels—of knowing self from not-self, who is in his proper place, and who, if unchecked, will endanger the safety of the organism. And a second great difficulty derives from the way in which specificity—the capacity to recognize—can only arise in a random fashion.

The Generation of Diversity

Ever since the publication of *The Origin of Species* in 1857 it has become more and more evident that evolution has found no way to introduce novelty other than to produce a wide diversity of inheritable patterns in some essentially random fashion, and then to expose those patterns to the test of competitive survival. This is just as applicable to microorganisms and to the mobile cells of the body as to the macroorganisms—the plants and animals—of Darwin's day. Clonal selection is an intensely Darwinian concept, and despite the controversies about the process by which a diversity of antibodies is generated, all the protagonists are seeking an interpretation concordant with evolutionary principles. To take one hypothesis, David Baltimore's theory of somatic mutation, mentioned in the introduction to the first section of this volume, we find that during development the subgenes responsible for constructing the L and H variable chains are subjected to a randomization procedure that influences what they code for the hypervariable regions. It is, like all such genetic procedures, completely random as far as the information that will be expressed on the resulting gene is concerned. The ultimate product is the complex configuration produced by the juxtaposition of L and H variable regions to form a combining site, on either an antibody or an immune receptor, to which antigen can attach. Many of those randomly produced combining sites will be reactive against antigens or antigenic determinants present in the body and are therefore unwanted and potentially dangerous.

The first requirement for an effective immune system is to ensure that the reactive lymphocytes, T or B, that unite with more than minimal affinity with accessible antigenic determinants within the body shall in one way or another be prevented from proliferating. Some of the possible ways by which this is achieved are described in my article on tolerance and unresponsiveness in Section III [see "Tolerance and Unresponsiveness," by Sir Macfarlane Burnet, page 114]. None of the interpretations that have been attempted in molecular terms are satisfactory. Probably the most useful statement—though it tells nothing about mechanism—is one due to Avrion Mitchison: that tolerance results whenever an antigen is constantly present in the animal and accessible to lymphocytes.

Recognition

In the day-to-day functioning of a system that depends almost solely on the outcome of random contacts between mobile cells, there are two basic requirements. These are, first, that the cells should possess capacities for mutual recognition, with the production of a signal of some sort when recognition is achieved; and second, that they should be capable of an appropriate repertoire of responses to suit each signal as it is experienced. The response that follows mutual contact between two cells may involve one or both of the participants. In addition to mobile cells, soluble or particulate materials, including hormones, antigens, immunoglobulins, complement components, and so on, provide a constantly changing background in the system. Less central to the system are the various phagocytic cells, which play important parts in mopping up excess antigen and eliminating it, but at the same time intervening in the preparation of antigen for presentation to immunocytes. The dendritic phagocytic cells of lymph nodules and germinal centers that were described by Nossal [see "How Cells Make Antibodies," by G. J. V. Nossal, page 22] are probably important in this respect.

Recognition at all levels depends on noncovalent union in various degrees of affinity between complementary molecular configurations. All patterns expressed either as receptor or effector that arise in the body are genetically controlled, though we might qualify this by remarking that antibody diversity is produced by some unique genetic mechanism not yet fully understood and that mutation—which is essentially random error in DNA sequences—when it occurs in stem cells, can produce aberrant populations of lymphocytes. Clinical examples of these pathological effects can be seen in acute and chronic lymphatic leukemia, various autoimmune conditions, and multiple myeloma. Probably the most interesting feature of the recognition function is how cells that have changed by one or the other of these "unorthodox" genetic methods can be recognized by others.

The appearance of a clone of B cells of new immune specificity automatically presents a heretofore unknown configuration of the combining site. The new molecular pattern will be present on specific Ig receptors and on the specific antibody, which may be in several functional states—in free molecular form, attached to cell surfaces, or aggregated as antigen-antibody complexes. The implications of this have been presented in Niels Jerne's article [see "The Immune System," by Niels Kaj Jerne, page 49]. In principle, any such configuration can serve as antigen to produce antiidiotypic antibodies which, in a fashion analogous to two mirror reflections, are immunologically equivalent to antigen, and it is obvious that antireceptor-receptors and antiantibodies could in theory be important reagents in controlling the immune system homeostatically. To carry out such experiments in the laboratory, however, usually requires the use of large amounts of monoclonal antibody as antigen, typically a myeloma protein with an antibody specificity toward a hapten such as phosphoryl choline. It may be doubted whether control obtained in this way is of any significance in healthy organisms. Most extrinsic antigens, such as pathogenic microorganisms, stimulate immune responses that are polyclonal and that include many distinct idiotypes, and the chance that a high-affinity clone will direct itself against any individual idiotype is probably very small. When for any reason there is an active proliferation of a single clone resulting in antibody production, the position is very different. Antiidiotype responses may then represent an important aspect of the partial control, accompanied by remissions and relapses, that is characteristic of many autoimmune diseases. Other aspects of the control of anomalous clones of immunocytes in pathological conditions are best left for a later section [see "The Nature of Autoimmune Disease," by Sir Macfarlane Burnet, page 254].

Lymphocyte Interactions

The undetermined nature of T-cell receptors is a problem that hampers every attempt at immunological generalization, particularly when one tries to visualize the immune system as a whole. At least three interpretations of T-cell receptors are not yet excluded: (1) T cells are essentially the same as B cells except that their immunoglobulin synthesis stops with the production of sufficient IgM1 to maintain an adequate number of surface receptors; (2) they synthesize and use as receptors a different type of macromolecule, conceivably a double-stranded RNA, capable however of expressing almost as wide a

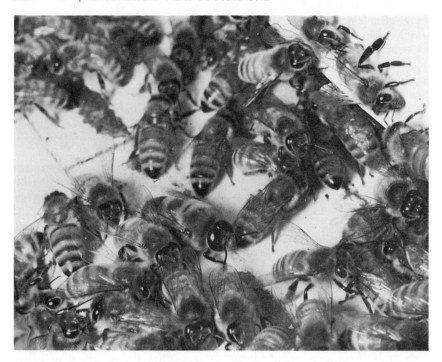

AT THE ENTRANCE TO A BEEHIVE (upper right corner of the photograph), communication between bees enables members of one colony to differentiate between fellow members of the colony and aliens from another colony. The photograph is reproduced through the courtesy of Edward Ross.

range of specificity as immunoglobulins; or (3) they carry a system of allogeneic recognition units complementary to the major histocompatibility antigens and in addition make use of passively obtained IgM1 as a set of receptors parallel to those of the contemporary B-cell populations. It seems unlikely that any alternative interpretation will be so different from one or some combination of features from more than one of the three interpretations just mentioned as to require a different overall approach.

It is of interest, therefore, to recognize that any of the alternatives cited are compatible with the picture that we are trying to develop of information transfer within a system of mobile units. One way to view that picture is to think of an immensely complex interacting network of mobile lymphocytes comprising thousands of distinguishable subpopulations. Control in such a network arises from the impact of patterned macromolecules carrying genetically coded information on receptors, which they can recognize and stimulate—depending on circumstances—to give synthesizing, proliferative, or destructive signals to the cell. (An example of such interactions in relation to autoimmune disease is illustrated in another article in this book [see page 257].)

The whole structure of the blood and lymph circulations and of the peripheral lymphoid tissues, and the processes by which lymphocytes move from one compartment to another—all of these work together to ensure the highest likelihood that any lymphocyte may make a tentative contact with any other lymphocyte, learning through that contact whether there are possibilities of mutual recognition and reaction. We can recall, as relevant to this, Mayerson's description of the general lymphocyte circulation, in which new cells arise by proliferation in the primary centers—bone marrow and thymus—and may undergo secondary multiplication in the germinal centers and diffuse lymphoid tissue of the spleen or lymph nodes as well as in Peyer's patches and other lymphoid accumulations along the gastrointestinal tract [see "The Lymphatic System," by H. S. Mayerson, page 123]. In general, new cells will pass via lymph vessels into the thoracic duct and from there into the circulating blood. From the general capillary circulation many move into the tissues, particularly of the gut wall, and are collected and moved from there through afferent lymphatics to the lymph nodes. Others pass actively into lymphoid tissue from the blood by passing through the cytoplasm of the cu-

boidal endothelial cells of post-capillary venules in the lymphoid tissue. Lymphocytes are actively motile, and in the lymph nodes one can picture a dynamic situation in which there is constant movement of cells in all directions but an overall trend from the peripheral sinuses toward the collecting vessels of the hilum. In life it would probably appear as a writhing "bag of worms," with more stable regions in the germinal centers and the plasma cells of the medullary cords. In the sheep, where a popliteal lymph node can be cannulated in both afferent and efferent trunks, it is possible, by infusing an antigen into the afferent channel and collecting everything that emerges from the efferent, to show that *all* reactive lymphocytes specific for the antigen in the whole of the body can be trapped in that lymph node. If, after a week, the experiment is terminated by excising the lymph node with its cannulated vessels, the animal can be shown to contain neither antigen nor reactive cells. Immunologically, it has been reconstituted as a virgin animal, in regard to that particular antigen. One could hardly have a more striking demonstration of the point I am making, that every lymphocyte has an opportunity to meet every other lymphocyte and that in this fashion countless effective interactions result which mediate the homeostasis and self-monitoring quality of the system.

The immune system is unique in that an intensely heterogeneous population of cells are capable of highly specific interactions among subpopulations without the necessity of any physical segregation. In terms of its functions, one can only conceive of it as a multidimensional universe presenting quite extraordinary difficulties to those who seek an effective understanding. There is no particular difficulty in devising experiments, and provided the conditions are rigidly standardized, reproducible results will be obtained. Yet most of those "good" experiments are best considered as making no more than two-dimensional sections of a multidimensional universe. We must never forget that the *sine qua non* for a definitive biological experiment—working with genetically uniform organisms or cells—just cannot from the very nature of the subject be applied to immunology. All that can be hoped for is that each new experiment will test a cross-section different from all the previous ones and make this or that conclusion a little more likely.

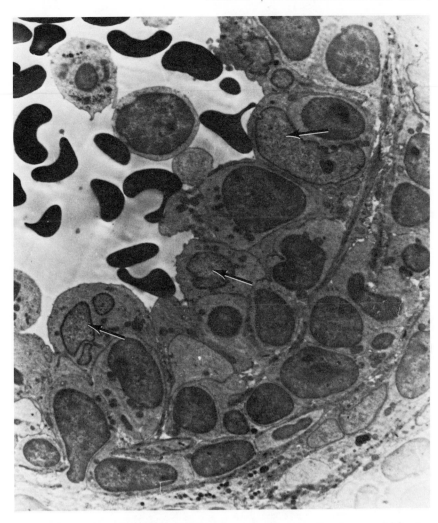

THE PASSAGE OF LYMPHOCYTES through post-capillary venules of a normal laboratory rat is shown in this electron micrograph. The nuclei of several lymphocytes (dark grey shapes) can be seen in the cytoplasm of endothelial cells, the larger, lighter nuclei of which are indicated with arrows (the darkest cells in the white lumen at the upper left are red blood cells). Most of the lymphocytes are outside the endothelium and are visible in the crescent extending from the upper right side of the picture down to the lower left. The micrograph, which shows a magnification of about 3240 diameters, is reproduced from V. T. Marchesi and J. L. Gowans, *Proceedings of the Royal Society*, Series B, 159:283–290 (1964).

Immunity in Relation to Medicine

VI

MANIFESTATIONS
OF IMMUNE DEFICIENCY

VI MANIFESTATIONS OF IMMUNE DEFICIENCY

INTRODUCTION

Almost more than any other area of biological research, immunology has always been strongly oriented toward its medical applications, and this section is the first of four all dealing with this topic.

I have divided this part of the book into four sections somewhat arbitrarily: (1) immunodeficiency diseases and immunosuppressive drugs; (2) transplantation; (3) immunity in relation to infectious disease; and to fill a gap not yet closed by a *Scientific American* article I have added what I hope will give a helpful outline of (4) autoimmune disease, to present a fuller picture of immunity in its bearing on disease.

It is true enough to say that most academic immunologists today are primarily interested in immunology because it is the area of human and mammalian biology where the application of new methods of molecular biology seems likely to yield the richest harvest of new understanding. But it is equally true, and perhaps more humanly important, that immunology is deeply concerned with all types of infectious disease and with the difficulties and successes of organ transplantation. In all probability, immune surveillance plays an important part in determining the age of incidence of malignant disease, and there is a significant group of gerontologists who see the immune system as controlling the rate of aging itself. In addition the immune system is primarily or secondarily subject to disease, usually of genetic or somatic genetic origin, and nowadays this forms one of the important areas of growth in pathology.

Probably the only major aspect of immunology demanding coverage supplementary to previously published *Scientific American* articles concerns the various conditions in which a man or an animal fails to show the capabilities for immunity that can be expected in a normal individual. Agammaglobulinemia, described in *Scientific American* by David Gitlin and Charles A. Janeway rather a long time ago, was only the first of a large number of medical conditions to be discovered in which inefficiency of some aspect of immunity seems to be primarily responsible for the symptoms and pathological changes. I have therefore tried to bring those medical conditions, including classical agammaglobulinemia, in which there is gross deficiency of one or more immunoglobulins, into line with modern concepts in the article that follows the one by Gitlin and Janeway. One of the most interesting features of these conditions is the high incidence of malignant tumors, particularly of lymphoid types, found in almost all of those diseases in which the patients survive beyond childhood. Since this is also seen in patients treated for years with immunosuppressive drugs, it is convenient to discuss these in the first section before moving on to the section dealing with transplantation; transplantation became surgically practicable in man only when immunosuppressive drugs had been discovered.

Agammaglobulinemia

by David Gitlin and Charles A. Janeway
July 1957

*This nonstop word refers to a disease in which the
blood lacks gamma globulin. Because antibodies are
found in gamma globulin, those who suffer from the
disease are prey to grave infections*

One day in 1951 a very sick eight-year-old boy was admitted to Walter Reed Hospital in Washington, D.C. His illness was not particularly unusual: bacteria had invaded his bloodstream to cause septicemia, or "blood poisoning." But the boy's medical history was distinctly unusual. Within the preceding four years he had suffered more than 20 grave infections, and in 10 of them bacteria had been found in his blood. On each occasion the bacteria had been identified as pneumococci.

Several attempts had been made to immunize the boy against the recurring infections. He had been injected with vaccines containing dead pneumococci and with substances manufactured by these bacteria. Ordinarily the injections would have stimulated his production of specific proteins, or antibodies, which would have increased his resistance to the pneumococci. The injections had been of no avail. Even when he had been injected with the vaccines of other bacteria, he had produced no antibodies against them. It seemed obvious that the boy suffered from a defect in his ability to make antibodies. But what sort of defect was it, and what could be done about it?

Antibodies are found in blood serum, the mixture of proteins that remains after the rest of the blood has clotted. Some 20 years ago Arne Tiselius of Sweden showed that the serum proteins could be fractionated by electrophoresis, in which an electric current is passed through a solution to separate one protein from another by the characteristic electric charge of its molecule. Tiselius separated the serum proteins into four main fractions: albumin, alpha globulin, beta globulin and gamma globulin. He noted that the antibody proteins were mostly in the gamma globulin fraction.

Colonel Ogden Bruton, the physician in charge of the boy's case, arranged to

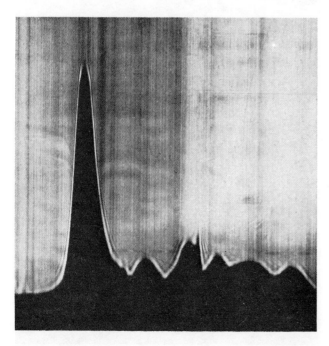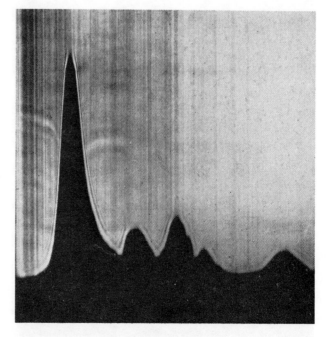

PROTEIN FRACTIONS of blood serum are separated by electrophoresis, in which one protein is separated from another by the electric charge at its molecule. The result is a pattern of dark peaks, one for each fraction. At left is the pattern of normal serum. The tall peak corresponds to albumin. Merging with the right side of this peak is a peak corresponding to alpha-one globulin. The second visible peak to the right corresponds to alpha-two globulin; the third, to beta globulin; the fourth, to fibrinogen; the fifth to gamma globulin. At right is the pattern of serum from a child with agammaglobulinemia; the gamma globulin peak is missing.

have the blood serum of his patient analyzed by electrophoresis. The analysis showed that the serum contained no gamma globulin! This was an astonishing result. It meant that the boy probably lacked antibodies of any kind.

At about the same time two other boys were under observation at Children's Hospital in Boston. They too had suffered from many severe bacterial infections, most of which would have undoubtedly been fatal if they had not been liberally treated with antibiotics. When the attending physicians heard of Bruton's case, they had the boys' blood serum analyzed by electrophoresis. Gamma globulin was absent in both patients.

Bruton named this newly recognized defect "agammaglobulinemia," which simply means "absence of gamma globulin in the blood." The story of the three boys was told by Leonard Apt of Children's Hospital at a pediatrics meeting in 1952, where the ensuing discussion indicated that the disorder had also been observed in other hospitals. Since then more than 40 cases of agammaglobulinemia in children have been reported.

This was not the end of the story; it was only the beginning. Agammaglobulinemia is a significant experiment of nature. Before the advent of antibiotics the disorder could not have been

detected, because without them most of its victims cannot survive the severe infections they contract early in life. Now it provided a unique means of studying the production of antibodies and their role in infections and other disease processes.

There were at least two possible explanations for the absence of gamma globulin from the blood of these children. One was that they were able to manufacture gamma globulin but destroyed it so rapidly that little or none remained in the blood. The other was that they could not make gamma globulin at all. To decide this question gamma globulin from normal individuals was injected into children with agamma-

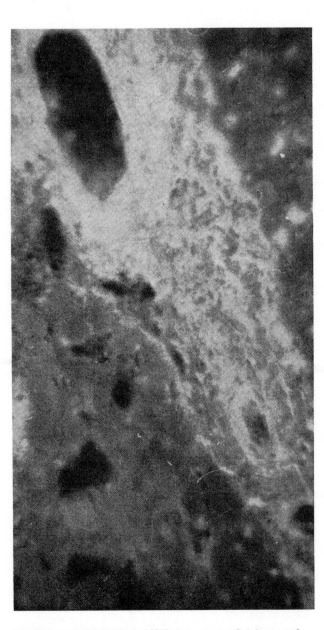
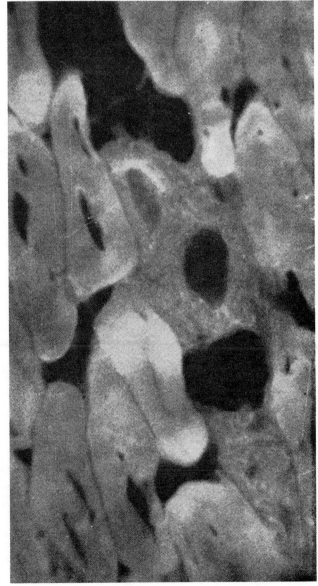

GAMMA GLOBULIN IN TISSUE shows up as a bright area when it is stained with a fluorescent antibody and photomicrographed under ultraviolet. At left is such a picture of connective tissue in the muscle of a normal person; the bright area runs from upper left to lower right. At right is similar tissue from a child with agammaglobulinemia; the tissue glows slightly but has no bright areas.

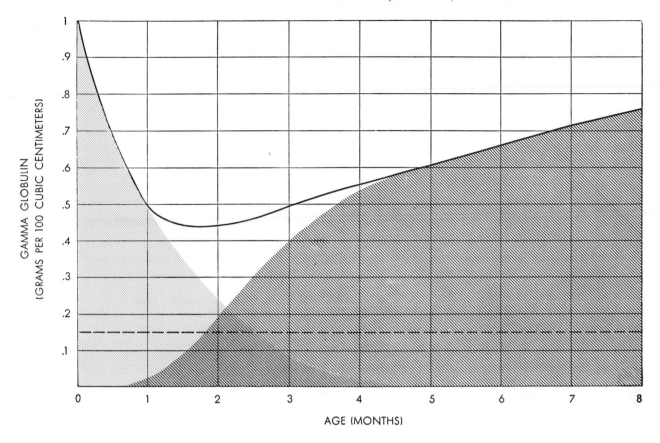

INFANT'S GAMMA GLOBULIN SUPPLY first comes from the mother's blood. This gift is gradually depleted (*colored area*) in the first four months of life. The normal infant starts to manufacture its own gamma globulin before it is one month old and gradu-ally builds up its store (*gray area*). The black line shows the actual concentration of gamma globulin usually found in an infant's serum during its first eight months. In agammaglobulinemia the concentration drops below the level marked by the dashed line.

globulinemia. It was found that, if anything, gamma globulin was destroyed more slowly in these children than in a normal child. Thus it appeared that the absence of gamma globulin was due to a defect in its manufacture.

This finding was now corroborated by another line of investigation. It had long been suspected that antibodies are made not by all cells but by certain kinds of cells found notably in the lymph nodes, the spleen and the walls of the large and small intestines. Recently Albert H. Coons and his colleagues at the Harvard Medical School, using an ingenious technique in which antibodies labeled with a fluorescent dye are used to locate substances in tissue sections, have shown that the ultimate source of antibodies is not certain kinds of cells but a single kind of cell: the so-called plasma cell.

Further studies showed that when a normal child had suffered from an infection, or had been injected with a vaccine or toxoid, large numbers of plasma cells appeared in its lymph nodes, spleen and intestinal wall. When a child with agammaglobulinemia had been similarly injected, practically no plasma cells were found in any tissue. Indeed, no plasma cells appeared after prolonged infection. This evidence supported the hypothesis that the plasma cell is essential to the formation of antibodies. It also indicated that the lack of antibodies in a child with agammaglobulinemia is due to the absence of the plasma cells by which they are normally formed. Finally, since antibodies constitute most, if not all, of the gamma globulin fraction, these findings substantiated the other evidence that the disorder is caused not by the destruction of gamma globulin but by a defect in its production.

It was now possible to investigate another question. It had been suggested that since antibodies were gamma globulins, specific antibodies might arise from the direct modification of gamma globulin already present in the body. To test this hypothesis several agammaglobulinemic children were injected with both gamma globulin and a vaccine. If the hypothesis were true, some of the gamma globulin should have been converted into an antibody against the vaccine. Subsequent tests of the children's blood gave no indication that any of the gamma globulin had been converted into

AUTHORS' NOTE

In preparing this article the authors have drawn upon their own work and upon information obtained by others. They would like to acknowledge their indebtedness to Colonel Ogden C. Bruton of the U. S. Army Medical Corps; their colleagues Drs. John Craig, Leonard Apt, Hans Habich, Walter H. Hitzig and Theodore C. Jewett, Jr.; and others in the U. S. and abroad, particularly Drs. Lee F. Hill of Des Moines, Conrad M. Riley of New York, Norman Kendall of Philadelphia, Robert A. Good of Minneapolis, Philip L. Calcagno of Buffalo, Nicholas Martin of London, Andrew Sass-Kortsak of Toronto and A. Hässig, S. Barandun and H. Isliker of Berne, Switzerland.

the antibody; thus it appeared that preformed gamma globulin is not readily made into specific antibodies, at least in the absence of plasma cells.

As physicians continued to study agammaglobulinemia they made new clinical observations. One was that although children suffering from the disorder were dangerously susceptible to infection by bacteria, their resistance to infection by viruses appeared to be relatively normal! For example, their medical histories frequently indicated that although they had been exposed to measles and chicken pox on numerous occasions, they had contracted these virus diseases only once. Moreover, the infections seemed to have been no more severe than usual. This observation demanded further study. If it could be substantiated, it would mean that factors other than antibodies are important to normal immunity to viral infection.

The cowpox virus, which confers immunity to smallpox, was admirably suited to test the observation. As almost everyone knows, when a person who is not immune to smallpox is vaccinated with cowpox virus, a blister surrounded by a red area forms on the skin; later the blister is replaced by a scab. When an immune person is vaccinated, no blister forms and there may be only a slight and transient area of redness. Children with agammaglobulinemia were vaccinated, resulting in the usual nonimmune response. When they were vaccinated again, their response was identical with that of normal immune individuals. Even when they were vaccinated a third

time on a patch of skin far removed from the site of the original vaccination, their response was normal. Despite their immunity, no antibodies against cowpox virus could be detected in their blood. The conclusion could only be that, although antibodies are necessary for immunity to at least some bacteria, they are not required for immunity to certain viruses.

How much antibody is necessary to prevent infection by bacteria? Here again children with agammaglobulinemia provided an answer. When the disorder was first discovered, a method had already been developed to isolate large quantities of gamma globulin from pooled blood plasma, thus concentrating the antibodies of all the individuals from whom the blood had been obtained. The children were immediately given large injections of the missing protein fraction, providing them with antibodies made by others. Because the disorder appeared to be permanent, it was necessary to administer the gamma globulin at regular intervals. It became apparent that to treat most cases of the disorder successfully it was necessary to maintain the concentration of gamma globulin at between 100 and 200 milligrams per 100 cubic centimeters of plasma. When the concentration fell below that level, infections occurred. The concentration of gamma globulin in a normal person is between 600 and 1,200 milligrams per 100 c.c. Since the gamma globulin given to the children came from the pooled plasma of hundreds of adults, this would seem to indicate that the average adult

has a safety factor of about six in his supply of antibodies to prevent infection by bacteria.

Antibodies are not always a blessing, as people with allergies can testify. For example, when some individuals inhale ragweed pollen, they manufacture a special kind of antibody which sensitizes them to the pollen instead of protecting them against it. In such a person a subsequent encounter with ragweed pollen causes a local reaction between the pollen and the antibody—an attack of hay fever. Other diseases which are not usually described as allergic may be due to a similar reaction. Rheumatoid arthritis, for example, may be caused by a chronic reaction between an antibody and a substance in the body tissues. The nature of the substance is not known: some investigators think it is derived from substances which enter the body; others, that it is a constituent of the body.

How does agammaglobulinemia fit into this problem? It was observed that at least a third of the children with the disorder developed chronic arthritis. Some years after the onset of the infections, their ankles, knees, wrists and the joints of their fingers began to swell. Although acute infection caused arthritis in some of the children, the chronic disease was not due to local infection. Surprisingly the chronic arthritis was accompanied by little pain; the generalized symptoms were few and less severe than would be expected were similar swellings to develop in a normal person. Under the microscope the tissues of the affected joints had some features characteristic of rheumatoid arthritis and others that were not.

Was this rheumatoid arthritis? The answer is still not clear. If it is rheumatoid arthritis, the implications are startling. For example, it may be that in a normal individual the generalized symptoms of rheumatoid arthritis are caused by a reaction between a specific antibody and the tissue of the joints, but that the arthritis itself is due to another process entirely. It is even possible, if these observations are correct, that antibodies made by the normal person protect him against rheumatoid arthritis. This cannot be construed to mean, however, that the administration of gamma globulin will prevent or ameliorate rheumatoid arthritis. A third of the children with agammaglobulinemia suffered from arthritis even though they had received large amounts of gamma globulin.

Periodic injections of gamma globulin have been very successful in preventing infections in children with agammaglob-

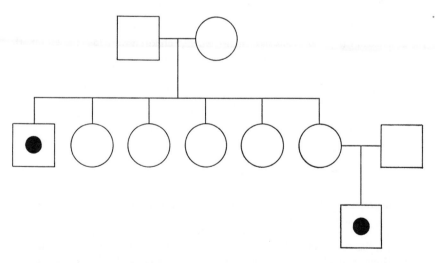

HEREDITARY TRANSMISSION of agammaglobulinemia is illustrated in this family tree based on an actual case. The disease (*black dot*) appears only in males (*squares*) but is transmitted by females (*circles*). The defective gene is carried as a sex-linked recessive trait by the mother. Daughters who receive the gene will also be carriers although they appear normal. Sons who receive the gene will show symptoms of agammaglobulinemia.

ulinemia; regular doses of antibiotics have also been helpful. Obviously these measures are expensive and inconvenient. Would it not be better to supply the missing plasma cells, so that the child could produce his own antibodies? Lymph nodes containing plasma cells have indeed been transplanted from a normal child to a child with agammaglobulinemia. Unfortunately the nodes failed to produce antibodies when vaccines were injected into the abnormal child. When the nodes had been stimulated with vaccines before they were transplanted, they manufactured small quantities of antibodies for a short time. When the nodes were transplanted from a normal adult and then stimulated, they manufactured antibodies, but again only temporarily.

Although these transplants were unsuccessful, much has been learned from other grafts between normal individuals and children with agammaglobulinemia. Skin cannot be successfully transplanted from one individual to another (unless the individuals are identical twins). When such a graft is made, the transplanted skin ordinarily degenerates in two or three weeks [see "Skin Transplants," by P. B. Medawar, the article beginning on page 182]. It has long been thought that the reason why the transplants do not "take" is that the individual who receives the graft makes antibodies against it. If this were the case, it should be possible to make successful skin transplants between a normal person and a child with agammaglobulinemia.

Robert A. Good and Richard L. Varco of the University of Minnesota Medical School have succeeded in making such grafts. In some cases, however, the transplants did not survive. The reasons for this are not clear. At this point it should be said that agammaglobulinemia is not a total absence of gamma globulin; it would be more accurate to describe the disorder as a severe deficiency of the protein fraction. Sensitive tests on children with agammaglobulinemia have indicated that some of them can make traces of gamma globulin. It may be that this small amount is sufficient to account for the failure of some of the skin transplants. It may also explain the immunity of the children to certain viruses. At the moment, however, these are pure speculations.

As more children with agammaglobulinemia were discovered, the fact that all of them were boys became more striking. It strongly suggested that heredity played a role in the disorder, and

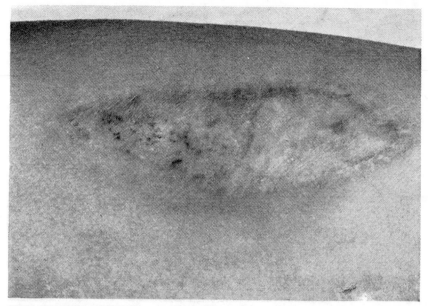

SKIN TRANSPLANTED from a 45-year-old woman to a boy with agammaglobulinemia has remained in place for three years. The graft was made by Robert A. Good of the University of Minnesota Medical School. This photograph is from the journal *Pediatrics*.

the families of the patients were accordingly studied. It was found that in many of the families brothers or maternal uncles of the patients had died of what appeared to be agammaglobulinemia. In several cases the disorder was diagnosed in a younger brother of the patient. In another it was found that a maternal nephew of the patient was affected. It is now clear that agammaglobulinemia is a hereditary disorder. Like hemophilia, it is a sex-linked recessive characteristic that is transmitted from mother to son. The mothers show no symptoms of the disorder, but half the sons will suffer from it. Because of this, and because the disorder begins in infancy or early childhood, it has been renamed "congenital agammaglobulinemia."

Agammaglobulinemia occurs not only in children. At present all those with congenital agammaglobulinemia are children; some day they will obviously be adults. But another form of the disorder has been recognized in both men and women. These patients appeared to be perfectly normal until they were adolescents or adults; then they began to suffer from repeated bacterial infections. In one case it was definitely shown that the blood of the patient had previously contained gamma globulin. It is not known whether this form of the disorder, like diabetes, is inherited as a tendency which is manifest only later in life. In any case it has been named "acquired agammaglobulinemia." There are certain differences between the effects of agammaglobulinemia in adults and

those in children. For example, the adults are less likely than the children to accept skin grafts. At least some of these differences may be attributed to the fact that the blood of the adults contains more gamma globulin than that of the children. The concentration of gamma globulin in the plasma of agammaglobulinemic adults may be as high as 100 milligrams per 100 c.c.

Agammaglobulinemia occurs in still another form which may be much more common than the congenital or the acquired. The gamma globulin in the blood of a newborn child was manufactured not by the child but by its mother. Normally the child begins to make its own gamma globulin at the age of four to 12 weeks; meantime the maternal protein gradually disappears. Sometimes, however, the development of the ability to manufacture gamma globulin is delayed. The result is the same as that of congenital agammaglobulinemia: the child may suffer from severe bacterial infections. Fortunately this type of agammaglobulinemia is temporary, and it can now be treated with injections of gamma globulin.

The study of agammaglobulinemia continues. Thus far it has made possible the successful treatment of the disease, and has clarified how normal individuals resist infection. It may yet provide significant evidence as to the nature of diseases such as rheumatoid arthritis, and shed further light on basic problems of immunity and allergy.

17 Immunodeficiency: Investigations since 1957

by Sir Macfarlane Burnet
An original article
1976

Studies of genetic or drug-induced deficiencies in the functioning of the immune system have thrown light on many aspects of immunology.

As is the invariable rule in medicine when a new form of disease is recognized and clearly defined, many examples are recognized by other workers; some of them are obviously examples of the prototype disease but others have only a limited resemblance, and rather often it gradually becomes apparent that the original disease was only a particularly "visible" example of a whole spectrum of disease conditions. This is what followed Ogden Bruton's recognition of agammaglobulinemia in 1951. Since then, many hundreds of patients have been observed with abnormally low amounts, or even apparent absence, of immunoglobulins, and it has proved difficult or impossible to sort these cases into well-defined disease entities. It seemed obvious that congenital sex-linked agammaglobulinemia should be but one example of a well-defined, readily diagnosable pattern of diseases. The combination of undue susceptibility to bacterial infection in early childhood, very low amounts of immunoglobulin, and therapeutic effectiveness of treatment with pooled human gamma globulin, taken with the characteristic inheritance as a sex-linked condition, is a striking one but it is far from defining a uniform pattern of disease.

Immunoglobulin Deficiencies Other than Agammaglobulinemia

Clinically and hematologically, cases show a considerable range of differences. Most cases represent a gross deficiency of B-cell function, though this is rarely, perhaps never, complete. The main weakness seems to be a regular failure of B cells to develop into plasma cells. It has been claimed that some patients have no B cells, but the ability of most or all patients to develop normal specific immunity against measles and other virus infections makes it highly probable that a proportion of B cells making monomeric IgM is present, and that what fails to occur is the further development of cells capable of liberating the standard pentameric IgM and then switching to IgG and IgA. On the other hand, some patients are said to have detectable amounts of IgE, the immunoglobulin associated with allergic disease.

The acquired type of immunoglobulin deficiency, now often called "common variable type of hypoglobulinemia," is even more variable in immunoglobulin levels. The factors responsible for the onset of these conditions are not understood, but genetic influences almost certainly play a part. In severe cases, B cells can be shown to be present and to synthesize IgM but these do not secrete more than minimal amounts.

Congenital Thymus Deficiency: Di George's Syndrome

In many ways congenital sex-linked agammaglobulinemia represents a human analogy to the chicken whose bursa is surgically removed immediately on hatching, inasmuch as both conditions represent a functional deficiency of B cells. Similarly, there is a human deficiency disease of congenital origin which is functionally nearly equivalent to the neonatally thymectomized mouse that has subsequently been heavily irradiated and "rescued," by an injection of normal bone marrow from animals of the same pure strain; both lack T cells but have essentially normal B cells. [See the table at the top of page 173]. The human condition, Di George's syndrome, is extremely rare and appears to be due to a genetic anomaly by which two derivatives of the branchial pouch region, the thymus and the parathyroid glands, fail to develop. Both organs are necessary for life and the condition is lethal in infancy if untreated. Some might feel that it is more humane in the long term to treat infants with such a gross defect only by sedation and control of symptoms, but at least three groups of immunologists have reported being able to control the parathyroid deficiency with parathormone and, by grafting thymus from a human fetus into infants with Di George's syndrome, to provide persistent immune function. At least one patient is recorded as surviving six years, and quite apart from humanitarian aspects, this success is of very great scientific interest.

Since genetically distinct thymus tissue can be grafted and accepted, to become fully functional, it is evident that patients with Di George's syndrome have no effective recognition of foreign histocompatibility antigens, with the implication being that it is a primary function of the thymus to provide the mechanism—the T-cell system—by which that recognition becomes possible. It follows also that when in due course the grafted thymus cells establish a functional recognition system, one must assume that both the patient's own cells and those of the functioning thymus will be accepted as "self"; the interesting possibility is that the patient will grow up with up to eight distinct HL-A antigens. There are, however, alternative possibilities, as suggested by the behavior of an abnormal mouse strain

	HUMAN DISEASE OR ANIMAL MODEL	B CELLS	PLASMA CELLS	T CELLS
B-DEFICIENCY CONDITIONS	CONGENITAL AGAMMAGLOBULINEMIA IN HUMANS	PRESENT BUT FUNCTIONALLY INHIBITED	NOT PRESENT	NORMAL
	COMMON VARIABLE TYPE OF HYPOGAMMAGLOBULINEMIA IN HUMANS	PRESENT BUT VARIABLY INHIBITED	NOT PRESENT OR FEW	NORMAL
	HORMONAL BURSECTOMY IN CHICKENS	NOT PRESENT	NOT PRESENT	NORMAL
T-DEFICIENCY CONDITIONS	DI GEORGE'S SYNDROME IN HUMANS	PRESENT	PRESENT	NOT PRESENT
	NEONATAL THYMECTOMY IN MICE	PRESENT	PRESENT	NOT PRESENT
	"NUDE" STRAIN OF MICE (nu/nu)	PRESENT	PRESENT	PRESENT BUT FUNCTIONALLY INHIBITED

AGAMMAGLOBULINEMIA is one of several immunodeficiency diseases in humans that have, as their counterparts, several animal models. In this chart, the human diseases and animal counterparts are divided into B-deficiency and T-deficiency groups. Notice that the presence of plasma cells is always associated with the liberation of antibody into body fluids.

which, for genetic reasons, fails to develop a thymus.

Recently there has been much interest in a mutant strain of mice originally recognized by its hairless character as "nude." Such mice are double recessives and are now often referred to as *nu/nu* mice. They survive poorly and fail to show functional T cells. B cells are present but antibody responses are poor and production is confined to IgM. The thymus is absent or extremely rudimentary, and in most respects *nu/nu* mice are analogous to children with Di George's syndrome. The nature of the lesion for which the genetic anomaly is responsible is unknown but, at the Basel Institute for Immunology, Berenice Kindred and Francis Loor have found that when a thymus from a normal mouse of a strain whose cells are recognizably different from those of the *nu/nu* race is grafted to a nude mouse, the cells with which the thymus is eventually populated are derived from the *nu/nu* recipient and not from the normal donor. Further evidence points to the existence in the spleens of *nu/nu* mice of lymphocytes that, on the basis of certain surface antigens, appear to be the progenitor T cells that become functional T cells in the grafted thymus environment.

Low-Grade Deficiency Diseases

Both the conditions described so far—immunoglobulin deficiency and congenital thymus deficiency—are regularly fatal in early childhood if untreated; as might be expected, those rare infants born without either B- or T-cell function (the so-called Swiss type agammaglobulinemia) die soon after birth and have never been successfully treated. There are, however, many forms of less severe immune deficiency, sometimes apparently alone but often associated with other anomalies, which allow relatively prolonged or even indefinite survival under good clinical surveillance and prompt treatment of infections. Two that show some points of special interest are Wiskott-Aldrich syndrome and ataxia telangiectasia.

Wiskott-Aldrich syndrome is, like the classical form of agammaglobulinemia, a sex-linked disease seen only in males. The symptoms appear early in life and include a tendency to skin hemorrhages associated with deficiency of platelets in the blood, eczema, and repeated infections of various types. Two that have been particularly noted are herpes simplex virus infections of the mouth and lips, which persistently fail to heal, and mucocutaneous infection with the fungus *Candida*. This produces a chronic induration of the skin, which may cover most of the body surface [*see the illustration at the right*]. Specific study of various immune functions points mainly toward a defect in T-cell function in these children, though they also have some deficiency in producing antibodies against polysaccharide antigens.

Most children with the disease die before three or four years of age, but with careful management some have survived into their teens. In their teens

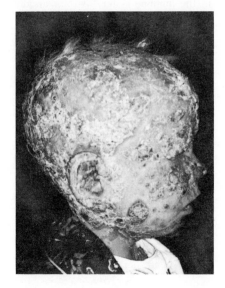

CHILD WITH T-CELL deficiency suffering from mucocutaneous candidiasis infection. The infection is a common sympton of Wiskott-Aldrich syndrome, a sex-linked disease seen only in males. However, in children of either sex, mucocutaneous candidiasis infection may occur in the absence of other symptoms of Wiskott-Aldrich syndrome. The photo is reproduced from R. J. Schlegel et al., in *Pediatrics*, 45:926–936 (1970).

nearly all afflicted patients die of malignant disease; most suffer from lymphoid cell tumors or leukemia, though several other types of cancer are also encountered. The incidence of any of these forms of cancer is vastly higher than in the general population of teenaged individuals.

Extensive mucocutaneous candidiasis can be seen in children of either sex in the absence of other signs of Wiskott-Aldrich syndrome, and there is a widespread opinion that a T-cell defect similar to that in patients with Wiscott-Aldrich syndrome is present also in these patients. There is much interest in recent claims that "transfer factor," an extract of human leucocytes from immune individuals, can help in the treatment of both types of patients.

The second disease, ataxia telangiectasia (AT), takes its name from two constant features, a progressive cerebellar ataxia and the appearance of dilated superficial blood vessels (telangiectases) on the conjunctiva of the eyeball and on the facial skin. It is a genetic disease transmitted in Mendelian fashion as an autosomal recessive condition. This has a puzzling implication: not only the two symptoms that give the disease its name, but also the others still to be mentioned, have a single genetic origin. All are agreed that these patients show defects in the immune system and are unduly susceptible to infection. However, the findings vary considerably. IgA is often absent, but by no means invariably, and T-cell function is depressed, as is shown by delayed rejection of skin grafts from other individuals and failure to show delayed hypersensitivity responses.

Malignant disease is quite exceptionally common and most frequently involves lymphoid tissues. In the period from 1957 to 1968, 23 of 29 fatal malignancies, including leukemia, studied in children or adolescents with AT were of lymphoid-cell origin. Three of the others were cancer of the stomach.

To add to the difficulty of identifying a single genetic abnormality responsible for the bizarre combination of signs and symptoms in AT, there is well-documented evidence of chromosome fragility.

Immunosuppressive Drugs

In 1958, Robert S. Schwartz and William Dameshek carried out an experiment that was to prove vital to the success of kidney transplantation as a lifesaving measure. They showed that if the chemical 6-mercaptopurine was injected along with an immunizing dose of a foreign antigen (bovine serum albumin) into rabbits, no antibody, or a greatly reduced amount, was produced.

The stimulus to the experiment came from the fact that active work was under way in many laboratories on the use of antimetabolites in the treatment of cancer. The structure of 6-mercaptopurine is basically similar to the biological purine bases adenine and guanine [see the illustration at bottom of page], and the rationale for its use as an antimetabolite is that its insertion in place of adenine in a DNA segment would render the cell incapable of division. This should only occur in actively growing and proliferating cells; hence it can be expected to have a much more toxic effect on an actively growing cancer than on normal body cells. Dameshek had been interested in autoimmune disease since 1938 and probably felt that the antibody-producing cells would be proliferating during the response and might therefore be as susceptible to an antimetabolite as cancer cells.

In the experiments, both the course of antigen removal and the rate of antibody production were measured. With an appropriate dose, no antibody was produced and the antigen was removed from the circulation at a steady rate without the sudden final disappearance that normally coincides with the appearance of antibody [see the illustration on the next page]. The experiment created much interest and shortly thereafter, in 1960, Roy Calne, an English surgeon interested in experimental transplantation, showed that the drug prolonged the survival of skin homografts. Within two years commercial drug manufacturers had produced a derivative of mercaptopurine, azathioprine ("Imuran"), which could be given by mouth and which has remained the sheet-anchor of renal transplantation ever since. Until then, success had been achieved only when a patient with serious kidney disease had an identical twin who showed no sign of kidney pathology, who was otherwise healthy, and who was willing to have one of his kidneys surgically removed. With the availability of azathioprine, and of corticosteroid and actinomycin to help deal with critical "rejection episodes," a substantial proportion of kidneys taken post mortem from accident victims could be used in transplantations with satisfactory acceptance and prolonged function. Within five years well over 50 percent of the operations were successful in the sense of providing a substantial extension of life without invalidism.

It soon became evident, however, that though a dosage of azathioprine could be reduced it could not be safely discontinued. A suitable maintenance dose having been found, the patient was advised to continue at that level indefinitely. In approximately 1 percent of persons accepting their transplants and surviving for more than a year, tumors have appeared which can reasonably be ascribed to the immunosuppressive effect of long continuation of the azathioprine dosage. Most of the tumors are the primitive B-cell tumors usually recorded as reticulum cell sarcomas. They have shown an unusual tendency to affect the brain and most have been fatal. Appropriate statistical comparison of the incidence of such tumors in populations of normal people of similar age and sex distribution indicated that there were 350 times the expected number of tumors in the patients under immunosuppression. There are figures to suggest an increased incidence of other tumors, especially the common forms of cancer of the skin and of the uterine cervix, but

ADENINE   6-MERCAPTOPURINE

THE CHEMICAL STRUCTURES of adenine and its competetive inhibitor 6-mercaptopurine. As an antimetabolite, 6-mercaptopurine was used in the treatment of cancer at the time it was discovered to be effective in suppressing production of antibody.

convincing proof of this has not yet been provided.

Other signs of immune depression might be expected; I shall mention three.

1. Herpes simplex (in the form of cold sores of the lips) takes an abnormally long time to heal and may become chronic.

2. Common warts appear frequently in these patients.

3. In Australia, solar keratoses on the back of the hand or the face are very common. In transplant patients under immunosuppression an exceptional number of these—five in one patient is the record—show the development of squamous epithelioma. This is not a common sequel in normal individuals of the same age range. Everything fits well enough with the hypothesis that the activity of immune response, particularly that of T cells, is damped down by the drug and that in most people infected this is adequate to allow symptomatic expression of low-grade viruses such as those responsible for herpes simplex and common warts. In others, initiated malignancies that in the normal person would be cut short by immune processes are enabled to develop into overt malignant tumors.

Some researchers have suggested that the tumors may represent a positive carcinogenic effect of the azathioprine and there seems to be no crucial way to eliminate this possibility. However, the results in chronic immunodeficiency diseases of genetic origin are so similar to those in patients with the drug-induced disease that the odds are strongly in favor of the first interpretation—that the tumors result from the failure of immune responses to deal with malignant disease at its initiation.

Immune Surveillance in Relation to Cancer

One of the main reasons for discussing the two chronic immunodeficiency diseases, Wiskott-Aldrich syndrome and ataxia telangiectasia, was to allow a consideration of the unusually high incidence of cancer, especially cancer of lymphoid cells, including acute lymphatic leukemia, in patients of an age group in which solid tumors of any sort are extremely rare. Clearly, two possibilities must be considered. The tumors may be a direct result of the underlying genetic anomaly or they may result from a failure of the process that I called immunological surveillance. The fact

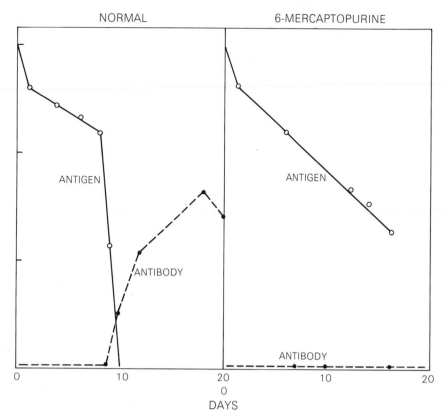

IMMUNOSUPPRESSIVE ACTION OF 6-MERCAPTOPURINE is evident in charts comparing the immune response in two rabbits. Both rabbits were immunized at the same time with a dose of radioactively labeled human serum albumin. One rabbit was a normal control (see the chart at the left) and the other was given an immunosuppressive dose of 6-mercaptopurine (chart at right). The course of disappearance of antigen is shown by the solid line. It measures the decreasing percentage of the initial radioactivity on a logarithmic scale. Notice that in the normal animal the fall accelerates sharply at the eighth day, with the beginning of antibody production. In the presence of the drug the fall continues at the same slope for at least sixteen days and no antibody is produced. The illustration is based on data from R. S. Schwartz and W. Dameshek in *Nature*, 183:1682–1683 (1959).

that a closely similar set of findings has been obtained in patients under long-term use of immunosuppressive drugs makes it almost certain that the factor common to both groups, an immune deficiency involving T cells particularly, is the important operative condition.

The intense concentration of malignant change observed on cells of lymphoid origin, both in chronic immunodeficiency disease and in patients under immunosuppressive therapy, obviously calls for some explanation. The most likely hypothesis is that malignant change in lymphocytes is more frequent than in any other human cell type but that the process of surveillance is correspondingly more effective in all normal individuals. This possibility has already been touched on in discussing the general quality of the immune system but can be expanded a little here, with the question of malignancy in the forefront.

With the recognition that most cancers and leukemias are monoclonal, there is a considerable measure of agreement that—aside from any preceding or predisposing factors—the actual initiation of a malignant cell clone is due to genetic error (somatic mutation), more often giving rise to a program change than a point mutation, which results in a structural change in the gene product. Of all the cells of the mature mammalian body, the lymphocyte is the one probably most subject to those normal developmental and functional changes during which error would be likely to occur. In addition to the process leading to diversity of antibody pattern we must take into account the switches of immunoglobulin from IgM1 to IgM5 to IgG to IgA. Every contemporary theory of T- and B-cell function calls for developmental changes as the cell matures to fulfill various types of executive function. All the changes must represent complex programmed reorganizations of genetic material in the course of which errors must inevitably occur. Many errors will be of no significance except to cripple the cell involved. The only common way by which errors can be manifested is by excessive proliferation of the cell concerned, and this, when intense enough, is seen as malignant disease.

In line with the general discussion of the nature of the normal functioning of the immune system, we can say it is axiomatic that cells of the system have the capacity to recognize, and react with, any cell carrying abnormal antigenic determinants on its surface and accessible to lymphocytic contact. Despite the inability to demonstrate a molecular mechanism for the purpose, it seems necessary to postulate that a homeostatic system must be able, when required, to recognize and control cells in each distinct functional state. Everything that has been said about how the "design" of the immune system allows exploratory contact of any lymphocyte with virtually every other lymphocyte in the body is also valid when we are considering a malignant lymphoid cell. There will be a very much greater chance of a malignant *lymphoid* cell making contact with a lymphocyte that can recognize and initiate a reaction against it than would be the case for any sort of cancerous *epithelial* cell.

This case for the effectiveness of immune surveillance against malignant lymphocytes is, in the eyes of several pathologists, strongly supported by what happens in that very curious disease, infectious mononucleosis. Without attempting to detail the reasons for so doing, we can regard infectious mononucleosis as a B-cell lymphocytic leukemia, caused or triggered by Epstein-Barr virus and provoking an active surveillance or suppressor response, predominantly by T cells, against the leukemia cells. Except under special conditions, when Burkitt's lymphoma may result, the surveillance is effective and complete.

VII

TRANSPLANTATION

INTRODUCTION

The successful transplantation of kidneys as a treatment for otherwise lethal kidney disease has been the most spectacular clinical achievement of applied immunology. Yet to me it is discouraging to recognize how little of that success was related to experimental work on the principles of immunological tolerance. Instead, it came as a result of the almost empirical use of immunosuppressive drugs whose modes of action are still incompletely understood. The only article on renal transplantation as such in the present volume, "The Transplantation of the Kidney," by John P. Merrill, dates perhaps quite appropriately from the period when it was believed that the only circumstances that justified a kidney transplantation was the availability of the patient's identical twin as donor of a healthy kidney. Such operations were based on the logical application of what was then known about graft acceptance and rejection in experimental animals and they were nearly all strikingly successful.

However, since Medawar's work in the 1930's there has been a continuing sequence of discoveries through experiments in transplantation, which have been almost as enlightening as those in any other area of immunology. In examining experimental progress it may be helpful to view the problems from the angle of their evolutionary origin and biological significance. This I shall attempt here in order to provide a context for the articles that appear in this section and because of my own special interest in the topics.

To the best of my knowledge every species of vertebrate, one partial exception being the golden hamster, shows a range of histocompatibility differences sufficient to ensure that skin grafted from one individual will be rejected by any other individual of the species taken at random, excluding first degree relations or members of homozygous strains artificially produced. This holds for lampreys, goldfish, chickens, mice, rats, rabbits, dogs, and humans, and presumably all vertebrates with a large and open gene pool.

There is no escaping the conclusion that the evolution of reciprocally reactive patterns fulfills some important biological need and that the appearance of a well-defined set of major histocompatibility antigens (MHCAs) is meaningless without the complementary allogeneic receptors (ARs) that were postulated in the introduction to Section II. Further, the number of MHCAs in any species appears to be within the range of from 10 to 100. This is small enough to make it likely that the allogeneic receptors are individually coded for in the genome and are not the result of a process of somatic diversification. Such a conclusion raises some interesting difficulties at the genetic level inasmuch as any change in MHCA is ineffective without the associated appearance of a complementary AR. The difficulty of accounting for the spread of such a change throughout a species makes it necessary, for the present, at least, to leave the genetic mechanism of their evolution out of consideration. Quite apart from the mechanism that was utilized, why vertebrates evolved the *need* for histocompatibility differences merits some brief discussion.

At various times I have considered three circumstances in which cells from other individuals of the same species could enter the body to the detriment of the individual's survival or reproductive efficiency:

1. By entry of fetal cells at some stage of viviparous reproduction. The pseudomalignant activity of trophoblastic cells in the early stages of implantation and the existence of chorionepithelioma probably point to the main potential danger.

2. As first suggested by P. A. Gorer, if the system of histocompatibility differences did not exist, malignant disease would be contagious. By analogy with the one spontaneous malignant disease that can override the histocompatibility barrier, venereal sarcoma in dogs, sexual transfer would probably occur particularly readily.

3. A more exotic suggestion is that if the semiparasitic mode of life of present-day hagfishes and lampreys was characteristic of the earliest vertebrates, some means of inhibiting parasitism on larger individuals of the same species might have become an evolutionary necessity.

The three suggestions are not mutually incompatible, but if we confine ourselves to mammals, the first two, which may turn out to be rather closely related, are the only ones that need be kept in mind.

In the articles by Rupert E. Billingham and Willys K. Silvers on transplantation in the hamster and by C. A. Clarke on the prevention of Rh disease, one can visualize some of the difficulties of handling the problems of genetically related but dissimilar cells within the body. Two approaches are possible and a combination of the two may be desirable. The first is to maintain the cells behind a barrier that will prevent antigenic materials from reaching sites where they can react with competent lymphocytes, thus preventing the development of antibody or populations of cytotoxic cells. The second approach is to use immunological means to deal with foreign cells that have not been held back by the barrier or for which no barrier has been developed.

Only a few comments need be made on the article by Billingham and Silvers on the immunology of the hamster. It is a unique laboratory animal, being wholly derived from one male and two females taken from the same nesting burrow in 1946, and perhaps for this reason the golden hamster shows only three histocompatibility types. There is incomplete evidence that other races of hamster also have very small numbers of histocompatibility types, which may suggest that special evolutionary processes, perhaps recurrent gross reductions and expansions of population, are needed to allow the progressive accumulation of new MHCAs and corresponding recognition sites. It would be of very great interest, though perhaps impossibly difficult and expensive, to undertake a comprehensive survey of the various species of mice, rats, and hamsters for the number and homologies of the MHCAs in each species. The only two species that are known in detail, man and the laboratory mouse, can hardly be regarded as representative of the whole range of mammals. In view of this, it is clear enough that we have a first-class problem in evolutionary biology to elucidate the real meaning of that laboratory artifact, the acceptance or rejection of skin transplants. Quite apart from the genetic mechanisms involved, we have still to find a compelling reason for the evolution of the system.

The curiously simple method of protecting against the occurrence of Rh disease in babies born to Rh-negative wives with Rh-positive husbands is a landmark of preventive medicine, but it has wider biological interest as well. In the first place the disease has nothing to do with histocompatibility antigens. The Rh group of antigens are quite distinct from the HL-A histocompatibility antigens on lymphocytes and most other nucleated cells, and the response they provoke in the mother is simply equivalent to that against any foreign antigen. The effect on the infant is determined only by the level of IgG antibody in the mother's blood, since neither IgM nor sensitized lymphocytes can accompany IgG across the placental barrier.

The protection afforded by antibody against immunization of the mother by fetal red cells may be due in part to blocking of the antigenic determinants on the fetal cells, but, as shown in Clarke's article, most of the protection depends on the rapid removal and destruction of the antigenic material.

18

Skin Transplants

by P. B. Medawar
April 1957

When skin from one man is grafted onto someone other than his identical twin, it soon drops off. The chemical mechanism which interferes with the graft is illuminated by animal experiments

Skin-grafting was introduced into medical practice by Jacques Louis Reverdin, a surgeon in Paris, about 90 years ago. In principle it is quite a simple operation. The skin has two layers: an outer epidermis, consisting of tiers of cells which are constantly replaced from the inside outward, and an inner dermis, or corium, consisting mainly of a latticework of tough connective-tissue fibers, to which skin owes its great strength [*see diagram on page 186*]. The portion sliced off for grafting is made up of the epidermis and the upper part of the dermis. Its transplantation amounts to little more than laying it in place over the area to be repaired and holding it there under light but firm pressure until the dermis becomes knitted to the graft bed below.

The early plastic surgeons supposed that skin could be grafted from one person to another; some of them—victims of heaven-knows-what enormities of self-deception—convinced themselves that even the skin of frogs and rabbits could be transplanted to man. It was not until 1911 that Erich Lexer, in a masterly address before a conference of German surgeons, showed conclusively that skin grafts exchanged between different persons, even between parents and their children, were invariably unsuccessful. The truth of what Lexer said was slowly and grudgingly conceded. Nowadays everyone agrees that skin transplanted from one individual to another will not survive permanently. After a week or so the transplanted skin becomes puffy and inflamed, and soon the graft is sloughed off or drops away. Ordinarily the only kind of graft that will work is an autograft—that is, a transplant of an individual's own skin from one part of his body to another.

One exception to this rule is that skin can be exchanged between identical twins. This test has provided crucial evidence in cases of disputed or uncertain parentage, as two stories will illustrate. The first story, which has the makings of an operatic libretto, is about three six-year-old boys called Victor, Pierre and Eric. Victor and Pierre were supposedly twin brothers, and would still be so regarded if their father (as he imagined himself to be) had not had his attention called to a third boy, Eric, who was the very image of his Victor. Inquiry showed that Eric had been born in the same maternity clinic and on the same night as Victor and Pierre. It seemed likely that Eric was Victor's real twin and that Pierre had been substituted for Eric by mistake. A very careful physical comparison (including a study of fingerprints, eardrum patterns and X-rays of the hands) made it virtually certain that Eric and Victor were identical twins. However, the mother to whom Eric had been allotted did not take kindly to the view that the boy whom she had brought up to the age of six was not in fact her son. Blood-group tests failed to exclude the possibility that Eric might be her son (though they did prove that Pierre could not be Victor's mother's son). It was agreed that a skin-grafting test would be decisive. A surgeon, Sir Archibald McIndoe, transplanted small squares of skin between Eric and Victor and between Victor and Pierre. The grafts exchanged between Pierre and Victor were sloughed off. But Eric and Victor accepted the grafts from each other, a result which proved that they

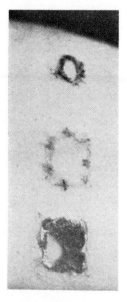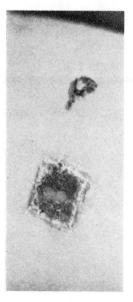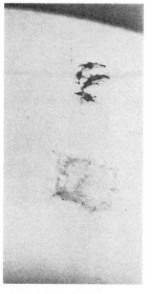

SKIN GRAFTS were made to determine whether two Swiss boys who closely resembled each other had been accidentally interchanged at birth. At left is the arm of Victor; on it are two square skin grafts, one from Eric (*top*) and the other from Pierre (*bottom*). The graft from Pierre has begun to slough off; the graft from Eric has "taken," indicating that Eric and Pierre are twins. In the middle is the arm of Pierre with a graft from Victor; the graft has not taken. At right is the arm of Eric with a graft from Victor; the graft has taken. The study was made by A. Franceschetti, F. Bamatter and D. Klein.

must be identical twins. So Eric and Pierre were restored to their rightful and now satisfied parents, and the story ends happily (which makes it unsuitable for an operatic libretto after all).

The second story is about a mother and daughter and a question of "virgin birth." Members of the staff at University College in London often give lunch-hour lectures which may be attended by the press and the public, and in the course of one such lecture a geneticist gave certain reasons for supposing that parthenogenesis (development of the egg without fertilization) occurred in guppies and might not inconceivably occur in man. (Later evidence indicated that the guppy births were probably a case of self-fertilization.) A section of the press, no doubt animated by a sense of public duty, instituted a campaign to find an authentic example of virgin birth in human beings. In response to an appeal 19 mothers presented themselves with daughters—daughters they must be, for genetic reasons—of allegedly parthenogenetic birth. Eleven who had not quite grasped the import of the idea of virgin birth were at once eliminated; seven more were disqualified by differences between the mother's and daughter's blood types. But there remained one mother whose daughter qualified on blood grouping and certain other grounds. To clear the matter up, skin grafts were transplanted from the mother to the daughter and vice versa.

Both grafts broke down and were sloughed away in a matter of weeks. The failure of the graft transplanted from the daughter to the mother proved that the child must have had a father.

The reaction which causes one individual to reject a graft from another is not a peculiarity of human beings. With the mysterious exception of the hamster, every species of vertebrate so far tested has exhibited this reaction against homografts (i.e., transplants between different individuals of the same species). Nor is the reaction confined to skin, though no other tissue shows it so clearly. W. J. Dempster of the Postgraduate Medical School of London has shown that it applies to a graft of a whole kidney, and it has also been shown to apply to the heart, the lung and even to grafts of tumor tissue. Some parts of the body will accept homografts—for example, the cornea of the eye and the brain—but in these cases special factors are at work.

Plainly the reaction against a graft is an immunological one; i.e., a reaction of the same general kind as that provoked in the body by foreign proteins, foreign red blood cells, or bacteria. This is easily demonstrated by experiments. After a mouse has received and rejected a transplant from another mouse, it will destroy a second graft from the same donor more than twice as rapidly, and in a way which shows that it has been immunologically forearmed. This heightened sensitivity is conferred upon a mouse even when it merely receives an injection of lymph-node cells from a mouse that has rejected a graft.

In most immunological reactions the body employs antibodies as the destroying agent—e.g., in attacking foreign proteins, germs and so on. Antibodies are formed in response to a homograft, but there are reasons to doubt that these are normally the instruments of the reaction against such a graft. Paradoxically enough, a high concentration of circulating antibodies seems if anything to weaken the reaction: it allows the graft to enjoy a certain extra lease of life.

The actual agents of attack on the graft seem to be not antibodies but cells produced by the lymph glands. Some skillfully designed experiments by G. H. Algire, J. M. Weaver and R. T. Prehn at the National Cancer Institute in Bethesda certainly point in that direction. In one experiment they enclosed a homograft in a porous capsule before planting it in a mouse which had been sensitized by an earlier homograft from the same donor. When the pores of the capsule were large enough to let cells through, the mouse destroyed the graft. But when the experimenters used membranes with pores so fine that they kept out cells and let through only fluid, the graft survived.

The hypothesis that the action against a graft is carried out by cells explains why grafts in the cornea are mercifully exempted from attack. The cornea

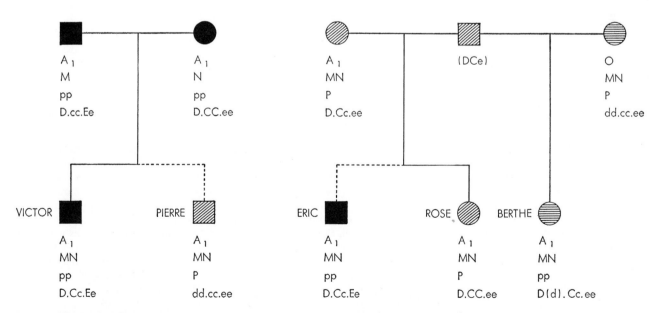

DIAGRAMS OF FAMILIES of the interchanged boys show the blood types of each person involved. The four major blood groupings (A, B, O; M, N; P, pp; and the Rh factors D, d, C, c, E, e) are indicated, with capital letters for dominant traits and small letters for recessive. Pierre could not have inherited dominant trait P from his supposed parents who both show the recessive pp, nor could he have the cc factor if he were the son of the mother (black circle) with two genes for the C trait. Pierre's blood groups are consistent with those of Eric's supposed mother (shaded circle, top center) and with what is known of the father. Eric's father had died, but certain of his blood factors were deduced from those of Berthe, his daughter by a previous marriage. Eric's factors fit with what is known of his supposed parents, but his blood groups are the same as Victor's and fit as well with those of Victor's parents.

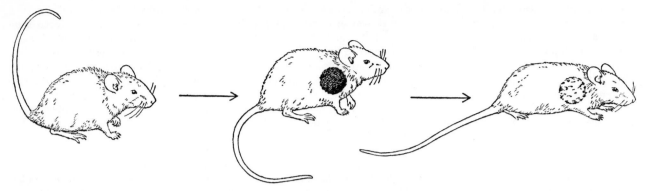

NORMAL WHITE MOUSE (*left*) which receives a skin graft from a brown mouse will reject it. The foreign skin disintegrates in about 10 days' time and falls off (*right*). Grafted skin from any other animal not an extremely close relative will also be rejected.

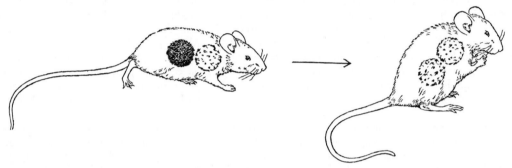

MOUSE WHICH HAS HAD A GRAFT will also reject a second one from the same donor. The second transplant and subsequent ones will disintegrate even more rapidly than the first. This occurs even when many months have passed between grafts.

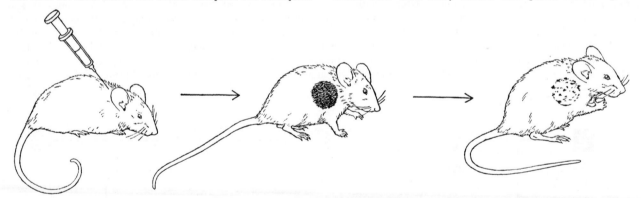

INJECTION OF LYMPH CELLS obtained from mouse which had earlier rejected a graft is administered to a normal mouse. If this mouse later receives a graft from a brown mouse, it will reject the graft as rapidly as the mouse which had had two grafts.

has no blood vessels; consequently blood-borne cells cannot reach the graft. In the brain, on the other hand, the converse of this situation obtains: the brain lacks a lymphatic drainage system, so that any antigens released by a graft there may not be able to travel to centers where they can stir up an immunological response. This probably explains why homografts can often be transplanted successfully into the brain.

For some years past at University College in London R. E. Billingham, L. Brent and I have been studying the cause of the reaction against homografts and steps that can be taken to prevent

it. Following up a clue provided by the work of R. D. Owen at the California Institute of Technology, we discovered that the power to react against homografts could be prevented from developing if we injected an animal at a very early age with cells from the donor strain —most conveniently cells of the spleen. In adult mice the injection of such cells increases the mouse's resistance to a graft from the donor. But if the spleen cells are injected in a mouse in the fetal stage or very shortly after its birth, the opposite happens: the mouse becomes tolerant of grafts from the strain that provided the spleen cells, though it remains intolerant of homografts from

mice of other strains. A tolerant mouse can be recalled to a sense of the fitness of things by injecting it with lymphnode cells from a normal mouse of its own strain. Its tolerance then slowly disappears. The operation seems to equip the tolerant mouse with cells which are competent to recognize and react against foreign substances issuing from the previously tolerated homograft.

This experiment, among others, shows that the tolerance of a homograft is due to absence of specific reactivity in the host, rather than to any change in the properties of the grafted tissue. The antigens are present in the graft, but the animal cannot react to them. The

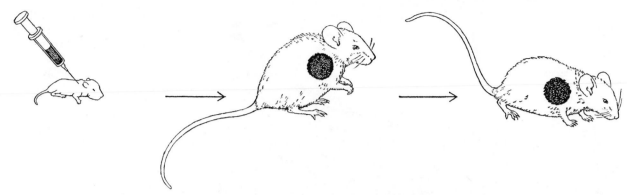

NEWBORN WHITE MOUSE is injected with spleen cells obtained from a brown mouse. If it is grafted later with skin from a brown mouse, the graft will "take" and remain intact for weeks or months just as if it had been taken from another part of the same mouse.

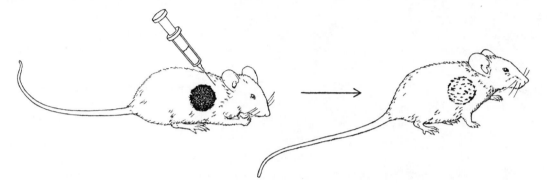

TOLERANT MOUSE, *i.e.*, a mouse which has accepted a graft after having been injected with spleen cells very shortly after birth, is injected with spleen cells from a normal mouse of its own strain. The mouse now rejects the graft it had accepted earlier.

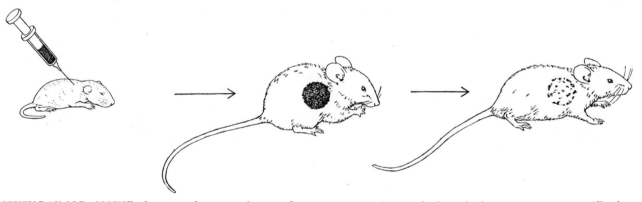

SEVEN-DAY-OLD MOUSE does not become tolerant when injected with spleen cells from a brown mouse. On the con- trary, it rejects grafts from the brown mouse more rapidly than usual. Adult white mice react in the same way to the injection.

phenomenon of tolerance of antigens cannot yet be explained by any chemical theory of the immunological reaction. No future theory will be acceptable unless it can take tolerance in its stride.

What are the tissue antigens that cause an animal to reject a homograft? When we began our work, it was known only that they are very numerous and that they are under the most exact genetic control. While the antigens could not be identified chemically, they could be separated by genetic methods, *i.e.*, by a combination of breeding and grafting tests. E. J. Eichwald and C. R. Silmser at the Deaconess Hospital in Montana have just made the remarkable discovery that, within certain inbred strains of mice, a female will accept a skin homograft from a female, a male from a male and a male from a female, but a female will not take a graft from a male. The discovery raises the possibility that the Y chromosome of male mice, hitherto thought to be concerned only with sexual differentiation, may actually control the formation of an antigen.

The study of the nature of the antigens that cause the homograft reaction is difficult and laborious. Their action cannot be investigated in the test tube but only by effects on living animals. Moreover, the antigens are highly un- stable. Cells which have been frozen and thawed or dried in the frozen state or heated to about 120 degrees Fahrenheit are no longer capable of eliciting a homograft reaction. Fortunately we have discovered ways of disintegrating cells without destroying their antigenic power. For example, with judicious use of ultrasonic radiation we have broken down cells into nuclear and cytoplasmic fractions and found that the antigenic power lies only in the nuclear material.

The antigenic substances in the nucleus are not soluble in water of the same salinity as the body fluid (*i.e.*, about 1 per cent sodium chloride). But they can be coaxed into solution in dis-

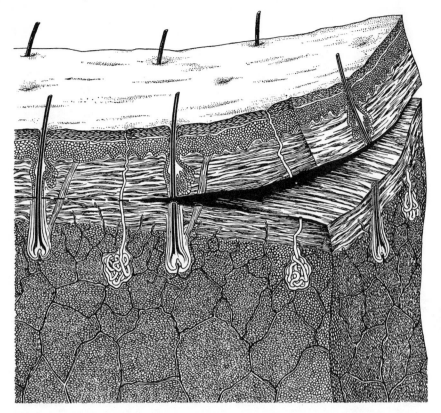

SKIN FOR GRAFTING is sliced off above the root of the hair, through the elastic fibrous tissue of the dermis. The graft then consists of the horny protective epidermis, the layer of growing cells and part of the connective tissue. The main portion of the sweat glands, the hair follicle and fatty tissue remain, and missing parts regenerate from them.

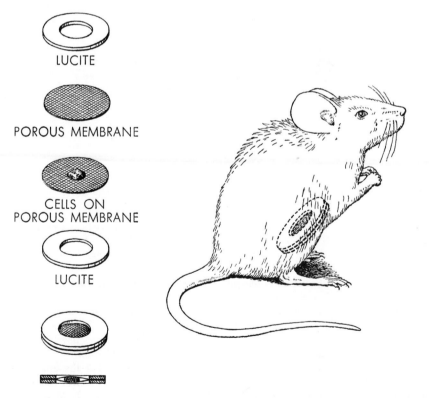

LUCITE

POROUS MEMBRANE

CELLS ON
POROUS MEMBRANE

LUCITE

PERMEABILITY CHAMBER to test the size of graft-rejecting substances is essentially a three-layered sandwich. Cells are placed between membranes of known pore size. Glue made of lucite and acetone holds the membranes together and fastens them to lucite rings. Cross section is shown at bottom left. The chamber is placed in the mouse's abdomen. If antagonistic substances in the mouse pass the membranes, the cells in the chamber are destroyed.

tilled water. After we learned the trick of dissolving them, we found by centrifuging tests that the active substances either were very large molecules or very small particles or were firmly attached to a large molecule or particle. The active matter can be precipitated from the water solution by adding a very small amount of magnesium chloride to the solution. It can be partly redissolved by raising the concentration of magnesium chloride and can then be precipitated again simply by adding water to dilute the solution. I mention these reactions because they have the crispness and clarity that one usually associates with schoolroom chemistry, and because of the commendable frugality of the reagents which we use—water and a number of simple salts.

Our experiments suggest, but do not yet prove, that the antigens responsible for the homograft reaction are compounds of desoxyribonucleic acid and protein—that is, chromosomal matter. Tests on the breakdown of the antigenic substances by specific enzymes support this interpretation. Furthermore, the idea that these antigens are chromosomal matter fits well with evidence that the antigens are present in all the tissues of the body, in embryos and (so it has been said) even in sperm.

Desoxyribonucleic acid itself does not act as an antigen. It is active only in combination with protein. Perhaps the protein part, like the protein coat of a bacterial virus, simply helps the nucleic acid to get into the cells from which it elicits a reaction—in this case, the lymphoid cells of the host. If that is so, the nucleic acid may be the part of the antigen that is specifically responsible for its power to sensitize an animal against the cells of a foreign graft. We have not yet proved this, but the evidence that desoxyribonucleic acid is the chemical embodiment of heredity makes it a plausible guess.

If our interpretation turns out to be true, the study of the antigens that cause the homograft reaction could be of decisive importance in working out the chemical structure of chromosomes, for it would provide a test to determine whether a chromosomal extract has been damaged by the process of extraction. At present no one can be sure, for only in microorganisms do we have biological tests that can guarantee that the nucleic acids are in working order. Our hypothesis has many other deeper and more exciting implications also, but there will be time enough to consider these when we have assured ourselves that the hypothesis is correct.

The Transplantation of the Kidney

19

October 1959

A kidney can be transplanted from one person to another, but the body is normally "immune" to the graft and rejects it. In certain special cases, however, the immune response of the body can be circumvented

If the human body were a simpler sort of mechanism, it might be possible to save many lives by replacing defective organs and tissues with healthy "spare parts" taken from the bodies of donors, either living or recently dead. The blood bank, of course, already functions as an approximation of this idea. Some hospitals also store corneas and sections of blood vessel, both of which can be transplanted by surgery. It is usually impossible, however, to transplant a whole organ such as a kidney, or even to graft skin successfully from one person to another.

The nature of this impasse is suggested by the familiar fact that blood must be "typed" and matched with care if transfusion is to be helpful and not disastrous. The tissue of each individual has its own chemical identity. Upon exposure to foreign tissue it rallies the most powerful defensive mechanism it possesses, the immune response, to destroy and reject the foreign tissue. The apparent exceptions—blood, cornea and blood vessel—each in its way proves the rule. Properly matched blood does not evoke the response, nor does the biologically rather inert corneal tissue. Transplanted blood vessels serve merely as "bridges" to guide the regeneration of the body's own tissue. The successful achievement of true "homografts" thus remains for the present a frontier of experimental surgery and of research in biochemistry and immunology. At the Peter Bent Brigham Hospital and the Harvard Medical School a group of us has been working at this frontier with

results so far that give promise only to the extent that they have added to general understanding of the underlying problems. We work with the kidney, an organ eminently suited for transplantation. Most individuals have two normal kidneys and can live perfectly well with one. The elective surgical removal of one kidney involves little risk, and the surgical connection of the blood vessels of the donated kidney to the vessels of the recipient is generally not prohibitively difficult. Many chronic kidney-diseases are progressive and cannot be arrested by any therapy. Kidney tissue destroyed by disease heals by scarring, and the fibrous scar-tissue in turn tends to destroy more functional units of the organ. Thus the only possible cure often seems to be a new kidney.

E. Ullmann of Vienna made the first attempts to transplant the kidney in experimental animals at the beginning of the century. He was able to remove a kidney from an animal and then restore it to the same animal (an autograft), but could not successfully transplant the organ from one animal to another of the same species (a homograft). In 1908 Alexis Carrel transplanted kidneys in both dogs and cats. He observed that the transplanted kidney was infiltrated with plasma cells, a species of white cell found in the bloodstream. All subsequent observers have noted infiltration by these cells and their next of kin: the lymphocytes. In 1923 C. S. Williamson of the Mayo Clinic attributed the infiltration of the grafted kidney to a "biological incom-

patibility" between donor and recipient.

In an extensive series of investigations beginning in the 1940's, W. J. Dempster, a British experimental surgeon, gave further substance to this concept of biological incompatibility. He knew that it had been demonstrated that a second transplant of skin from one animal to another of the same species was much more speedily rejected than the first. He extended these observations and found that if the animal had been made "immune" to a donor by a skin graft, it would react in the same way to a kidney transplanted from the same donor. By this time it was believed that an important role in the immune response is also played by the so-called antibodies: molecules that are produced by the blood-forming tissues and perhaps also by the white cells and that react with great specificity to foreign molecules. In his microscopic studies Dempster found indications that not only did the host react against the graft; in some cases the kidney graft itself was evincing an immune reaction against the host.

The first attempt to transplant a kidney in man is recorded in Russian medical literature of the 1930's; the effort was not successful. In this country unsuccessful attempts were reported in 1950. In France somewhat later healthy kidneys taken immediately from guillotined criminals failed to survive transplantation into patients chronically ill with uremia.

Our work at Peter Bent Brigham dates from the attempt by Charles A. Huf-

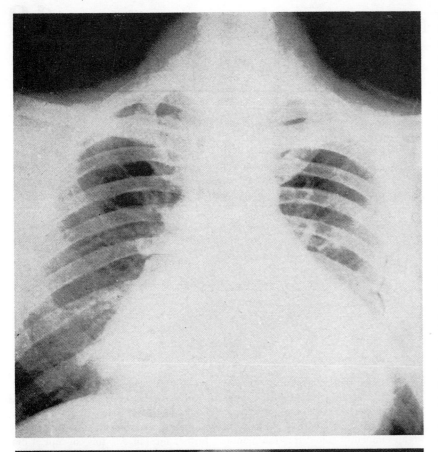

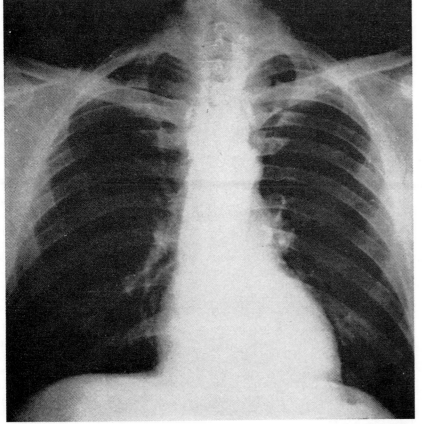

ENLARGED HEART AND FLUID IN CHEST, visible in top radiograph, are signs of severe high blood-pressure and heart failure resulting from kidney disease. The pressure of the fluid interferes with heart action. Bottom radiograph shows return to normal in same patient three weeks after he had received a graft of a kidney from his identical-twin brother.

nagel and Ernest K. Landsteiner to attach a kidney to the arm of a patient acutely ill with uremia. The kidney secreted a few drops of urine but never developed measurable function. The patient, however, recovered from her attack of acute kidney failure. In 1955 David M. Hume, Benjamin F. Miller, George W. Thorn and I reported our experience in nine similar procedures. All of the patients were terminally ill and required treatment with artificial kidneys. Indeed, without the artificial kidney we could not have undertaken this procedure in patients as sick as these. The transplanted kidneys came from patients who had died of chronic heart disease. In eight cases we grafted the kidney into a "pocket" fashioned in the skin on the middle of the upper thigh. We connected the blood vessels of the kidney to the vessels of the thigh. The ureter, the tube that drains urine from the kidney into the bladder, was led to an opening in the skin. Three considerations prompted the placing of the kidney in this bizarre position: the surgical procedure was somewhat less extensive than placing it in the abdomen; we could measure urine as it came directly from the kidney, thus avoiding the complicating factor of the output of the two defective kidneys; and we could more easily remove the kidney if the procedure failed or if the kidney became infected, leaving the patient certainly no worse than before. Four of the nine transplanted kidneys functioned; two did so well that the patients had some relief of symptoms. In one of the two patients, a South American physician with severe uremia and high blood-pressure, the kidney functioned for five and a half months before it failed; the patient was even able to leave the hospital for three months.

These results in human patients were far more encouraging than experiments with animals had led us to expect. In dogs grafted kidneys had functioned for only five to 12 days; then blood appeared in the urine and the kidneys suddenly failed. Moreover, microscopic examination revealed that the changes in the transplanted human kidneys were much less drastic than those in the dog. At first we thought that the species difference between dogs and men might account for the difference in behavior of the transplants.

In 1953, however, I was fortunate enough to be in Paris to observe a case in which a kidney had been transplanted. A healthy young man had fallen from a roof and severely injured a kid-

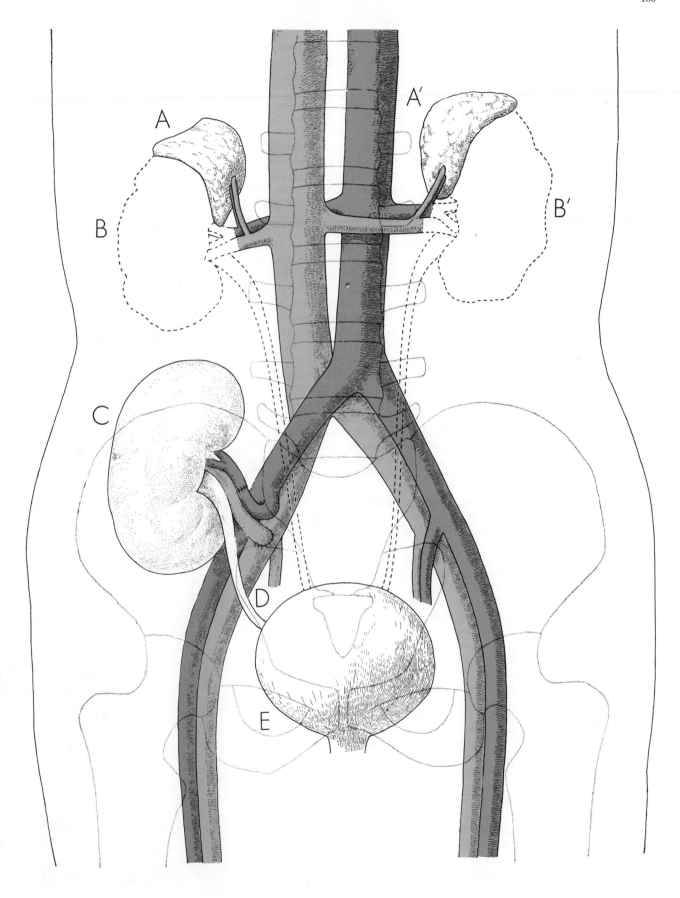

TRANSPLANTED KIDNEY (C) is placed in the abdominal cavity as shown in this diagram. Its blood vessels are attached to nearby vein and artery. Ureter (D) is implanted in bladder (E).

The defective kidneys (B and B′), indicated by broken lines, are removed, while the adrenal glands (A and A′), normally located on top of the kidneys, are left in place in the patient.

ney, which was then removed by a surgeon in a hospital outside of Paris. Unfortunately the kidney turned out to be the only one the patient possessed. A week later surgeons in Paris transplanted a kidney into the young man from his mother. The immediate results were striking. The kidney began to form urine and functioned well for three weeks, greatly decreasing uremia and improving the patient's condition. But on the 21st day blood appeared in the urine and soon the kidney stopped functioning.

In the post-mortem examination we found that this kidney, transplanted from a healthy donor into a previously healthy recipient, had behaved very much like the grafted dog kidneys. The microscopic picture was almost identical. We now realized that the difference between grafted dog and human kidneys that we had observed had stemmed not from any species difference but from the fact that we had transplanted kidneys from chronically ill individuals into other chronically ill individuals. Our sick subjects apparently did not react as violently against sick kidneys as healthy subjects (or dogs) do against healthy kidneys. Skin grafts to chronically ill uremic patients confirmed this deduction; the grafts survived seven to 10 times as long as those on normal healthy recipients. Apparently the general depression of body function in these patients also depresses the immune response to the homograft.

At this juncture we listed our accomplishments: We had acquired a good deal of technical experience in transplanting kidneys and in the care of critically ill uremic patients, and we had learned that the immune response was not so violent in chronically ill people.

In 1954 we were confronted with a unique opportunity to apply this experience. David Miller, an alert physician in a nearby U. S. Public Health Service hospital, was caring for a young veteran who was dying of severe kidney failure and high blood-pressure. A daily visitor to his bedside was his apparently identical twin. Miller knew of our work on kidney transplantation. He also knew that biological incompatibility was the reason transplantation of tissues generally failed. He reasoned that if the two young men were identical twins, their tissues might not be biologically incompatible. As is well known, identical twins develop from a single fertilized egg; they not only resemble each other in appearance but also have a high degree of bio-

logical identity. What is more, skin transplants between identical twins have succeeded. With these considerations in mind Miller referred the patient and his brother to the Peter Bent Brigham Hospital.

To be sure that these twins were identical we transplanted skin from each to the other. Knowing that such a transplant might "take" for a prolonged period (though not permanently) in the sick twin, we were especially concerned to observe the result in the healthy twin. Both grafts took normally. Although this was the critical test, we thoroughly investigated other significant similarities that might confirm identical inheritance. A geneticist carefully compared the boys' facial features, iris color and pattern, hair color and form, shape of the ears and even taste similarities. A hematologist found their blood groups identical in all the major categories and in 20 separate subcategories. Extensive examinations convinced us that the healthy twin was free from all kidney and other diseases. Thus we had adequate medical and genetic bases for proceeding with the transplantation.

On the other hand, we had no precedent for the removal of a perfectly normal kidney from a healthy individual, and this consideration weighed heavily in our deliberations. Meanwhile the sick twin grew sicker. His uremia became so bad that it required treatment with an artificial kidney; his blood pressure continued to rise, with dangerous effects upon his heart and blood vessels. Finally, two days before Christmas, 1954, a normal kidney was removed from the donor twin by J. Hartwell Harrison and transplanted by Joseph E. Murray into the sick recipient.

Murray placed this kidney not in the thigh but in the hollow of the pelvis, inside the abdominal cavity, where its surroundings resembled its normal habitat [see illustration on page 189]. He connected the kidney's artery to a branch of the large iliac artery and its vein to a vein in the pelvic cavity through which blood flows from one leg. The operation cut off the blood supply of the healthy kidney for almost an hour. In spite of this delay, when the clamp was released from the artery to which the grafted kidney was attached the kidney became a healthy pink, and within minutes urine began to drip slowly from the end of the ureter. Murray thereupon implanted the ureter directly into the bladder so that the urine would drain normally. In this case we wanted no possibility of technical failure to compromise our very real

chance to avoid the immunologic barrier.

By the time the patient had left the operating room, urine was definitely flowing, and over the succeeding days and weeks the kidney gradually improved its function. The patient's uremia cleared up; his appetite and mental processes improved. Then—and this was beyond our expectation—we observed a drop in blood pressure. Six weeks after the transplantation we performed two operations, the first to remove one of the patient's diseased kidneys and the second to remove the other kidney. Following the second operation the blood pressure at last fell to normal, where it has remained ever since. All signs of heart

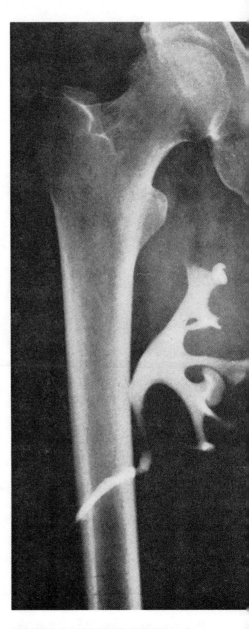

KIDNEY GRAFT INTO THIGH is shown in radiograph and diagram. The femur, the

strain and hemorrhage from smaller blood vessels soon disappeared.

This was a dividend we had not fully anticipated. The role of the damaged kidney in causing high blood-pressure had been investigated in experimental animals for many years. This case provided the first opportunity to study in a human subject the kidney's role in high blood-pressure by first adding a normal kidney in the presence of two diseased ones and then removing the diseased kidneys in separate operations. We have now been able to make the same observations in six successful kidney transplants between identical twins; in each

case the sick twin was a victim of severe hypertension.

Since 1954 we have transplanted a total of 13 kidneys between identical twins. Each of the 13 recipients had been terminally ill with uremia; 10 are alive and healthy today.

The kidney is of course one of the most complex organs in the body. It not only disposes of wastes but also delicately regulates the content and balance in the blood of salts and other substances. Our 10 successful transplants show that it can continue to do so in a totally different location in a different individual. Furthermore, the kidney functions even though its nerve connections are sev-

ered. This was indicated some time ago in animal-kidney autografts, and has been proved by our successful human transplants.

The moral problem of taking a healthy kidney from a healthy donor is acute, we feel, when the twins are minors. In such cases we have asked court permission to perform the graft. Permission has been granted on the ground that the healthy child would suffer more from the psychical loss of his twin than from the physiological loss of a kidney that can be spared.

The graft failed in one of our 13 cases because a congenital abnormality of the blood vessels in the donated kidney pre-

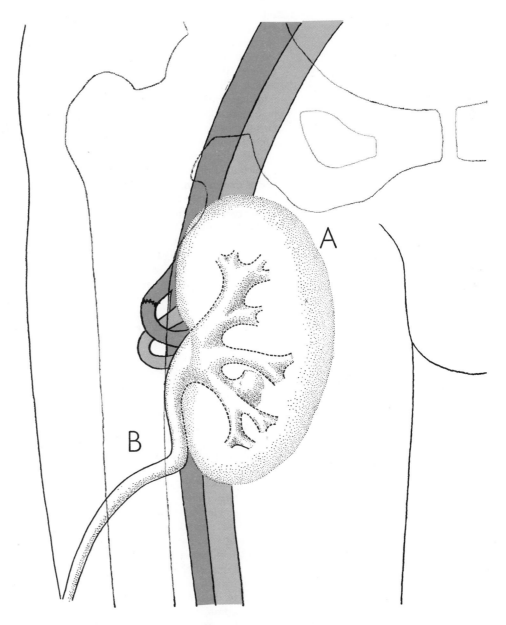

ureter and the kidney's pelvis and calyxes are visible in the radiograph. Diagram shows the ureter (B) and the renal cortex (A) as well as the blood-vessel connections of grafted kidney. Eight early grafts were done in this way in case grafted kidney had to be removed.

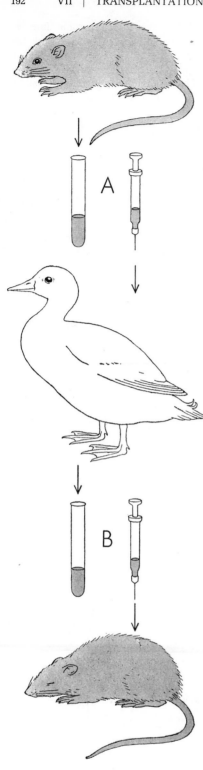

BRIGHT'S DISEASE IN RAT is produced by injecting extract of rat kidney (A) into a duck, which produces antibodies against this foreign tissue. Duck antibodies (B) injected into the rat now mask rat's kidneys; rat's antibody system attacks its own kidneys because they seem to be "foreign tissue."

vented them from fitting the vessels of the recipient. The other two deaths, following initially successful transplantation, gave us a critically important insight into the working of the immune response.

We found that these two patients had died because their transplanted kidney developed the nephritis (Bright's disease) from which they had suffered before the operation. Why was this finding important? For many years workers have been able to produce in animals a disease that appears to be the equivalent of human nephritis. To do this they make a serum from ground-up rat kidney and inject it into a rabbit. The immune response in the rabbit produces antibodies against this foreign material. When serum from the rabbit's blood is injected into the rat, the antibodies attack the rat's kidneys, causing the disorder that so resembles nephritis. A condition even closer to human nephritis is produced by injecting the ground-up rat kidney into a duck. When the duck serum is injected into the rat, the duck antibodies somehow mask the rat's kidneys so that the rat's tissues no longer "recognize" them. The rat then produces antibodies that act against its own kidneys.

Such investigations had strongly suggested that in human nephritis the body has formed antibodies against the kidneys. Proof of this hypothesis, however, had been lacking. Now we had transplanted normal kidneys into patients with nephritis, and had seen these kidneys contract the disease. Apparently in man, as well as in the rat, either antibodies circulating in the blood plasma or sensitized lymphocyte white cells had attacked the grafted kidney. Since skin grafts had taken in both of our cases, we knew that the attack upon the transplanted kidneys was no ordinary immune reaction to a graft.

The identical-twin grafts have demonstrated that where an immunological barrier does not exist kidneys can be successfully transplanted to cure otherwise incurable kidney and vascular disease. This limited success in surgery furnishes an additional motive for investigation of the immunological barrier, which is a problem of great fascination in itself. From long experience with skin grafts, investigators have a clear picture of the normal course of the immune response. A piece of skin from one person transplanted to the forearm of another will assume a firm, healthy appearance for several days as blood vessels grow into it. Four to five days after transplanta-

tion, however, the small vessels begin to be plugged, the skin becomes discolored in a patchy fashion and the skin cells become necrotic and die, to be overgrown by the epithelial cells of the host's skin. After this the host will react much faster in rejecting a new skin transplant from the same donor. This acceleration in the reaction suggests that the recipient's tissues have in some way learned to "recognize" as foreign the tissue from the donor.

The recognition system involves the reticuloendothelial tissues of the body, which are found in the bone marrow, in the lymphatic system and spleen and in the liver. These are the blood-forming tissues and also the generators of the immune response, as the source both of white cells and of antibodies. In some way contact with antigens produced by a graft of foreign tissue "teaches" the reticuloendothelial system to recognize the foreign material. After the "lesson" by a first graft from a particular individual, the system is sensitized and the rejection of any subsequent graft of any kind of tissue from that individual is speeded up.

One tortuous detour around the immune response is suggested by the fact that the response is not fully developed in many animals until after birth. Thus day-old chicks may tolerate skin grafts from other chicks. In rats this neutral period when skin grafts may be accepted can extend to as late as 10 days after birth. The maturing reticuloendothelial system of the young animal is still learning to recognize the tissues of the animal; a hypothetical "self-marker" in these tissues presumably tells the reticuloendothelial system not to develop antibodies to them. R. E. Billingham and P. B. Medawar of University College London have injected the spleen cells of brown mice into embryonic white mice and found that as adults these white mice tolerated skin grafts from brown mice [see "Skin Transplants," by P. B. Medawar, the article beginning on page 182]. The immature recognition system of the embryonic mice apparently accepted the foreign cells as having the "self-marker."

In solving the problem of tissue transplantation in man, however, we do not expect to make popular the injection of cells from a prospective donor into the human fetus. There is another approach that is receiving consideration. This is the destruction or incapacitation of the crucial centers of the reticuloendothelial system by means of total body irradiation, followed by the transplantation of bone marrow. The idea is to obliterate the patient's own recognition system and replace it with one compatible with the tissue to be grafted. The feasibility of this admittedly heroic procedure has been supported by limited success in terminal cases of leukemia, in which the massive irradiation is, of course, directed to the destruction of malignant cells. In experimental animals destruction of the bone marrow by radiation has made it possible to graft marrow and other tissues not only from other animals but from animals of a different species!

We have attempted to use this procedure in two terminal cases of kidney disease to condition the patient for transplantation of a kidney. In both cases the bone-marrow transplant eventually failed. Indeed, there is no evidence from the world's medical literature that transplanted bone marrow has ever functioned in man for more than a few weeks.

Recently we have attempted another experiment that combines experience both with irradiation and with the reduced intensity of the immune response in chronically ill patients that we had noted in our first series of kidney grafts. This experiment also applies the knowledge, gained from more recent work with experimental animals, that a large dose of antigen introduced into the bloodstream may produce tolerance to foreign tissue where a small dose excites the immune response. We transplanted a kidney from a healthy man to his critically uremic brother. Though the men were probably not identical twins, we hoped that their relationship might make for some immunologic compatibility. The recipient was chronically and dangerously ill, and he was given a total dose of X-rays large enough to depress his reticuloendothelial tissues severely. Immediately after the last irradiation, the kidney was transplanted. A transplanted kidney of course introduces a large dose of antigen directly into the bloodstream. As the patient's reticuloendothelial system recovers from the radiation, it may be forced to become familiarized with the antigens of the transplanted kidney and accept them as carrying a "self-marker," after the precedents in research with animals. It is as yet too early to evaluate the results of this transplant, but initially it appears to be successful. Obviously the combination of circumstances favoring its success is unusual. The general principles, however, are universal, and give us some idea of the way in which not only kidneys but other living tissues may eventually be routinely transplanted.

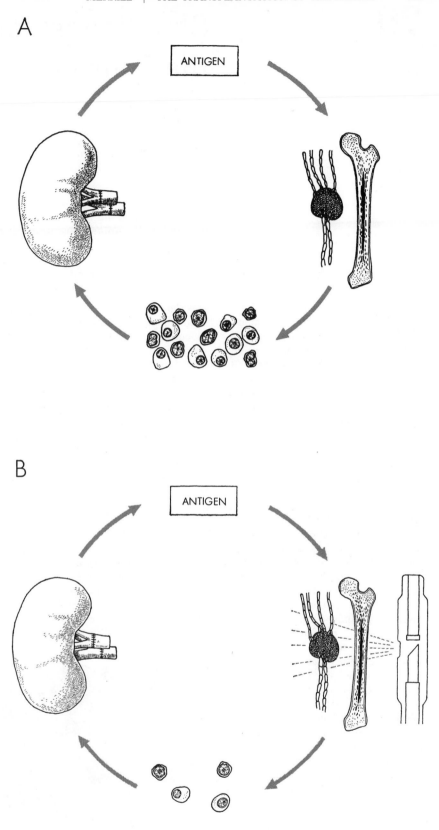

IMMUNE RESPONSE TO GRAFTED TISSUE is diagrammed. The transplanted kidney in diagram A produces large quantities of an antigen that arouses and "teaches" the antibody and white-cell system to recognize this foreign tissue. Then antibodies and scavenger cells attack grafted tissue. Diagram B indicates that X-rays suppress antibody system of bone marrow and lymph nodes (right), reducing the immune response to the transplanted kidney.

20

Skin Transplants and the Hamster

by Rupert E. Billingham and Willys K. Silvers
January 1963

This familiar laboratory rodent is an anomaly of the animal kingdom in several respects, not least of which is the unique hospitality it shows to many kinds of foreign-tissue grafts

A fairly recent addition to the select number of small mammals that have been domesticated for laboratory use is the Syrian, or golden, hamster. About midway between the mouse and the rat in size, reasonably placid, clean and prolific, it is easy to maintain and handle. These virtues alone would account for its growing population and numbers, now estimated at 100,000, in laboratories around the world. The hamster does special service, however, in those lines of investigation that involve the transplanting of tissue from one animal to another: studies of cancer, aging, endocrine function and, of course, the immunological reaction that ordinarily brings about the rejection, or "sloughing off," of a tissue graft. To make other species serve this purpose requires the mating of brothers to sisters over many generations to produce at last a stock of individuals with the genetic compatibility of identical twins; decreasing fecundity of the breeding line is only one of the hazards that can bring such an inbreeding program to a halt. Among the members of any laboratory colony of hamsters, in contrast, one usually finds that a high proportion of individuals will exchange tissue grafts. In addition, it is fairly easy to inbreed a strain for full compatibility. More remarkable still, the cheek pouch of the hamster, in which it collects and transports food in nature, will accept grafts not only from other hamsters but also from other mammals and even from animals as alien as the frog.

Plainly the hamster is deserving of investigation in its own right. At the Wistar Institute of Anatomy and Biology in Philadelphia we have over the past several years established the genetic basis of the animal's remarkable receptivity to homografts—grafts from genetically unrelated members of its species. Our findings show that the hamster presents one of the simplest instances of the working of one of the many different genetic mechanisms that underlie the uniqueness of the individual at the biochemical level. The cheek pouch is another matter entirely. The receptivity of this tissue environment to heterografts—grafts from members of other species—as well as homografts is not yet explained in full or with certainty. It may hold a clue to the nature of the barriers that insulate tissues and glands that have distinctive biochemical constituents from one another in the body—barriers that break down in certain rare cases of autoimmunological disease.

Although the Syrian, or golden, hamster has come to be known as "the hamster," it is one of three species—along with the European black-bellied hamster and the Chinese gray hamster—that have been brought into the laboratory. In nature it is one of 66 varieties or subspecies distributed over the Eurasian continent. Belonging to the mouse group in the large order of rodents, hamsters are formally designated as the family Cricetidae. They dwell in deep, chambered burrows in which they hoard grain and other vegetable foodstuffs foraged from the field at night. As a result of their short gestation period of 16 days, the large size of their litters and the early sexual maturation of the female, at four weeks, these animals have a remarkably high rate of reproduction and are considered a pest in agricultural lands.

Of all the hamsters, the Syrian is one of the most narrowly restricted in natural habitat, being confined to the Mediterranean side of Asia Minor. It was first identified as a species (*Mesocricetus auratus auratus*) in 1839 by the British naturalist George R. Waterhouse, who obtained a single characteristically fawn-colored specimen from Aleppo in Syria. It was not until 1930, when I. Aharoni

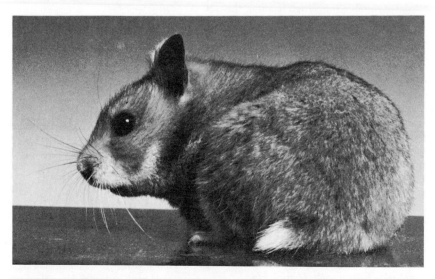

GOLDEN HAMSTER is a relative newcomer to the laboratory. All domesticated hamsters are descended from a single litter found in Syria in 1930. As a result of their recent common ancestry different laboratory stocks of hamsters may be very closely related genetically.

of the Hebrew University in Jerusalem captured a litter from a deep burrow, that this hamster began to attain a more cosmopolitan distribution. All the domestic stocks of the animal are descendants of one male and two females of Aharoni's original litter.

The Adam-and-Eve-like origin of the laboratory hamster suggests itself as the first explanation for the animal's acceptance of homografts. As recent successes in surgery have advertised, tissue grafts and even organ grafts have been successfully exchanged between identical twins [see "The Transplantation of the Kidney," by John P. Merrill, the article beginning on page 187]. Identical twins, in consequence of their derivation from a single fertilized egg cell, have exactly the same genetic and biochemical constitution. Grafts exchanged between them are more properly termed isografts. Foreign tissue in the form of a homograft or heterograft, on the other hand, elicits the build-up of a state of specific resistance in the host's body—an immunological reaction—and the total destruction of the graft as a living entity follows. Not being represented in the host's own body, certain constituents of the foreign tissue are antigenic, just as foreign blood proteins and pathogenic organisms are. The tissues of the host—specifically the tissues of the host's lymphatic system—respond by producing the complementary proteins, called antibodies, that neutralize the antigens.

In the case of the heterograft the foreign proteins are more diversely and powerfully antigenic and provoke a correspondingly powerful antibody response. Skin grafts exchanged between adult mice and rats or between hamsters

and rabbits normally heal in feebly, acquire a poor and transient blood supply and suffer complete cell death within a week. Although homografts also provoke antibodies in the host, these do not appear to play any significant role in the destruction of the graft. The transplanted tissue develops a better blood supply and gives the appearance of "taking" before it breaks down. The agents that attack and destroy the homograft seem to be lymphocytes: white cells produced by the lymph nodes and carried to the site of action in the blood. In this respect homograft immunity appears to be related to the similar immunity (here meaning sensitivity) that is built up in the human body in response to poison ivy and certain chemical agents [see "Delayed Hypersensitivity," by Alfred J. Crowle, the article beginning on page 81].

Recent research indicates that the transplantation antigens liberated by homografts are lipoproteins—proteins with a lipid, or fatty, molecular constituent—and that they are associated with membranous structures of the cell. Furthermore, like the antigens involved in blood-group incompatibilities, transplantation antigens are determined by multiple dominant genes, termed histocompatibility (tissue compatibility) genes. The tedious and uncertain process of inbreeding, which must be carried through at least 20 consecutive generations, is necessary to produce uniform populations for transplantation experiments. In such a stock, or strain, every member has the same genetic constitution, including, of course, identical complements of histocompatibility genes. Obviously the distinctive genetic consti-

tution of an inbred strain will depend on the genetic constitution of the particular base-line breeding pair from which it was initially derived. Thus members of different inbred strains of entirely independent origins may differ from one another just as much as do randomly selected individuals from an outbred, or wild, population.

The discovery that members of an ordinary breeding colony of hamsters would exchange tissue grafts successfully was made quite by accident in 1939, when the animal was still a newcomer to the laboratory. Investigators at the Imperial Cancer Research Fund Laboratories in London were surprised to find that they could transplant tumors from one animal to another with a high degree of success. Independent studies by Richard A. Adams and his colleagues at Boston University and by William H. Hildemann and Rupert E. Billingham, coauthor of the present article, confirmed that homograft rejection occurred far less frequently in the hamster than in other species. They found, in fact, that the majority of grafts exchanged among members of noninbred stocks were usually accepted for long periods, if not permanently, in perfectly healthy condition. It looked almost as though the hamster's immunological machinery for reacting against homografts was not fully developed. This possibility was set aside, however, by the observation that homografts exchanged between some donor-recipient combinations were rejected in a prompt and orthodox manner. The high degree of compatibility to homografts displayed by these animals was therefore to be regarded not only as a

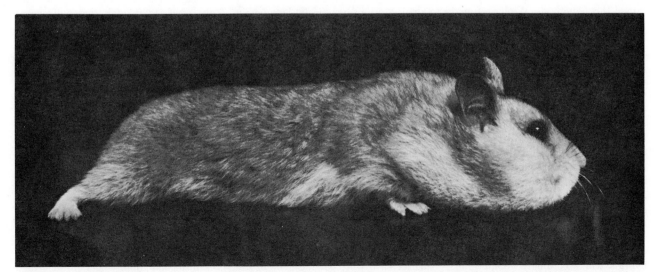

CHEEK POUCHES of the hamster in this photograph have been stuffed with cotton wool to demonstrate their great storage capacity when fully distended. Normally the pouches are used to transport large quantities of food to the rodent's elaborate underground burrow. The hamster's parsimonious habits are the source of its common name: *hamstern* in German means "to store or to hoard."

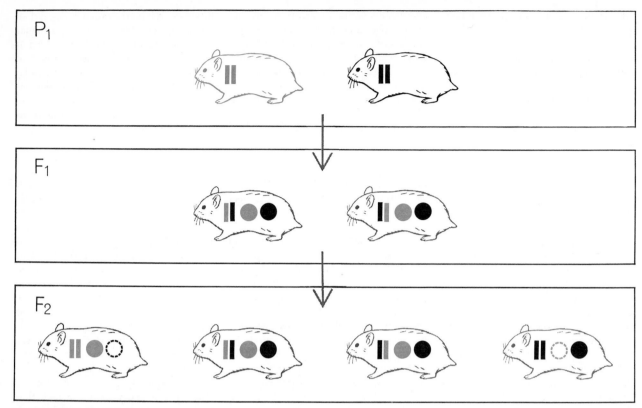

DIFFERENCE OF ONE GENE between an original (P_1) breeding pair will result in four possible genetic combinations in the chromosomes of the second-generation (F_2) hybrids. Of these, three will receive at least one specific antigen-producing gene from one of the P_1 grandparents and consequently will tolerate a skin graft taken from any member of the inbred strain to which that grandparent happened to belong. The fourth will reject such a graft, since the antigens received from it would be foreign to this hybrid's own genetically determined set. The same situation of course holds true for grafts taken from the other P_1 strain. Regardless of the number of genes by which any P_1 pair differs, all first-generation (F_1) offspring will accept a graft donated by a member of either P_1 strain.

convenience for the investigator but also as a question for investigation.

The most obvious hypothesis was that the genetic constitutions of the laboratory hamsters are differentiated at relatively few histocompatibility loci—these being locations on the chromosomes at which alternative histocompatibility genes may occur in different individuals. Work in our laboratory has recently confirmed this hypothesis. We have found, in fact, that the laboratory hamsters, at least, have only three such loci.

The making of such a determination for any laboratory animal begins with the crossing of two isogenic lines. The members of each such line have two identical sets of chromosomes (44 chromosomes in all), so that each histocompatibility gene is present in duplicate. When the lines are crossed, the first-generation hybrids (F_1) inherit one complete set of chromosomes, including all the histocompatibility genes, from each parent. Since these genes are codominant, the histocompatibilities of both lines are expressed in the make-up of the offspring. The F_1 hybrids will accordingly accept grafts from either parental strain. When the F_1 hybrids produce their sperm and egg cells, however, they likewise pass on only a single set of chromosomes (22 altogether). Each chromosome of this set will be an exact replica of each of the chromosomes present in one or the other of the original isogenic parental strains, but which chromosome will come from which strain is a matter of chance. The second-generation offspring (F_2) produced by the matings of the F_1 individuals are thus genetically heterogeneous, in particular bearing all possible combinations of the histocompatibility genes present in the two original parental strains. Some percentage of F_2 offspring will inherit all the histocompatibility genes of one or the other original strain. This percentage is predictable and depends on the number of histocompatibility genes by which the strains differ from each other. If they differ by only a single gene, as, for example, when one is AA and the other A'A', then out of the four possible combinations into which the original pairs of genes can be reassorted, half will bear the codominant histocompatibility genes of both parental strains (AA') and a quarter each will bear the gene of one or the other (AA or A'A').

As a result 75 per cent of the F_2 generation will accept grafts from either strain—a different 75 per cent in each case. If two loci are involved, 56 per cent will show histocompatibility with one or the other strain. Provided that each gene is passed on independently and provided that the antigen determined by each is singly sufficient to elicit the immune reaction to the homograft in a host that lacks this gene, the percentage of F_2 individuals that will accept grafts from one or the other parental strain can be shown by the laws of probability to be equal to $(.75)^n$. The exponential n is simply the number of histocompatibility loci at which the parental strains differ. By challenging a fairly large number of F_2 animals with grafts from their parental strains and determining the percentage that accept them, the value of n can be calculated from the equation. Since $(.75)^2$ equals .56, for example, the finding that 56 per cent accept grafts from one or the other strain can be taken as an indication that two histocompatibility loci are involved. It is apparent that this procedure can only give some idea of the minimum number of histocompatibility loci present in a species. Experiments conducted with inbred strains of mice and rats have indicated that these species have at least 15 such loci.

For our work with hamsters we inbred three strains, bringing each in a few generations to complete histocompatibility, as evidenced by the consistent, long-term acceptance of intrastrain homografts. What is more, the invariable rejection by each strain of grafts from the other two showed that these strains differed from one another with respect to their histocompatibility genes.

When we carried out grafting tests of F_2 hybrids in different combinations of these strains, the results indicated that tissue-graft incompatibility between the three strains depended on differences in genes present at no more than three loci. The alternative genes at only one of these loci appear to be of major importance in that they determine the production of antigens strong enough to cause the rejection of a graft within two weeks.

One obvious explanation for the paucity of histocompatibility genes in the hamster is that Aharoni's original breeding trinity was almost, if not completely, uniform at least with respect to their

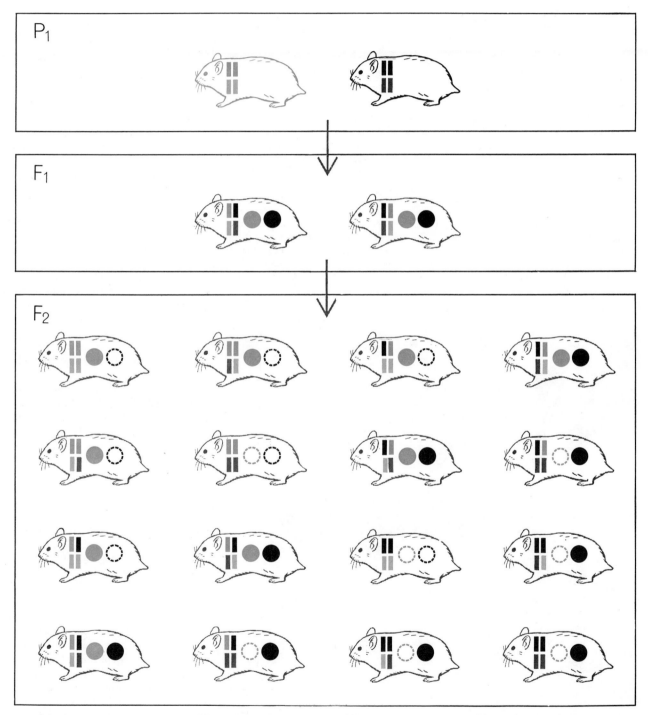

DIFFERENCE OF TWO GENES between P_1 progenitors will result in 16 possible genetic combinations in the F_2 generation. In this case nine of the 16, or 56.2 per cent, will accept a graft from one of the P_1 strains. Four will accept a graft from either P_1 strain and two from neither. The F_1 generation will again accept either P_1 graft. By working backward from the observed percentage of successful P_1 to F_2 transplants, the authors have been able to determine a maximum possible histocompatibility gene difference between random combinations of P_1 hamsters equal to only three factors. By contrast, mice and rats differ by at least 15 factors.

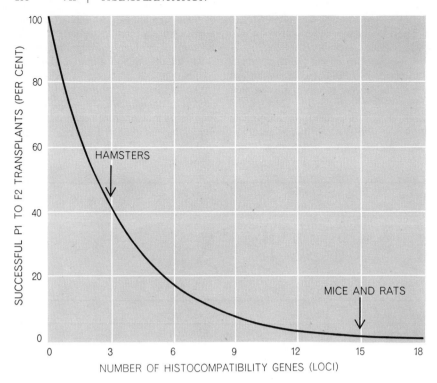

DISPARITY between the hamster's homograft compatibility and that of some closely related rodents is illustrated in this graph. At least 40 per cent of the hamsters tested accepted P_1 to F_2 transplants, whereas no more than 1 per cent of such grafts succeeded in the case of mice and rats. All higher mammals, including man, differ by more than 15 histocompatibility gene factors and accordingly accept fewer than 1 per cent of all P_1 to F_2 transplants.

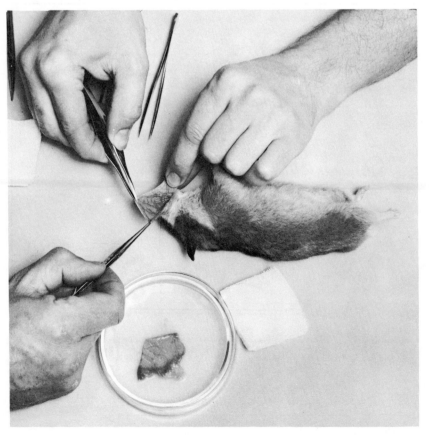

CHEEK POUCHES ARE EVERTED by grasping their deep ends with a pair of forceps and withdrawing them through the hamster's mouth. In this position they are useful for studies of their rich blood circulation and also as convenient graft sites. Excised pouches, such as the one shown in the dish here, can also be test-grafted onto the bodies of other hamsters.

complement of these genes. Even if this were the case, however, one might have expected that a number of histocompatibility mutations would have occurred during the domestic history of the species. An appreciable number of mutations affecting eye and coat color have been observed in laboratory colonies. Current experiments with hamsters of a different subspecies, *Mesocricetus auratus brandti,* captured for us in Kurdistan, suggest that a high degree of compatibility to homografts may be a characteristic of this subspecies as well as of *M. auratus auratus* and perhaps of other members of the Cricetidae family too. The paucity of histocompatibility genes in the domesticated Syrian hamsters would thus reflect the situation in wild populations. The only other mammal that is known to show a tolerance approaching that of the hamster is the Mongolian gerbil (*Meriones unguiculatus*), a rodent only recently recruited to the laboratory.

From early in the hamster's laboratory career investigators were attracted by the potential usefulness of its cheek pouches. These are tubular prolongations of the animal's cheek cavities that run backward beneath the skin of the shoulder regions. They are lined by a continuation of the mucous membrane of the mouth and have a rich blood supply. When empty, they are three to five centimeters long and a centimeter wide, but they can be distended by food to more than twice this size. Because of the loosely packed, highly elastic connective tissue that unites the wall of the pouch to the adjacent tissues of the cheek, one can easily evert the pouch by grasping its "blind" (inner) end with forceps. Stretched out on a block of glass and transilluminated, the relatively thin sheet of hairless skin provides an excellent preparation for studies of the blood circulation in its rich plexus of vessels. Indeed, it is almost as useful for such purposes as the web of the frog's foot, the wing of the bat or the tail of the tadpole. When released, the pouch returns to its normal position by muscular contraction.

Investigators soon found that the pouch tissue is a hospitable site for tissue grafts. Small pieces of tumor tissue from other hamsters rapidly acquire a blood supply and begin to grow upon insertion in a tiny incision in the pouch. Such grafts can readily be inspected *in situ* under the microscope, and specimens can be removed for study or transplantation to other hamsters. Even small numbers of dissociated tumor cells may give rise to a solid tumor mass upon simple injection into the pouch wall.

In the course of such experiments it was found that the pouch will invariably accept homografts without regard to the strain of the donor hamster and will not infrequently accept heterografts for experimentally useful periods of time. Since grafts of either type were rejected from other sites in the same animal or in others of its strain, some factor other than the hamster's paucity of histocompatibility genes was indicated. The cheek pouch was somehow immunologically privileged. It was clear that foreign-tissue grafts in this environment either were insulated from the consequences of the immunological response or failed to evoke a fully effective response. Examples of such immunological privilege are well known. Cartilage typifies privilege of the first sort; because it requires little by way of a blood supply and enters into minimal exchanges with the body of the host, a cartilage homograft is protected from whatever response it evokes in the host. The brain is an immunologically privileged site of the second kind. Grafts implanted in the cerebral cortex derive a rich blood supply from it but often fail to elicit an immune response. The reason for this, apparently, is that the brain has no lymphatic drainage system. In the absence of the pathway that carries the antigenic stimulus from other sites in the body to the lymph nodes— the seat of the immunological response —a graft in the brain does not excite the production of antibodies and immunologically activated lymphocytes.

Upon reflection we decided that the situation here might resemble that in

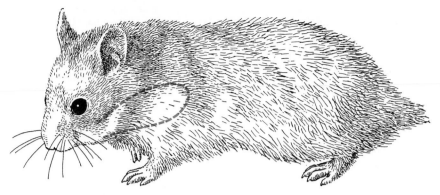

LOCATION OF EMPTY CHEEK POUCH is indicated in this drawing by the broken line. When full, as in the photograph on page 195, the volume of the pouch is more than doubled.

the brain. We quickly found confirmation of this hypothesis. Homografts from an incompatible strain that had become well established in an animal's pouch could be destroyed by challenging the animal with a skin graft on the chest or simply with an injection of cells from the same strain. Furthermore, prior immunization of an animal by the same means would prevent a subsequent graft from becoming established in the cheek pouch. Once a state of immunity has been evoked, in other words, it can express itself just as effectively in the pouch as elsewhere in the body. The hospitality of the pouch to foreign tissue must therefore depend on some barrier that keeps the antigens liberated by a graft in the pouch from gaining access to the host's seat of immunological response.

In search of insight into the specific nature of the barrier, we now prepared relatively large grafts of pouch "skin" and transplanted them to prepared sites

on hamsters' chests. The grafts from donors to recipients of the same strain healed in rapidly, acquired a rich blood supply (indicated by their healthy pink color) and were permanently accepted, as one might anticipate. To our gratified surprise, pouch skin grafts between strains known to be incompatible for ordinary skin grafts healed in just as promptly. The majority outlived the ordinary grafts, some of them remaining alive and healthy for as long as 100 days after operation. As in the case of grafts to the pouch, these grafts could be destroyed by challenging the immunological mechanism of the host by "proxy": with a skin graft or an injection of cells from the donor strain. This was evidence again that the pouch skin barrier works in one direction only and by some means blocks entry into the host's system against whatever antigens the pouch cells liberate, or against antigens liberated by grafts placed in the intact pouch wall.

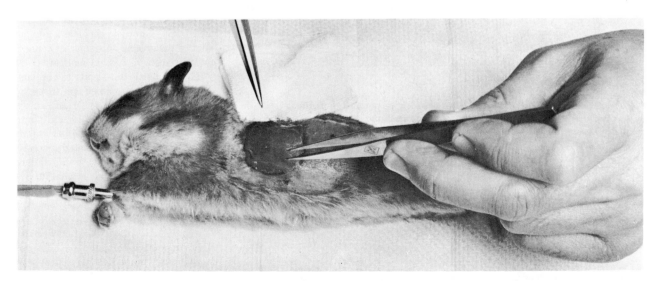

POUCH SKIN GRAFT is shown being applied to a prepared site on the side of an anesthetized hamster. The unusually high degree of success attained with such grafts lends support to the authors' **"barrier hypothesis," which was originally postulated to account for the behavior of the pouch as an immunologically privileged site for the transplantation thereto of many kinds of foreign tissue.**

Microscopic inspection of the structure of the pouch skin suggested a possible candidate for the barrier. Most of the living cells in the skin and so most of its biochemical activity are located in the epithelial, or outer, layer. It therefore occurred to us that the antigens liberated by these cells and, to a lesser extent, by the more sparsely distributed cells of the inner connective tissue layer might conceivably be prevented from reaching the host's body as a result of some sort of absorptive activity in the connective-tissue matrix. We explored this possibility in two series of experiments. From the centers of long-established isografts of pouch skin we excised the outer layer of epithelial cells, leaving intact almost the entire thickness of the pouch-skin connective tissue. We then fitted small grafts of body skin from an incompatible strain into these prepared defects. The results were most encouraging. Instead of undergoing rejection within two weeks, as they would have done if placed in direct contact with host tissue, many of these "inlays" lived for a long time, regenerating crops of hair of normal density. Even heterografts of rabbit skin manifested some tendency to survive when grafted in this manner.

We then put the barrier hypothesis to a more direct test by stripping sheets of the rather slimy, elastic connective tissue from freshly excised pouches and spreading them over graft beds on the sides of hamsters' chests. On top of this layer of connective tissue we placed grafts of skin from an incompatible strain. The skin grafts soon acquired a normal blood supply without any apparent interference from the layer of connective tissue. The layer of connective tissue did, however, interfere with the capacity of the graft to elicit the immunological response of the host. This was evidenced in the prolonged survival of many of the grafts. Whether the cell population of the connective tissue was alive or not at the time of grafting did not appear to affect the outcome. Sheets of the tissue that had been repeatedly frozen and thawed under conditions known to be lethal for cells of hamster skin continued to demonstrate the barrier effect that protected the overlaid skin grafts. The barrier did not, of course, afford protection from the immune response of the host elicited by proxy.

The postulated one-way barrier is supported by still another series of experiments. We have attempted by various means (by the topical application of chemical irritants and by mechanical irritation) to stimulate the release of effective amounts of antigen from long-established pouch skin homografts. All of these efforts—including even superficial injection with hyaluronidase, an enzyme known to dissolve a component of the ground substance of connective tissue—have proved ineffective.

The evidence thus leads to the conclusion that the connective tissue of pouch skin presents a barrier to the escape of antigens from the graft into the body of the host. Whether this is due to some enzyme-mediated reaction, to absorption or simply to the failure of the host's lymphatic system to establish drainage vessels through the connective-tissue barrier are questions that remain to be investigated.

It is difficult to see what benefit hamsters can derive from the peculiar immunological properties of their cheek pouches. The barrier it presents to antigens may be merely a secondary consequence of the anatomical plan of these organs, which has been revealed by the unnatural act of grafting. The principles

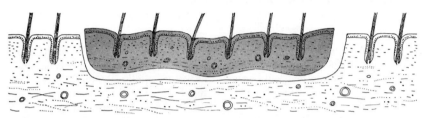

ORDINARY SKIN HOMOGRAFT, exchanged between two hamsters known to be incompatible, is promptly rejected. Antigenic stimulation of the host's immune mechanism results in the total destruction of the foreign tissue by an attack force of native lymphocytes.

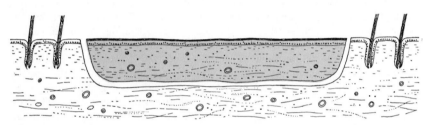

POUCH SKIN HOMOGRAFT is accepted. Antigens emitted by the epithelial cells at the surface of the graft are prevented from entering the host's body by some sort of physiological barrier located near the upper face of the loose-fibered areolar connective-tissue layer.

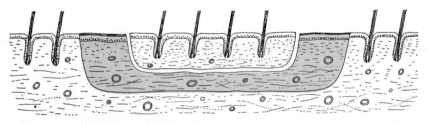

SUPERIMPOSED SKIN HOMOGRAFT is isolated from the host by the long-established pouch skin graft underneath. Incompatible antigens from the inlaid skin cannot penetrate the pouch's protective barrier to provoke an immune response and both grafts are accepted.

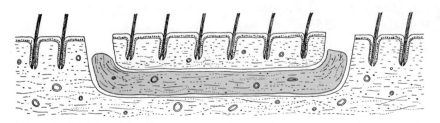

SIMULTANEOUS APPLICATION of a skin homograft over a sheet of cheek-pouch connective tissue also results in the long-term survival of both. Any subsequent introduction of antigenic material by proxy into the host body will cause the rejection of all the above grafts.

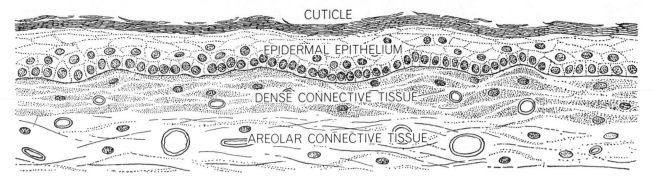

CUTICLE

EPIDERMAL EPITHELIUM

DENSE CONNECTIVE TISSUE

AREOLAR CONNECTIVE TISSUE

CROSS SECTION OF POUCH SKIN reveals its typical three-layer construction. Antigen-producing epithelial cells constitute the uppermost layer, which is covered by a very thin and compact cuticle. Underlying this is an intermediate layer of densely packed muscle fibers. Eversion of the pouch is made possible by the great elasticity of the loose areolar layer, which connects the pouch directly to the inside of the hamster's cheek. Antibodies and lymphocytes are able to, circulate freely through the numerous blood vessels present in both connective-tissue layers, but lymphatic vessels, the ordinary avenues of antigenic dispersal, have not been detected in either.

underlying the action of the barrier may nonetheless have general biological implications. May not such barriers play an important role in keeping individual organisms from reacting against certain substances in their own systems that are known to be potentially antigenic to the organism itself? Certain diseases of the thyroid gland, for example, appear to be the outcome of an immunological reaction against specific products of this organ that may have escaped as a result of the compromise or breaking of some sort of barrier. It is tempting to put another question: Is there any hope of finding a source of similar connective-tissue sheets in the human body or of being able to produce synthetically a material that has similar properties? Such a material, natural or synthetic, might facilitate the acceptance of human homografts in reparative surgery.

The hamster's contribution to a general understanding of the genetics and physiology of the immune reaction as it relates to the transplantation of tissues does not exhaust its interest for experimental biologists. Another curious faculty of the species may derive from an adaptation to its native habitat in Asia Minor. This is its high resistance to colchicine, a drug that inhibits cell division. The lethal dosage of colchicine is about one milligram per kilogram of body weight in rodents and eight milligrams per kilogram in man. But for the Syrian hamster it is nearly one gram per kilogram. This effect, first noted in 1952 by Margaret Ward Orsini and Ben Pansky at the University of Wisconsin, has recently been exploited by Alvin Midgeley, Barry Pierce and Frank J. Dixon at the University of Pittsburgh to investigate the arrest of cell division in

human tumors planted in the cheek pouches of hamsters. It may be that the Syrian hamster acquired this tolerance because plants of the genus *Colchicum*, which are the source of the drug, have their center of distribution in Asia Minor and may form part of the hamster's diet.

As hibernators, hamsters have also contributed to knowledge of the physiological mechanisms that enable some animals to withstand reduction of their body temperature to low levels. Finally, they have proved to be highly susceptible to the polyoma virus, a mammalian cancer virus, and to some adenoviruses, which cause respiratory disease in man. Altogether it appears that the position of the hamster in the laboratory is established, with tenure.

21

Markers of Biological Individuality

by Ralph A. Reisfeld and Barry D. Kahan
June 1972

The rejection of transplanted organs has focused attention on the body's ability to distinguish foreign cells from its own. The cells of each individual are uniquely marked with protein

It is often observed that every human being is unique. Our superficial differences, however, scarcely hint at the differences to be found at the level of the genes and the chemistry of the cell. It is now becoming clear that these differences play an important role in enabling living organisms to distinguish between "self" and "not self" and to reject cells that are not labeled with the appropriate recognition markers. The advances in surgery that make it possible to transplant organs from one person to another have stimulated an intensive study of the factors that cause the recipient to reject foreign tissue unless the donor is a close relative. Criteria for matching unrelated donors and hosts have proved extremely difficult to establish. The reason, we now see, is precisely the genetic and chemical uniqueness of each individual. Where organ transplants have been successful it is usually because ways have been found to suppress the rejection mechanism that normally operates. The techniques of suppression, however, still depend more on good luck than on fundamental understanding. Here we shall try to summarize what has recently been learned about the unique markers of individuality carried by each cell.

Individual differences are readily apparent in anatomy and physiology. "Normality" can only be defined by statistical methods involving many individuals, from which one can arrive at mean values with limits of variation. Any given individual, however, must possess many physical characteristics that are outside the normal range but that are not necessarily pathological. Functional differences are subtler; for example, individuals commonly exhibit large differences in the ratios of the electrolytes present in blood serum or in the structure and function of the various enzymes that mediate specific biochemical reactions. It is clear that such differences are innate: they are demonstrable over periods of years and are only slightly influenced by the environment.

Individual peculiarities are sometimes tragically illustrated by the idiosyncratic reactions of patients to particular drugs. Fifty years ago Sir Archibald Garrod, in his pioneering book *Inborn Errors of Metabolism*, noted that "these [pathologic defects of enzyme chemistry] are merely examples of variations in chemical behavior which are probably everywhere present in minor degrees, and that just as no two individuals of a species are absolutely identical in bodily structure, neither are their chemical processes carried out on the same lines."

Since these individual differences can be preserved from generation to generation only by the maintenance of a complex polymorphic gene pool, that is, a pool of genes with many alternative expressions, they must serve some important purpose. Unless they contributed to the survival of the species they would have been eliminated long ago by the pressures of natural selection. Moreover, it is clear that individuality is not confined to higher organisms. As Thomas Humphreys and Aron A. Moscona of the University of Chicago have shown in their studies of specific aggregation of sponge cells, even primitive species can distinguish their own cells from others. Genetic variability enhances the ability of members of a species to survive changes in their external and internal environments. Thus by studying the factors that determine and express individuality one can hope to acquire insight into basic biological phenomena relevant not only to the role of isolated characteristics but also to the functioning of the organism as an integrated collection of cooperating processes.

One of the most valuable techniques for studying individuality pits the distinctive factors of one organism against those of another. It is easily achieved by transplanting a bit of tissue from a donor to a host. The host is then required to distinguish its own unique biological markers from those of the interloper. One might regard this as a test of parasitism: What prevents one individual from becoming an integral part of another?

Humans are not good subjects for transplantation studies because the uniqueness of each individual precludes getting a "typical" response. One would have to conduct many experiments with many individuals and interpret the results statistically, which would of course tend to obscure the individual factors one was setting out to study. The alternative is to use inbred strains of laboratory animals such as mice or guinea pigs, so that one has a better chance of isolating the chemical and biological determinants of individuality. In the 1920's Sewall Wright and Clarence Cook Little showed independently that by repeated brother-sister matings one can develop animal lines possessing a common pool of genes. This does not mean that each newborn individual contains the same set of genes but rather that each set is derived from the same limited pool. Wright and Little demonstrated that tissue grafts between members of the same line survived longer than grafts between members of two different lines.

Little's colleague George D. Snell, working at the Jackson Memorial Laboratory, went further and showed that tumors obtained from one line of mice are rejected by hosts that differ from the donor strain by a factor subsequently designated H-2. The gene controlling the H-2 set of factors is transmitted by simple Mendelian laws [*see illustration below*]. Grafts of normal tissue exchanged between members of the same inbred line (isografts) are accepted. Grafts exchanged between members of two different lines (allografts) are uniformly rejected within 14 days. Grafts transferred from parental lines to the first-generation hybrids of those lines are accepted, but grafts transferred from the hybrid offspring back to the parents are not.

Moreover, if the grafts are tumors rather than normal tissue, the response generated by the *H-2* gene is strong enough to destroy the graft when the donor and the host possess different *H-2* genes. Evidently the *H-2* gene gives rise to strong markers on the surface of the cell that are readily recognized by cells of a different strain. In the absence of such a strong response tumors grow rapidly and outstrip the host's defenses. Snell also observed that when the grafts consist of normal tissue, they can be rejected by genetic factors weaker than those supplied by the *H-2* gene.

Furthermore, working with congenic lines of mice (inbred lines differing from one another at a single genetic locus), Snell found that a number of weaker factors, distributed as loci in the genetic material different from the *H-2* locus, could initiate the rejection of normal-tissue grafts, although rejection could take as long as 200 days. Differences at a second genetic site are not capable, however, of stopping the growth of tumor grafts when the donor and the host possess the same *H-2* gene. The strong markers placed on cells by the *H-2* gene in mice have their counterpart in man in markers traceable to the human leukocyte locus *A* (HL-*A*) gene. Thus transplantation experiments have revealed a number of discrete genes that control the production of markers, or distinctive factors, that determine the fate of foreign grafts.

Genetic markers of this type have long been exploited in the typing and matching of red blood cells for transfusions. The individuality markers that have to be accounted for when tissues are transplanted from one organism to another, however, are much more numerous and harder to classify because many genes are involved. When studies of tissue transplantation were extended to outbred populations of mice, it was shown that the number of alternative gene expressions associated with the strong factors that control rapid rejection of transplants in mice is probably no smaller than the number observed in man. A comparison of the data obtained in mice with observations in human populations led Jean Dausset of the University of Paris to suggest that the genes controlling the strong transplantation factors are collected in a single genetic region. This hypothesis was subsequently supported by the work of Ruggiero Ceppellini of the University of Turin and Jan van Rood of the University of Leiden. Ceppellini demonstrated that the rapid rejection of grafts exchanged between two human subjects depends on a single genetic locus; van Rood then found that the locus controls the production of factors that can be detected with HL-*A* antibodies. The region seems to be divided into two subregions, each of which determines a series of allelic, or alternative, factors. There are multiple alternatives in each subregion: the *D* and *K* regions in mice each have at least 10 alleles; in man the L-*A* region has at least 11 alleles and the region known as "Four" has at least 17. Thus a simple biological test, the acceptance or rejection of transplanted tissue, has uncovered a richly polymorphic genetic system in mice and men, providing a tool for attacking the problem of biological variability.

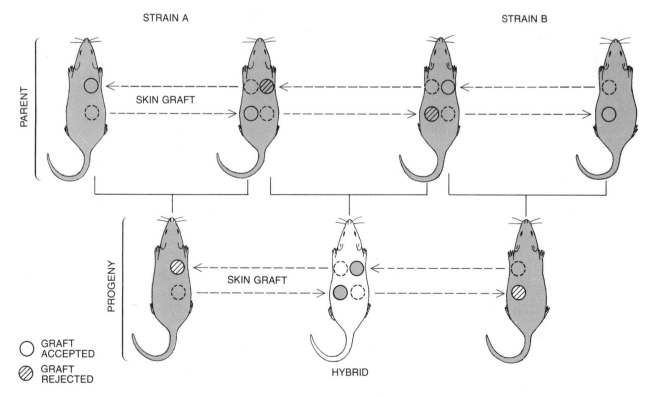

STRONG RESPONSE TO TUMOR TRANSPLANTATION in mice depends on factors controlled by a specific gene known as *H-2*. George D. Snell of the Jackson Memorial Laboratory demonstrated in the 1940's that the *H-2* gene obeys simple Mendelian laws of inheritance. Tumor grafts exchanged between inbred lines of mice, such as between two mice of strain *A* or two of strain *B*, are accepted. Tumor transplants between mice of different strains, however, are vigorously rejected, being destroyed within two weeks. Hybrid offspring will accept grafts from either of the pure parental lines, but grafts in the reverse direction are destroyed.

The polymorphic marker system protects an individual from invaders that otherwise could not be distinguished from the self. Although data from human populations originally suggested that one out of every 10,000 unrelated individuals might possess the same strong transplantation genes, it has since been demonstrated that the frequency of identical genes is far rarer. In fact, Leo Loeb proposed many years ago that the possible combinations are infinite and that no exact matches can exist. The results of human transplantations offer little to refute Loeb's conjecture. Clinical success in organ transplants seems related less to genetic similarities between donors and recipients who are unrelated than to the impaired ability of the host to react to foreign markers.

What is the mechanism that enables the host to recognize and destroy foreign cells? There are many conceivable possibilities. For example, the host might provide a local environment in which foreign cells were deprived of essential nutrients. Plants are able to resist certain parasites by depriving them of substrates, for example polysaccharides, they need for growth. A parasite's success might depend on its ability to break up whatever such molecules may be provided by the host and to utilize their fragments. Another possibility, envisioned by Loeb, is that the growth of foreign tissue may result in the generation and release of specific substances that are toxic to the host. This might lead in turn to a nonspecific inflammatory response that would destroy the invader.

These and other hypotheses were finally ruled out some 20 years ago when P. B. Medawar and his colleagues at University College London demonstrated that the host's response to foreign tissue involves an immunological mechanism similar to the one that provides resistance to bacterial and viral infections. In his first group of experiments Medawar showed that the recipient of a graft develops a resistance that is specific for the donor: when the recipient is challenged with a second graft from the same donor, the transplanted tissue is destroyed even more rapidly than it was the first time. Medawar called this the second-set reaction [see "a" in illustration on opposite page]. Furthermore, the "memory" of the initial experience can be evoked by a second challenge graft no matter where it is placed on the recipient; in other words, the second-set response is system-wide, not local. Medawar then found that specific individuality markers are associated with every nucleated cell of an organism. Thus an animal can be "immunized" against foreign skin grafts by first injecting it with cells derived from other tissues of the same donor, for example cells from the spleen [see "b" in illustration on opposite page].

Finally, Medawar and two of his colleagues, Rupert E. Billingham and Leslie Brent, drawing on observations made by Ray D. Owen and a theory proposed by Sir Macfarlane Burnet, demonstrated that an animal of strain A can be made tolerant to tissue grafts from an animal of strain B by injecting the strain-A animal soon after birth with a suspension of spleen cells from the strain-B animal [see "c" in illustration on opposite page]. With this experiment Medawar and his colleagues proved that resistance or lack of resistance to foreign tissue is not a localized phenomenon but an immunological one. They later showed that the host's capacity to reject foreign tissues can be reconstituted by lymphoid grafts, which are known to restore immune reactions. This set of experiments left no doubt that the factors previously identified by genetic studies were those re-

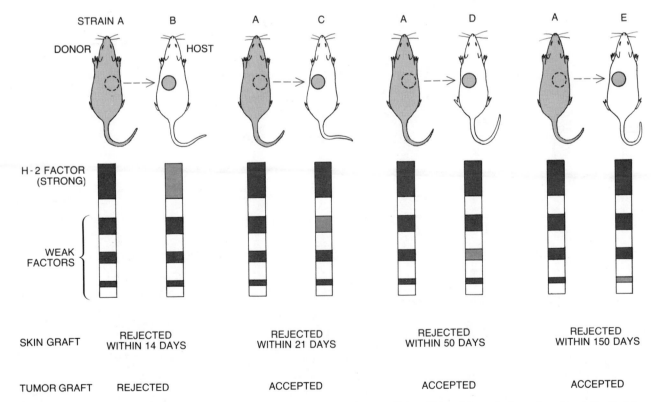

ADDITIONAL GENETIC FACTORS determine the survival rate of normal skin grafts but not the survival rate of tumor grafts. If an animal of strain A and an animal of strain B differ in H-2 (that is, strong) individuality factors, each will vigorously reject tumor grafts as well as ordinary skin grafts from the other. Animals that share the same H-2 factors will accept tumor grafts from one another. Because animals C, D and E differ from A in weaker transplantation factors they reject normal skin grafts at various rates.

sponsible for graft rejection, since alteration of the host's responses toward these factors made it unable to react against grafts.

To account for these findings and related ones Medawar proposed that all nucleated cells possess surface markers that act as "antigens" when the cells are transplanted to another organism. The antigens trigger an immune response in the host that makes it specifically resistant to the donor's tissues. Evidently these markers are functional components of the outer membrane of every nucleated cell, although the role they play remains to be elucidated. Presumably the host becomes alerted to their presence when they perform their natural functions, perhaps as cell receptors or as factors involved in growth and development.

James L. Gowans of the University of Oxford has shown that foreign grafts are met by "wandering" lymphocytes, white scavenger cells produced in the lymph glands; the lymphocytes "check" cell surfaces like watchmen in order to ensure that all constituents of the host organism bear its own markers and not those of an invader [see illustration on next page]. When the wandering lymphocytes discover foreign markers in a graft, they carry the alarm back to the lymph nodes and stimulate an immune reaction. The reaction consists in the proliferation of lymphocytes with receptor sites that can engage the markers of foreign cells as a key engages a lock and thus interfere with their functioning, ultimately causing the death of the grafted cells. There is also evidence that whole cells or fragments from the graft tissue are detached and find their way into the drainage channels of the lymphatic system, where they eventually reach the lymph nodes and directly trigger the proliferation of suitably designed lymphocytes. Presumably the transplant markers have a role in the metabolism of the cell that requires them to occupy an exposed position on the cell's surface, so that a reaction against them is lethal to a cell transplanted in a foreign host.

Working with crude subcellular fractions, a number of investigators obtained evidence some years ago that nearly all the strong antigens of the cell are located on the surface of the cell membrane. Goran L. Möller of the Royal Caroline Institute in Stockholm found that serums produced in a host by challenge with intact foreign cells contain antibodies that react with cell surfaces [see illustration on page 209]. That these

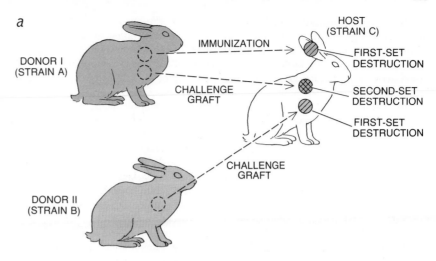

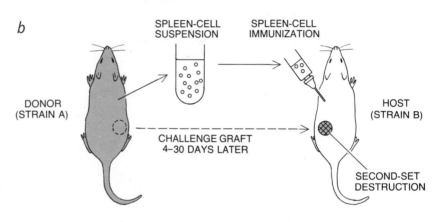

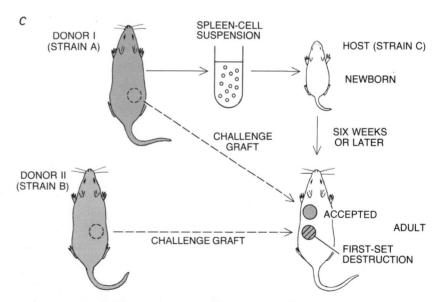

IMMUNOLOGIC NATURE OF TISSUE REJECTION was demonstrated by P. B. Medawar and his colleagues at University College London. His early studies showed (a) that a second graft from the same donor is destroyed more rapidly than the first. Medawar called this the second-set reaction; it shows that the host develops an "immunity" to a specific foreign donor. He then showed that immunization is not specific for the tissue involved (b). Animals exhibit a second-set reaction to a skin graft if they have previously been injected with cells derived from the donor's other tissues, such as the spleen. Finally Medawar and his group demonstrated that animals can develop immunologic tolerance (c). A mouse of strain C will accept a skin graft from a mouse of strain A if the strain-C mouse has been injected soon after birth with spleen cells from the mouse of strain A. The strain-C mouse, however, still retains its ability to reject challenge grafts from an animal of another strain, say strain B.

surface sites are indeed transplantation markers was proved in our laboratory at the Scripps Clinic and Research Foundation in La Jolla, Calif., by Soldano Ferrone, who recently demonstrated that solubilized and purified human individuality markers stimulate the production of antibodies that react with surfaces of intact cells.

Workers in a number of laboratories have been exploiting various techniques to isolate the individuality markers in a water-soluble form from the cell-membrane matrix with which they are associated. The task is complicated because the cell membrane consists of a lattice of lipoprotein molecules in which are embedded a variety of carbohydrates and proteins in addition to the individuality markers [see top illustration on opposite page]. Some of the proteins serve as structural components; others

regulate the passage of nutrients, respond to environmental stimuli and effect the cell's associations with neighboring cells. Whereas the architectural components of the cell membrane tend to be fixed, some of the functional proteins probably float like icebergs in a "sea" of membrane lipids, so that they are at least partially exposed to the external environment. Michael A. Edidin of Johns Hopkins University has inferred that transplantation markers are among those in a dynamic state from the way they spread rapidly between membranes when two unlike cells fuse.

One current model of the cell surface visualizes membrane components held together either by strong covalent chemical bonds or by weaker noncovalent interactions, such as those provided by hydrogen bonds and salt linkages. Since the individuality markers appear to be

mobile, it seems likely that they are associated with the architectural proteins and with other functional proteins through noncovalent interactions. One can only speculate on the role of these interactions. For example, by altering the expression of the individuality markers the interactions may protect the host against environmental agents that might alter the cell's identity. Fortunately it turns out that the antigenic activity associated with the individuality markers is independent of secondary interactions with other membrane components and depends solely on the marker's primary structure. Therefore it was possible for us to remove the markers from the membrane in water-soluble form and study their biological activity with a minimum of interference from other membrane components.

There are two general methods for re-

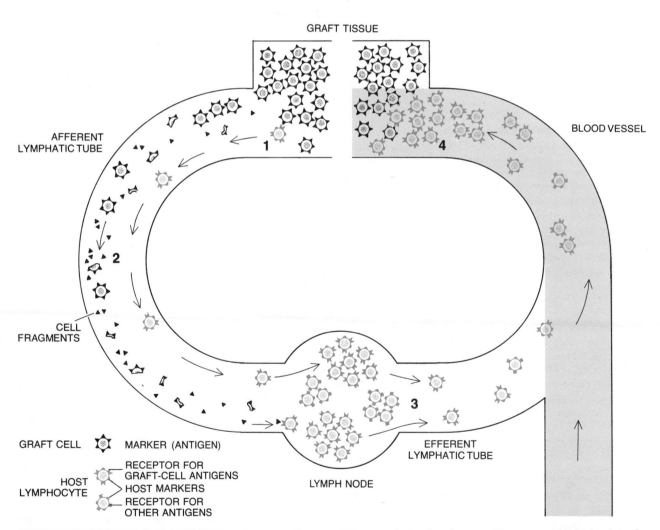

THEORY OF IMMUNOLOGIC RESPONSE to tissue transplants, proposed by Medawar, visualizes that cells carry individuality markers that another organism perceives as "antigens." Here the markers, or antigens, carried by the cells of a foreign graft are represented by black spikes. These are detected by the host's "wandering" lymphocytes, some of which are equipped with receptors that interact with the foreign markers in a lock-and-key fashion. These wandering lymphocytes (1) carry an alarm signal to the host's lymph nodes, stimulating the proliferation of more lymphocytes (3) equipped to destroy the invading cells (4). Cells detached from the graft, together with fragments carrying antigens, also enter the lymph drainage system (2) and carry the alarm message directly to the lymph nodes. Evidently lymphocytes are equipped with a variety of "keys" to engage any number of antigen "locks."

leasing markers from their membrane matrix [*see bottom illustration at right*]. One method uses proteolytic enzymes, for example papain, that randomly break the covalent bonds holding proteins together, thereby releasing an array of antigenic materials from membranes. Some of these fragments represent broken markers; others contain extraneous materials, such as carbohydrates, that apparently are not involved in the recognition of foreign cells in transplantation.

A gentler method of disruption, which leaves the markers more or less intact, involves exposing cells to low-intensity sonic energy. Noncovalent bonds are disrupted by a combination of cavitation (the rapid expansion and violent collapse of air bubbles trapped in the medium), mechanical agitation, foaming, shearing and local heating. The treatment produces a complex mixture of markers, other solubilized membrane components and soluble proteins that are released from the interior of the cell by the disintegration of its surface membrane.

Noncovalent bonds can also be dissociated by a simple salt, potassium chloride, which acts as a weak chaotropic agent, decreasing the orderly arrangement of water molecules in the medium surrounding the cell membrane. Irving M. Klotz and his colleagues at Northwestern University have postulated that a decrease in the ordered structure of water makes it possible for hydrophobic parts of membrane-embedded proteins to become detached from their lipid environment and to become dispersed in an aqueous one. Thus by subjecting cells to a strong solution of potassium chloride for about 16 hours one can obtain a crude extract containing a variety of cell components, including intact membrane proteins in solubilized form. Since the protein markers of cell individuality represent only a minor fraction of the entire crude mixture, their extraction and purification present a challenging task.

One separation technique that has proved successful is polyacrylamide-gel electrophoresis, originally developed by Leonard Ornstein and Baruch J. Davis of the Mount Sinai School of Medicine. Its usefulness has been considerably enhanced by a computer program based on theories developed by Andreas Chrambach and David Rodbard of the National Institutes of Health. With this program we have been able to exploit subtle differences in the molecular size and net charge of various components in the crude mixture of solubilized surface materials so that the transplantation mark-

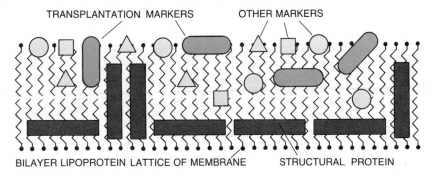

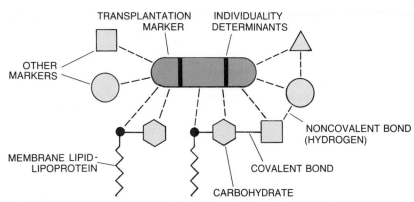

INDIVIDUALITY MARKERS that trigger a strong immunologic response in tissue transplantation are proteins (*dark color*) distributed in the surface membrane of virtually all nucleated cells. The black stripes represent determinants that vary from individual to individual. The membrane also contains other proteins that act as weaker surface markers. The matrix of the membrane is a bilayer of lipid molecules. The strong transplantation markers are bound to other membrane units (*bottom diagram*) largely through noncovalent bonds, which are more easily broken than the covalent bonds that hold molecules together.

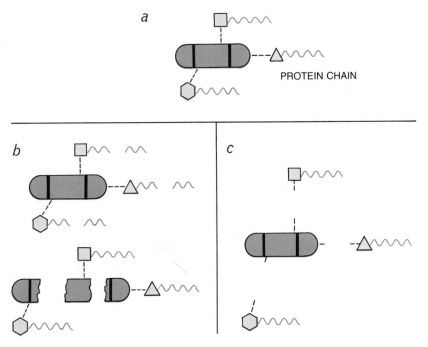

RELEASE OF MARKERS FROM CELL MEMBRANE can be accomplished by treating cells with proteolytic enzymes, which break covalent bonds, or by using milder methods that disrupt mainly noncovalent bonds. A marker is shown before treatment in *a*. Two possible results of treating cells with proteolytic enzymes are shown in *b*. In one case (*top*) the enzyme breaks the bonds of proteins loosely attached to the marker; in the other case (*bottom*) the enzyme breaks up the marker itself. The marker remains intact (*c*) if cells are subjected to low-energy sound or to solutions of certain simple salts, such as potassium chloride.

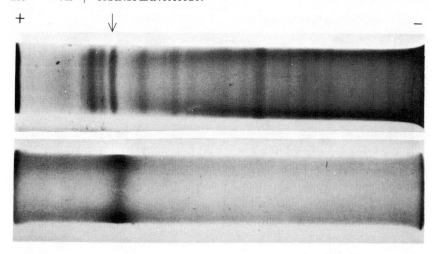

PURIFICATION OF MARKER ANTIGENS can be achieved by subjecting a crude membrane extract to polyacrylamide-gel electrophoresis. The separation exploits differences in size and charge affecting the rate at which proteins and other cell components move through a gel medium of defined pore size in response to an electric field. The image at the top shows the electrophoretic pattern of a crude extract containing a human transplantation marker (*arrow*) known as HL-*A* antigen. At the bottom the highly purified antigen isolated from a cultured human lymphoid cell line, designated RPMI 1788, is clearly separated.

ers separate clearly. In this way the markers carried by the cells of guinea pigs and the cells of humans have been extracted as homogeneous substances with high biological activity [*see illustration above*].

The purified markers turn out to belong to a family of proteins that differ from one another in their specific amino acid composition. It was exciting to find that individuality differences heretofore undetectable except by transplantation between two strains of guinea pigs or two unrelated human subjects could be predicted by specific differences in the amino acid composition between their isolated protein surface markers. Our findings supported earlier work by An-

drew A. Kandutsch of the Jackson Memorial Laboratory showing that the specificity of antigens arrayed on membrane fractions was destroyed by chemicals that attacked proteins. Thus antigenic activity resides entirely in membrane proteins and not, for example, in carbohydrates that might be associated with them. This was confirmed by Stanley Nathenson of the Albert Einstein College of Medicine in New York, who demonstrated that the carbohydrate fraction of solubilized *H-2* antigens seems to be devoid of antigenic activity.

Transplantation markers are therefore simple proteins consisting of about 300 amino acid units strung together in a linear chain. Chemical studies show, however, that the markers of unrelated individuals have major differences in amino acid composition at five sites in the chain. As is well known from studies of the genetic code, a sequence of three bases in DNA, the genetic material, is needed to specify a particular amino acid in a protein molecule. In the case of at least four of the five variable amino acids a change in only a single base in one of the coding triplets is enough to account for the observed differences in the marker proteins.

In addition there are amino acid sequence differences involving the ordering of units in individual chains. When Michele Pellegrino in our laboratory subjected marker molecules to a proteolytic enzyme (trypsin) that attacked the covalent bonds adjacent to specific amino acids (lysine and arginine), he obtained 24 fragments, as determined by "fingerprinting" analysis [*see bottom illustration on this page*]. This is a technique in which a treated sample is placed in the corner of a square of filter paper; fragments are separated by chromatography in one direction and by electrophoresis in a direction at right angles to the first. The first separation reflects the rate at which fragments are carried across the paper by solvents; the second separation reflects the rate at which fragments move in an electric field. The resulting pattern provides a "fingerprint" of the protein.

The fingerprint of markers of two unrelated human subjects showed only six differences in the location of 24 fragments. This means that the amino acid composition of 18 of the fragments was the same in both subjects. The other six fragments exhibited amino acid differences. These findings suggest that transplantation markers are superimposed on a backbone of constant amino acid sequence but that interspersed along the

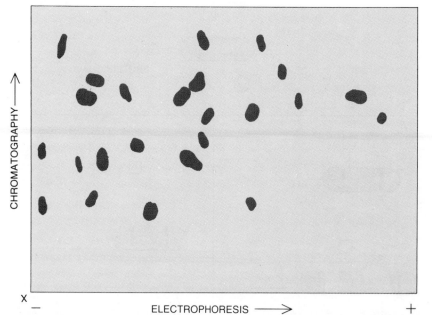

FINGERPRINT OF HUMAN ANTIGEN is produced by a technique that combines electrophoresis with chromatography. The purified protein antigen isolated from cell line RPMI 1788 is treated with a proteolytic enzyme that breaks the molecular chain wherever it contains amino acid subunits of lysine or arginine. The chain is cleaved at 23 places, yielding a total of 24 fragments. The mixture is spotted at one corner (*X*) of a square of filter paper; the fragments are separated by chromatography in one direction and by electrophoresis in another. From such studies it appears that the amino acid differences in protein markers obtained from unrelated individuals are confined to six regions of the molecule.

backbone are small regions within at least some of which the amino acid sequence is varied to establish the organism's individuality.

Since transplantation markers are simple proteins, it should be possible in time to work out the complete base sequence in the structural gene that controls their synthesis. Direct gene-mapping is not possible for other strong individuality systems in mammals, such as blood-group substances, because their antigenicity depends on carbohydrates inserted in a supporting protein molecule by enzymes.

The limited variability of transplantation markers makes them much more tractable for detailed study of individuality than the immunoglobulins, the proteins that act as antibodies in blood serum, where they exhibit recognition and inactivation functions similar to those performed by cell-surface markers. The immunoglobulin molecule consists of a "constant" region whose amino acid composition varies among different individuals of the same species. This variation, known as allotypy, is not related to the molecule's recognition function in its role as an antibody. That difference is provided by the "variable" region of the molecule; each individual has the capacity to produce a vast number of different immunoglobulins (perhaps several hundred thousand) each containing a slightly different amino acid sequence in the variable region. It is not yet known how much of the far more limited variability detected in fingerprints of transplantation markers represents allotypy, or transplantation individuality differences, and how much represents functional variability.

The human marker studied by Pellegrino is known to be the product of the HL-A, or human leukocyte locus A, gene. The HL-A, gene product, which may be the primary determinant of whether a human graft will be tolerated or rejected, is now available for use in clinical transplantation.

The distribution of transplantation markers in the general population can be studied with the methods of "tissue-typing." Individuals can be immunized against foreign tissue in several ways: by skin grafting, by organ transplants or by the natural transplant represented by the fetus in pregnancy. Immunization produces antibody that reacts not only against the particular donor's cells but also against the cells of unrelated individuals. To perform the typing, blood serum containing antibody

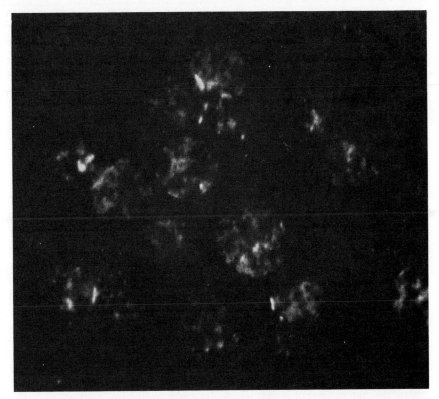

LOCATION OF INDIVIDUALITY MARKERS, the cellular proteins that help to establish each organism's identity, can be visualized by fluorescent microscopy. Target lymphocytes bearing the HL-A, or "strong," antigenic markers of one individual were first reacted with specific HL-A antibody from another individual. The resulting antigen-antibody complex on the lymphocyte surface was made visible by adding a fluorescein-labeled antibody to human gamma globulin produced in a goat. The micrograph, prepared in the authors' laboratory at the Scripps Clinic and Research Foundation by P. G. Natali, shows that the antibodies recognize and affix themselves to specific antigenic sites on the cell's surface.

is taken from the host and is mixed with white blood cells taken from another person [see illustration on next page]. Everyone whose cells are killed by the serum shares a factor foreign to the host and thus forms a tissue type.

Tissue-typing has been intensively studied during the past decade, but it is still in a period of flux. It has been found that human hosts can respond to multiple antigens in the challenge graft and not solely those related to transplantation. Furthermore, the reaction of a given individual against a set of determinants is highly complex. The reaction depends on the individual's capacity to respond to a given amount of marker, on his previous exposure to related materials that may have shared the same determinants, to say nothing of his own genetic constitution. As a result the superimposition of the individuality of immune responses on the vast genetic variety in transplantation markers and other markers yields a bewildering array of results, restricting the present value of typing in predicting the best unrelated donor for a given patient in need, say, of a kidney transplant.

An important advance in typing has recently come out of Ferrone's work in our laboratory. Ferrone finds that when solubilized human antigens (individuality markers released from cell membranes) are administered to rabbits, the animals' immune system can recognize individual differences it cannot discern when it is confronted with whole human cells. The explanation is that intact cells carry species-specific markers that are much stronger than the markers that vary from individual to individual. The purified soluble material evidently does not possess the species markers. As a result the rabbits respond to the individuality markers rather as another human being would. Studies involving many rabbits have shown that some animals respond to only a limited number of leukocyte locus A markers, and in some cases to only a single marker. These studies promise to improve tissue-typing and so lead to more successful organ-matching.

Other potential clinical applications of solubilized transplantation markers will be investigated in our transplantation unit at Northwestern University. The markers may provide an index to measure the patient's response to grafts so that the surgeon can regulate the amount of drugs necessary to suppress the patient's immune response and thereby enable the graft to survive. Another approach, which is now being tested in animals, is to pretreat the host with purified solubilized individuality markers obtained from the prospective donor. The host normally confronts such markers on the donor's intact cell surfaces; there is evidence that his immune system may be confounded and respond less vigorously or erratically when the markers are first presented in solubilized form. Under the circumstances his body may accept the markers as his own and fail to react at all, thus exhibiting immunological tolerance. He may develop a response that actually protects the subsequent graft rather than destroying it, a response termed immunological enhancement. Or his response may be an impotent "deviant" reaction that neither destroys the graft nor protects it. Whichever the case, experiments with animals demonstrate that the survival of a graft is significantly prolonged by pretreating the host with a solubilized individuality marker. Immunotherapy with these substances may well provide a major step in controlling the rejection of tissue transplants and break the barrier that has so far limited the clinical transplantation of organs.

As we have observed, individuality markers are present on virtually all nucleated cells and hence must play an essential role in the cell's economy. Since they spread freely across cell surfaces, it seems unlikely that they are involved in the cell structure itself. Conceivably they help to regulate the permeability of the cell membrane. Another possibility is that they may assist cells of the same type to form aggregates. Thus they may facilitate the adhesion of cells in the architecture of tissues or enable cells to exchange information. These functions might be a property of the structurally constant regions of molecules that also possess localized regions of individuality. It seems reasonable to suppose natural selection would have endowed marker molecules with one or more functions in addition to providing an identification label unique for each organism.

One puzzling observation is that cells from individuals never previously exposed to foreign markers in grafts often act as if they had encountered the markers before. H. Sherwood Lawrence of the New York University School of Medicine has suggested that such individuals may have encountered the markers, or close copies of them, in molecules carried by bacteria or viruses. This idea is supported by the fact that grafts, like intracellular bacterial and viral parasites, are destroyed by a cellular immunological mechanism. It seems entirely possible that each person is characterized not only by his innate individuality markers but also by an entire menagerie of infectious agents to which he has been exposed and whose markers he carries around throughout his life. This suggests in turn that a person's own markers may either help to protect him from certain disease processes or increase his susceptibility to them. In other words, in order to attack a cell successfully a bacterium or a virus might have to play a molecular game of wits with the individuality markers and with the immune potentials of the host that stand in its way. The hypothesis is supported by the observation that certain anti-HL-A antibodies that block leukocyte locus A marker sites also interfere with the infectivity of viral agents, thus suggesting that the agent shares the determinants.

There is evidence that various diseases are associated with leukocyte locus A factors, indicating that individuality markers are indeed related to the inception, development and pathogenic reaction to disease. On the other hand, the host's life might be prolonged if he were fortunate enough to harbor a para-

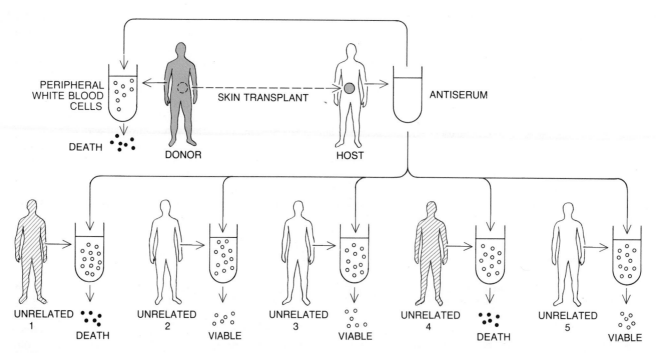

TISSUE-TYPING has been used to study the distribution of transplantation markers in the general population. An individual ("host," top) who has been immunized against an unrelated person ("donor"), for example by a skin graft, produces antiserum, a serum that contains antibody. The antiserum will destroy not only the donor's white blood cells but also the white cells of other unrelated individuals (1, 4). All the individuals whose cells are so destroyed are considered to belong to a common tissue type. Tissue-typing has been helpful in selecting related donors for organ transplants but is only modestly useful with unrelated individuals.

site that supplied markers he lacked. For example, it has been reported that leukemia and Burkitt's lymphoma have regressed after a patient had contracted measles. One might say that the perfect parasite is one that succeeds in lengthening the life of its host—but then should it still be called a parasite?

The individuality-marker system may protect the species against viral infections in another way. When some viruses that contain RNA rather than DNA as their genetic material infect a cell, they form buds and carry a portion of the cell's surface membrane along with them. If the cell's individuality markers thereby end up in the coat of the virus, they could elicit a "graft" rejection when the virus attacks another unrelated individual of the same species as the original host. The possibility that transplantation individuality markers can determine the host's response to viruses is potentially important in clinical diagnosis, prophylaxis and immunotherapy.

Recently Burnet has elaborated on a suggestion made earlier by Lewis Thomas of the Yale University School of Medicine to construct a comprehensive hypothesis of an immune surveillance system. Early in evolution primitive organisms developed a class of wandering cells capable of recognizing and destroying foreign cells or parasites. This mechanism, Burnet points out, would be able to act not only against agents of external origin but also against mutated cells of the host organism that exhibited new individuality markers. This would tend to make the individual resistant to new growths, that is, tumors and cancers in general. Functional surface markers on the host's own cells would serve as local recognition sites for the wandering surveillance cells; in addition markers released from cell membranes in the normal course of cell repair and replacement would telegraph subcellular messages to draining lymph nodes, keeping them informed of their constituency. Natural selection would favor such a system because it enhances the viability of the organism. Burnet suggests that the aging process involves a depletion in the number and vigilance of the "wanderers," allowing such abnormalities as cancer and immune responses to the host's own tissue to develop. Therefore markers of biological individuality provide an excellent tool for probing the most intimate functions of the cell. Knowledge so obtained cannot fail to be useful in meeting the challenges of human transplantation and disease.

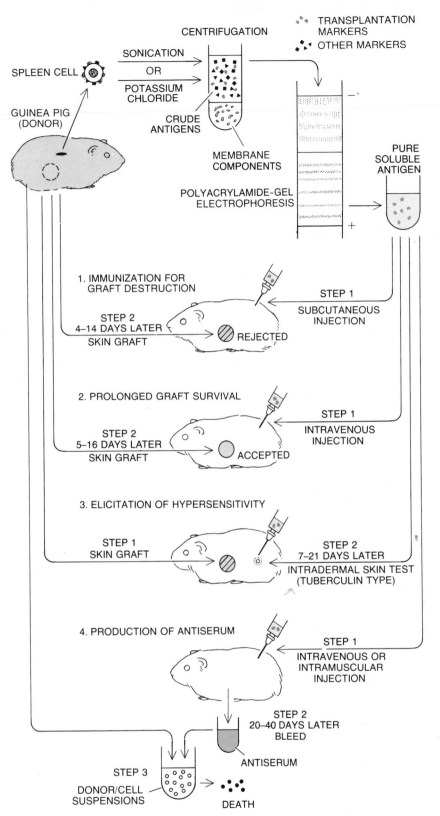

RESPONSE TO SOLUBLE INDIVIDUALITY MARKERS can take a variety of forms. Here pure markers, or antigens, obtained from guinea pig spleen cells are administered to four unrelated individuals. Subcutaneous injection of the antigens (1) will normally immunize an animal against a subsequent skin graft from the animal that supplied the antigens. On the other hand, an intravenous injection of antigens (2) will often prolong the survival of a skin graft made from five to 16 days later. One can tell if an animal is hypersensitive to the donor's tissue (3) by applying antigens from the donor in the form of an intradermal injection from one to three weeks after the skin graft. Finally, one can produce antiserum by injecting the antigens subcutaneously in an unrelated host (4). After a few weeks the host's serum will contain enough antibodies to destroy the donor's white cells.

22

The Prevention of "Rhesus" Babies

by C. A. Clarke
November 1968

The problem of Rh incompatibility can now be solved by giving an Rh-negative mother an anti-Rh antibody that inactivates any Rh-positive fetal blood cells that may pass into her circulation

As a child I was fascinated by butterflies, particularly a yellow swallowtail butterfly that flies in a marshy area of the east coast of England known as the Norfolk Broads. After World War II, I wanted to breed these insects but found it easier said than done. Swallowtails usually will not mate in a cage, as they need an elaborate courtship flight to stimulate pairing. My interest in the insect did not wane, and by persevering I learned a simple trick to make captive swallowtails mate. Holding the female in the left hand and the male in the right, one brings the pair close together, pries open the male's claspers with the nail of the left-hand middle finger and thereby induces the male to lock onto the female, after which mating follows naturally.

The happy acquisition of this technique in 1952 led me on to experiments in crossbreeding butterflies that turned up some surprising results and fruitful genetic findings. Thus, by the pleasant route of pursuing idle curiosity, my colleagues and I were led unexpectedly to a solution for the well-known medical problem having to do with the inheritance of the Rh factor in human blood! A clue suggested by the butterfly work has enabled us to develop a successful method of preventing the anemia hazard for babies born of an Rh-positive father and an Rh-negative mother. The method can best be explained by describing both the butterfly work and the blood-group investigation from the beginning.

In 1952 I happened to acquire a female butterfly of a black swallowtail species common in America (*Papilio asterias*), and in an idle moment one Sunday afternoon I hand-mated her to a male of the yellow British species (*Papilio machaon*). Since the two species are related, the mating was successful, and their first-generation offspring turned out to be like the American parent (showing that black and American were dominant to yellow and British!). When the hybrid was back-crossed to the recessive yellow parent species, however, the new (second) generation segregated for the ground color again: half of the offspring were black and half were yellow. Clearly, then, the ground color of the wings must be controlled by a single gene. A butterfly that inherited the dominant gene for black from either hybrid parent would have black wings, whereas an offspring that received yellow genes from both parents (each of which possessed the yellow as the recessive gene) would be yellow.

It was this experiment that aroused my interest in genetics. Soon afterward I met P. M. Sheppard, who is now a colleague of mine at the University of Liverpool but then was at the University of Oxford. We decided to use the mating technique to investigate the genetic aspects of mimicry in certain butterfly species. In wing coloring and form the mim-

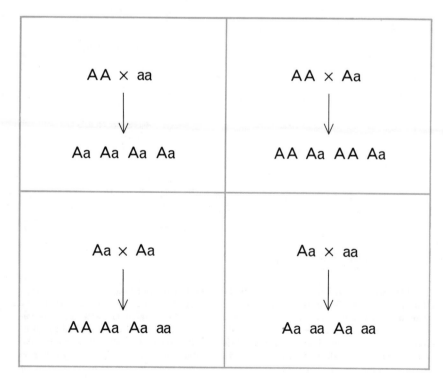

DOMINANT AND RECESSIVE GENES figure in the Rh problem. Each box shows in the top line a parental arrangement of dominant genes (*capital letters*) and recessive ones (*small letters*) and in bottom line the combination of genes to be expected in offspring.

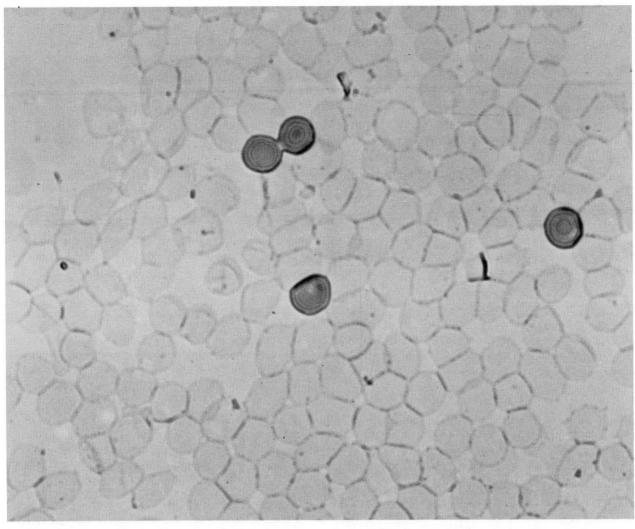

BABY'S CELLS in the mother's circulation give rise to the Rh problem. In this photomicrograph, made by Flossie Cohen of the Child Research Center of Michigan, the red blood cells of the baby are darker than the mother's red blood cells because of a technique that has washed the hemoglobin out of the adult cells while leaving hemoglobin in the fetal cells that are more resistant to the technique. The steps whereby fetal cells in the maternal circulation can create an Rh problem are shown at top of next two pages.

icking butterflies copy butterflies of different species or genera and even of different families. The "model" butterflies are nauseous to predators (particularly birds), and thus the mimics avoid attack although they are themselves edible. A single species of mimic may have several different forms, each imitating a different model; such a species is said to be polymorphic. In formal terms polymorphism refers to distinctly different types (such as blood types in human beings) that persist in an interbreeding population living in the same habitat, and that occur in frequencies such that the rarest form could not be maintained by recurrent mutation. In both mimic butterflies and their models the relative proportion of edible and inedible species in any one area is kept in balance by natural selection. For example, if the edible species mimicking a particular wing pattern comes to outnumber the inedible species, that pattern becomes attractive to predators. The pressure of natural selection is then unfavorable to the mimic species instead of being favorable to it.

How does the mimicry arise in the first place? Does it come about by the mutation of a single gene, causing a butterfly to acquire a mimetic pattern at one jump? This seemed to us a tall order, considering the complexity of colors and configurations in a butterfly's wings. For an answer to our question we investigated an African butterfly (*Papilio dardanus*) and one from southeast Asia (*Papilio memnon*). In both cases we found that the "gene" controlling the wing pattern is really a group of closely linked genes behaving as a single unit—what is known as a supergene. We found evidence for this in crossovers (exchanging of genes) within the genetic group. For example, in a southeast Asian butterfly we bred we were able to see a crossover in the chromosomal unit responsible for the change in wing pattern [*see illustration on page 217*].

There is another significant point about these two species of butterfly that is relevant to the blood-group work. In these species mimicry occurs only in the female; in both species the males do not show mimetic patterns although they carry the genes that are responsible for the patterns in the female. Evidently there is an interaction between sex and the mimetic supergene, so that the supergene is somehow switched off in the male.

By the time we had got this far in the genetic research on butterflies we could not help noticing certain striking parallels between the inheritance of their wing patterns and the inheritance of blood types in man. In man the blood-

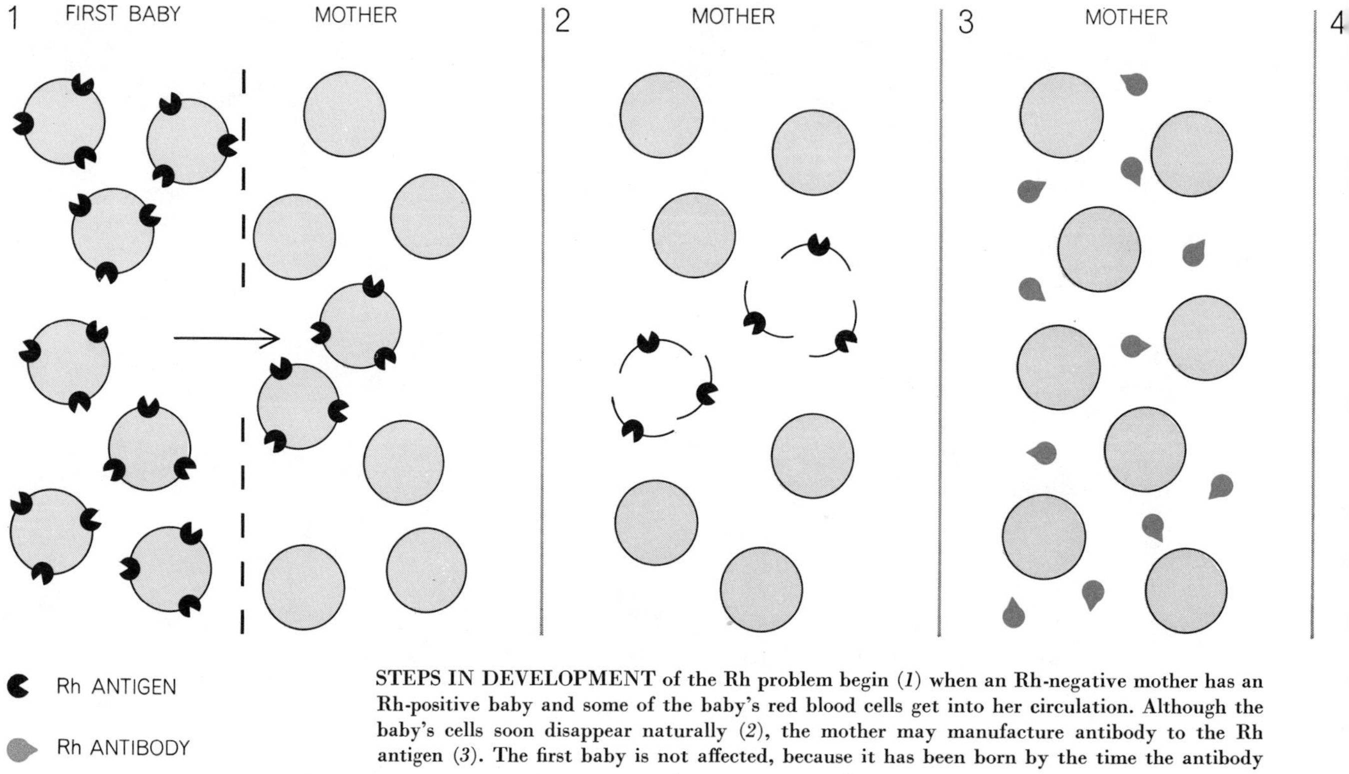

C Rh ANTIGEN

🬀 Rh ANTIBODY

STEPS IN DEVELOPMENT of the Rh problem begin (*1*) when an Rh-negative mother has an Rh-positive baby and some of the baby's red blood cells get into her circulation. Although the baby's cells soon disappear naturally (*2*), the mother may manufacture antibody to the Rh antigen (*3*). The first baby is not affected, because it has been born by the time the antibody

group differences between individuals —Rh-positive, Rh-negative, O, A, B, AB and so on—are genuine manifestations of polymorphism. The Rh genetic units are supergenes, composed of three closely linked genes, with alternative recessive forms in many different combinations. Moreover, as in the male butterfly, in man there is an interaction whereby another blood-group system can interfere with the formation of antibodies against the antigens controlled by the Rh supergene. To appreciate the significance of these facts we must take a fresh look at the particulars of the Rh problem.

About 85 percent of the population in Britain and in the U.S. are Rh-positive, which means their red blood corpuscles contain the "rhesus" factor or substance, so named because it was originally detected in rhesus monkeys. The Rh factor is an antigen; if Rh-positive blood gets into the bloodstream of an Rh-negative individual, the person may produce an antibody (called anti-Rh or anti-D) that destroys the Rh-positive red blood cells. Therein lies the hazard for babies of an Rh-negative mother. The hazard, when it arises, usually comes about in the following way. If an Rh-positive father and an Rh-negative mother produce an Rh-positive baby (inheriting the Rh factor from the father), and if some of the baby's Rh-positive red blood cells get into the mother's circulation at the time of delivery, the mother may subsequently manufacture the Rh antibody. The

antibody does not harm the mother, and a first baby is not affected because the antibody is produced after the baby's birth. The antibody in the mother's blood remains as a threat, however, to any subsequent Rh-positive baby, because it will enter the circulation of the fetus in the womb and destroy red blood cells, thereby causing possibly fatal anemia. The baby may be stillborn or be born with hemolytic disease.

The risk of this happening is not very high; although 15 percent of women are Rh-negative, among the 850,000 births each year in Britain, for instance, the number of "rhesus" babies is probably not more than about 5,000. Several factors operate to limit the risk. First, leakage of the baby's blood through the placenta into the mother's circulation in sufficient quantity to stimulate the production of Rh antibodies does not occur often. Second, some women do not produce antibodies even though there is leakage. Third, when the Rh-positive father is heterozygous (having received an Rh-negative gene from one of his parents), there is only a 50 percent chance that the baby will be Rh-positive. Fourth, and this is what particularly interested us, in about 20 percent of all the potential cases the formation of antibodies is prevented by the protective mechanism arising from interaction with other blood-group genes.

As an example, the mechanism operates in cases where the blood of the Rh-

negative mother is of the type known as Group O. Blood of the O type always contains naturally occurring antibodies against A-type or B-type blood. The antibodies, called anti-A and anti-B, attack the red cells in blood of Group A or Group B. Thus if a Group O Rh-negative mother bears an Rh-positive baby whose blood is of the A type, her anti-A will rapidly get rid of any red cells that leak into her circulation from the baby at delivery, thereby removing the stimulus for the production of anti-Rh antibodies [*see illustration at right*]. This situation, technically called ABO incompatibility between the mother and the fetus, is almost always effective in preventing immunization of an Rh-negative mother against an Rh-positive baby.

Here, then, was an intriguing analogy to our findings about butterflies. The mode of inheritance of the blood groups and the interaction of the Rh and ABO systems were remarkably similar to what we had observed in the insects, particularly the interaction of sex and the mimetic supergene that in male butterflies prevents wing mimicry. Could we somehow devise a protective system for unprotected Rh-negative mothers, that is, for cases where there is no ABO incompatibility between the mother and the fetus?

For months I puzzled over the problem with my colleagues Sheppard and Richard B. McConnell. One night my

SECOND BABY   MOTHER

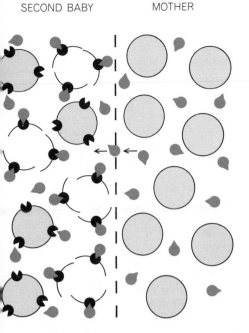

appears. If the mother has a subsequent Rh-positive baby, however, the antibody may attack the baby's red blood cells (4), thereby giving rise to a possibly fatal anemia.

wife, who had taken a keen interest in our work, woke me from a sound sleep and said: "Give them anti-Rh." Now, nothing is more irritating to a physician than to be awakened in the middle of the night and told how to manage his medical affairs. In a huff I replied, "It is anti-Rh we are trying to *prevent* them from making," and turned over and went to sleep again. In the clear light of morning, infuriatingly, the idea began to make sense. Giving the mother antibody to get rid of incompatible Rh-positive cells before her own antibody machinery went into production was obviously similar to the way nature accomplished the same objective, for instance in Group O mothers with a Group A baby or Group B one. I discussed the proposal with my colleagues, and we decided to test it.

The first experiments consisted in injecting Rh-positive red blood cells, labeled with radioactive chromium atoms, into Rh-negative male volunteers and then giving anti-Rh to half of the subjects, the other half serving as controls. We put Ronald Finn in charge of the experiments, and Dermot Lehane, director of the Liverpool Blood Transfusion Service, provided and injected the radioactively labeled infusions. The immediate results were exciting: the injected anti-Rh did indeed knock down a high proportion of the Rh-positive cells. Alas, the initial effect did not stand up. After six months we found that instead of suppressing the formation of antibodies the treatment had actually enhanced it. Confident nonetheless that our reasoning was basically sound, we persisted and discovered that we had given the wrong type of anti-Rh: the "complete" form of the antibody (which acts

in saline solution). This material, we found, destroys the Rh-positive cells but still leaves the residue antigenic. We therefore did a second series of experiments with "incomplete" anti-Rh, which coats the antigen so that it does not make contact with the antibody-forming cells. These injections were much more successful: they prevented the production of Rh antibody in most of the subjects.

We now proceeded to find out if the treatment would work in Rh-negative mothers who received the antibody injection after delivery of their first baby. First of all, Finn and Joseph C. Woodrow of our group determined that the likelihood of production of Rh antibody by mothers generally depended on the number of Rh-positive cells that had leaked into the maternal circulation from the fetus: the more such cells in the mother's blood just after delivery, the greater the risk she would produce antibody. On the strength of this information we felt justified in testing the preventive effect of antibody injection in Rh-negative mothers who, after delivery of their first baby, showed a fair number of fetal red cells in their blood (five or more per 50 fields in a low-power microscope). Our obstetrical liaison was with Shoma H. Towers of the department at Liverpool headed by T. N. A. Jeffcoate. In these clinical trials we used a new form of the antibody preparation that was similar to one that had been

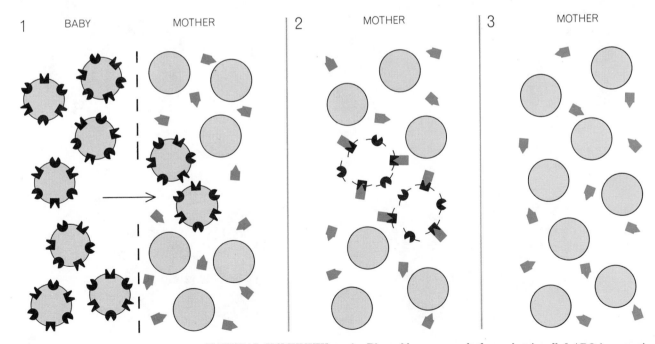

Rh ANTIGEN

TYPE-A ANTIGEN

TYPE-A ANTIBODY

NATURAL IMMUNITY to the Rh problem can result from what is called ABO incompatibility. Blood of the O type always has antibodies against blood of the A and B. Hence if an Rh-negative woman with O-type blood has an Rh-positive baby with A-type blood (1), her anti-A factor will attack any fetal red blood cells that enter her circulation (2). The cells are thus made nonantigenic, and the mother's body does not make antibodies against them. As a result she is not immunized against Rh-positive blood, so her subsequent Rh-positive babies will not be harmed.

developed by a team at the Sloane Hospital for Women in New York: John G. Gorman, Vincent J. Freda and William Pollack, who had arrived independently at the anti-Rh concept. The preparation consists of anti-Rh gamma globulin instead of anti-Rh serum; its great advantage is that it avoids the risk of jaundice, which is always a potential danger in blood transfusions. Employing anti-Rh gamma globulin prepared for us from the serum of our immunized male volunteers by William d'A. Maycock and his colleagues at the Lister Institute in London, we gave the antibody to 131 selected first-baby mothers within 48 hours after delivery of the baby. Six months later W. T. A. Donohoe and his staff, who have carried out all our serological tests, assayed the mothers' blood for the presence of Rh antibody. Only one of the 131 mothers produced this antibody, whereas in a comparable control group of 136 first-baby mothers who had not received the anti-Rh injection 21 percent proved to be anti-Rh producers at the six-month examination.

This result, suggesting that the treatment gave almost complete protection, was far better than we had anticipated on the basis of the anti-immunization results in our male subjects. Furthermore,

clinical trials of essentially the same method in the U.S., Canada, West Germany, Australia and elsewhere produced similarly successful outcomes for first-baby mothers. Critics objected that the six-month test was not necessarily conclusive as to protection: the treated mothers might start to make anti-Rh antibody under the stimulus of a second pregnancy. This objection proved to be groundless: subsequent tests at various centers on treated women who had a second Rh-positive baby showed that these mothers very rarely produced anti-Rh antibody. Immunologically speaking, the treated mothers entered their second pregnancy as if it were their first. The possibility remains, of course, that a "bleed" from the baby across the placenta at the second delivery or any subsequent one may stimulate the mother to begin producing antibody. In such cases the mother will require a new injection of the protective treatment whenever her blood after the birth carries fetal Rh-positive cells.

We are currently conducting studies to settle on a standard, minimum effective dose of antibody for the treatment. Tentatively it appears that about 200 micrograms of anti-Rh (about a fifth

of what we gave in the original trials) is effective in most cases.

We have, of course, given a great deal of study to the possible risks involved in the anti-Rh injection. Occasionally we have noted a local swelling afterward at the site of the injection (made intramuscularly), but this disappears within a day or two. Will the injected gamma globulin produce harmful effects later? It disappears from the blood after a few months, but some women (about 5 percent in our trials) do produce antibodies to the gamma globulin that perhaps might cause a reaction to an anti-Rh injection given after a later pregnancy. This, however, does not appear to be a substantial hazard, as is evidenced by the fact that after a person has received an ordinary blood transfusion (which can generate gamma globulin antibodies) it is not considered necessary as a general practice to test the person for sensitivity before giving him a second transfusion. All in all, it appears that the risks of giving anti-Rh gamma globulin to an Rh-negative mother after her first pregnancy are negligible.

On the other hand, there is some risk for the donors of the anti-Rh: the male Rh-negative volunteers who must be injected with whole Rh-positive blood to

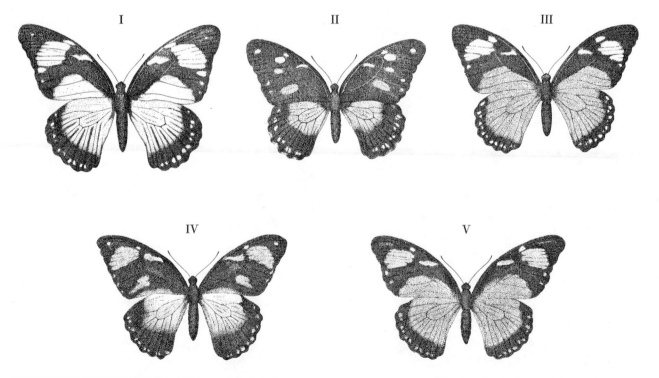

I   II   III

IV   V

WORK WITH BUTTERFLIES provided a lead to the solution of the Rh problem. The work involved an investigation of mimicry, in which a form of butterfly that is palatable to birds comes to resemble a form the birds find distasteful. Mimicry occurs only in females. A single difference in genes can turn one mimetic pattern into another. Here five female forms of the South African butterfly *Papilio dardanus* are arranged in order from the bottom recessive (*I*) to the two top dominants (*III and IV*), which form a recognizable heterozygote (*V*). The human blood types equivalent to these mimetic patterns are respectively O, B, A₂, A₁ and AB.

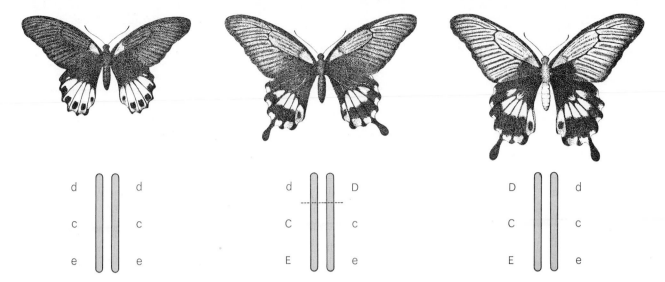

BREEDING EXPERIMENTS involving a nonmimetic (*left*) and a mimetic form (*right*) of the butterfly *Papilio memnon* of southeast Asia produced a crossover insect (*center*). At bottom are the respective chromosomal arrangements; *D* is yellow body color, *C* is small white wing window, *E* is long tails, *d* is black body color, *c* is large white wing window and *e* is absence of tails. The patterns are controlled by a group of closely linked genes called a supergene. There is interaction of sex and the mimetic supergene, reflected by the fact that mimicry does not occur in male butterflies. The Rh factor in human genetics is also controlled by a supergene.

manufacture the antibody. This risk is the possibility of the virus of jaundice being present in the injected blood. It can be minimized by making sure that the blood is obtained only from donors whose contributions have never induced jaundice in recipients. We have used blood from a few carefully selected donors and so far have not had a case of transmitted jaundice. There is, of course, the possibility of using serum from Rh-negative women who have been naturally immunized by an Rh-positive pregnancy; the Canadian workers use this source exclusively. The number of volunteers can also be greatly reduced with the new technique called plasmapheresis, which makes it possible to bleed the donors of anti-Rh every few weeks; a liter of blood is taken, the plasma containing the anti-Rh is skimmed off, and the red blood cells are reinjected into the donor.

Some authorities feel that, because of the jaundice risk to the donors and possible long-term harm to the women who receive anti-Rh, it is unwise to administer the antibody on a wholesale basis to all Rh-negative mothers who conceivably might have "rhesus" babies. Considering the small proportion of cases in which this actually happens, they suggest that anti-Rh should be given only to mothers who show a high probability of producing Rh antibody. The trouble is that it is impossible to identify these "high risk" cases with precision. The number of red cells from the baby found in the mother's circulation after the birth

is not always a reliable measure of the risk. Many women produce antibodies after receiving only a very tiny bleed from the baby, and the indications are that the cell-count basis for selection of women to be treated would catch only about a third of the risky cases. It seems to us that if proper precautions are taken, the hazards involved in the treatment are so small, for the donors as well as the mothers, that they are far outweighed by the benefits. All vaccination programs entail giving the injection to great numbers of people who do not necessarily need it but who take it nonetheless for safety's sake. In this case the inoculation would banish anxiety for Rh-negative women, who would no longer need to worry about the possibility of endangering their babies.

The discussion of the risks has, however, called attention to the fact that the need for anti-Rh treatment could be obviated in some cases by doing more than is now done to keep the baby from bleeding into the mother's circulation in the first place. It appears that the situations most likely to produce this untoward happening (called transplacental hemorrhage) are the following: peeling the placenta off the womb by hand when the afterbirth is delayed, attempts to turn around a poorly positioned baby in the womb before it is delivered, an excessive number of abdominal examinations of the pregnant mother, toxemia of pregnancy, Cesarean delivery and abortion. Therapeutic abortions are particularly likely to give rise to transpla-

cental bleeding, and when this occurs in an Rh-negative mother with an Rh-positive fetus, all the Rh-positive children she may deliver subsequently are apt to be exposed to anti-Rh attack. It therefore seems prudent to give anti-Rh to all Rh-negative women who have had an abortion even if the husband is Rh-negative, as one cannot always be absolutely certain that the husband is the father.

Among the thousands of mothers who have received the anti-Rh treatment since the trials began in 1964, there have been a few failures—cases in which the mother produced antibody in spite of the treatment. Two interesting possible explanations suggest themselves. The general rule has been to select for the treatment only women who apparently are not immunized, that is, who do not show evidence of producing Rh antibodies. One can suppose, however, that the antibodies may be present in the blood but not detectable by the usual methods, and that they manifest their presence only by going into action against Rh-positive cells when the woman becomes pregnant with an Rh-positive child. This may happen in the case of a mother who had a previous Rh-positive pregnancy but showed no sign of immunization afterward. In short, she may have been "primed" by the earlier pregnancy. We have actually encountered a case of priming in an Rh-negative man who volunteered for one of our experiments. After testing his blood and finding no evidence of the presence of

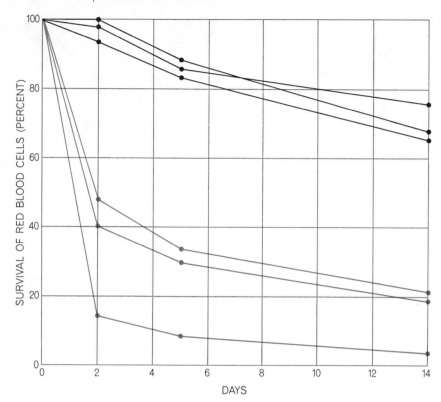

FIRST TEST of plan to attack the Rh problem by administering Rh antibody produced these results. Male volunteers were injected with Rh-positive cells and then half of them (*color*) were given anti-Rh. Technique produced the same result as natural ABO incompatibility.

Rh antibodies, we injected five milliliters of Rh-positive fetal blood. Within 48 hours all the fetal cells disappeared from his circulation, and we found traces of Rh antibodies in his blood. Since they could not have been produced so soon after the injection of the Rh-positive blood, we had to assume that he had been primed earlier. We then learned that the subject, who was 70 years old, had received a blood transfusion in World War I, which evidently was the source of his immunization against Rh-positive red cells.

This clear case of unsuspected priming suggests the exciting possibility that the anti-Rh treatment may work even for some mothers who are immunized, that is, whose antibody-producing mechanism has already been set in motion. It may be that a number of the mothers who have been given anti-Rh in the trials had actually been primed by previous exposure to Rh-positive cells although they showed no sign of being immunized when they were accepted for the treatment. If that is the case, the nearly perfect success in eliminating immunization in the thousands of women who have received anti-Rh is all the more remarkable.

Undetected priming is one of the two interesting explanations that have been offered for the few failures. The other is that occasionally the Rh-positive fetus's red cells may get into the Rh-negative mother's circulation early in her pregnancy, in which case the mother may develop the antibody-producing capacity before the baby is delivered and treatment with anti-Rh at that time will be too late. We believe such cases must be very rare, because first babies are seldom exposed to antibody from the mother. Bruce Chown and his colleagues at the University of Manitoba have, however, found evidence of the presence of Rh antibodies in some mothers during the first pregnancy or immediately after delivery. They have therefore begun giving anti-Rh to the mother during pregnancy and find that in the doses they use it does no harm to the baby. In cases where a bleed is known to have occurred early in pregnancy this method may be extremely valuable.

So, starting with experiments in the breeding of butterflies, the research has grown into a project that has enlisted the enthusiastic interest of a large team at Liverpool, stimulated workers in other laboratories around the world and produced a helpful advance in medicine and that may be found to have still wider applications.

VIII

IMMUNITY AND INFECTIOUS DISEASE

VIII

IMMUNITY AND INFECTIOUS DISEASE

INTRODUCTION

In an earlier introduction, I noted that immunology as an experimental science began with Jenner's work and was reopened by Pasteur, who was concerned with applying the Jennerian method to the prevention of infections from which bacterial pathogens had been cultivated. Essentially, immunology followed the course so laid down till the end of the nineteenth century, at which time a wider interest was generated by the recognition that red blood cells of another species were as effective as any microorganism in provoking an immune response. The application of immunology to the prevention of disease can be thought of as having been completed in principle by 1955 with the first effective large-scale use of the Salk vaccine. Since then there has been much more widespread application of preventive immunization but relatively little work that introduced any new principles. Modern advances in the field of immunity as applied to infectious disease have come mainly from efforts to understand the highly diverse quality and effect of the immune responses seen in different types of infection. The articles in this section on rheumatic fever, tetanus, and the laboratory studies of lymphocytic choriomeningitis in mice are characteristic of these efforts, and an additional article on measles has been included. Several other infectious diseases could probably have been at least equally illuminating; tuberculosis, malaria, and infectious hepatitis A and B represent important immunological topics still under active study that will in due course uncover new manifestations of interaction between pathogens and the immune system.

During the period when vaccine development was at its peak, the main guide to the development of immunizing agents was their capacity to produce antibody, either the type of antibody that seemed most relevant, as in diphtheria and tetanus, diseases in which antitoxins were measured, or, *faute de mieux*, the antibody most convenient to measure. Diphtheria and tetanus toxoid were developed and proved effective in large-scale tests, but the vaccines against typhoid and cholera, though very widely used, are still regarded with a certain skepticism. When interest moved to the prevention of viral diseases—yellow fever, poliomyelitis, and measles, for example—serological assessments of the response to immunization remained necessary but the basic philosophy changed. The objective had become to imitate the subclinical infection that, particularly in yellow fever, poliomyelitis, and influenza, played a major part in the epidemiology of the natural disease. If a strain of virus could be found or developed which regularly induced infection and involved all the processes that were responsible for a firm subsequent immunity but gave rise to trivial symptoms or no symptoms at all, then one could hope for a fully satisfactory immunization. This practice was very much strengthened by the considerable technical difficulties encountered in producing large enough amounts of virus to prepare killed vaccines for general use. One major difference between the two types of vaccine—the living attenuated and the killed—is that a killed virus preparation must supply the whole amount of antigen for the immunizing process, whereas living attenuated virus induces an infection resulting in viral proliferation and the production of much more antigen in the same situations and sequences as a normal infection by the epidemic virus. So it is that the currently used vaccines against smallpox, yellow fever, poliomyelitis, measles, mumps, and rubella all contain living virus as the immunizing agent.

Living virus vaccines, as would be expected, can be dangerous to children with congenital deficiency in T-cell function, but such children are so extremely rare and so unlikely to survive the inescapable infections of childhood that this danger is not regarded as justifying a veto on the use of living virus vaccines.

As with so many other aspects of immunology, much will remain obscure about immunity and infectious disease until the controversy on the nature of the T-cell receptor concerned with immune responses to extrinsic antigens is resolved. As long as living vaccines are used, we can reasonably assume that whatever is the normal relationship of T and B responses will persist in the subclinical infection produced by a live vaccine. This does not necessarily hold with a killed vaccine, which produces no infection, and in measles an apparent inadequacy of killed vaccine to stimulate T-cell function is already on record, as I show in my article concluding this section.

23   Vaccines for Poliomyelitis

by Jonas E. Salk
April 1955

*There has been some discussion as to whether one
made of "killed" viruses can be as effective as
one made of live viruses. A brief account of the
matter by an investigator of killed-virus vaccine*

We shall soon learn the results of last year's extensive field test of the vaccine against poliomyelitis. Whatever the analysis of that test shows, the type of vaccine that is being tested will continue to be an issue among virologists, because an immunological principle is under test as well as a vaccine. The vaccine in question is made of a "killed" virus, that is, a virus rendered noninfectious by treatment with formaldehyde. Many virologists believe such a vaccine can never be

as effective as one containing live virus, and that the best hope of conquering poliomyelitis is to develop a safe live-virus vaccine. The question has been discussed at a number of recent meetings. I share the view that a killed-virus vaccine not only avoids the hazards of live virus but, if properly prepared and used, may be just as effective in producing immunity. This article will present some findings that bear on the questions involved.

Many authorities have long held the

view that "there is no immunity like convalescent immunity," meaning the immunity a person acquires after recovery from infection. Poliomyelitis is considered a particularly good illustration of this principle, because infection with the virus seems to give lifelong immunity to those who recover. Pursuing this reasoning further, proponents of the live-microbe approach point to the success of the live-virus vaccines against smallpox and yellow fever, and observe that no human virus disease has yet been brought under control by a killed-virus vaccine.

In reply it is possible to point out that convalescent immunity is not always permanent or absolute. The smallpox vaccine, made of a modified virus, usually does not confer lifelong immunity, one indication of which is that travelers abroad must be revaccinated if they have not been vaccinated within three years. And there is no lasting immunity after infection by a virus of influenza or the common cold. In the case of poliomyelitis we have strong reasons to seek a solution which will avoid the risk of putting the live virus in human beings. On the basis of studies of both poliomyelitis and influenza, there is every reason to believe that a killed-virus vaccine can work, and that the failures of such vaccines hitherto have been due not to inherent limitations but to the way they were prepared or used.

The theory of the killed-virus vaccine rests on the well-established fact that an inactivated virus, though it has lost the power to infect or multiply, may still act as an antigen stimulating the body to produce antibodies against the specific virus. That the present vaccine can evoke these antibodies has been proved abundantly. The chief question

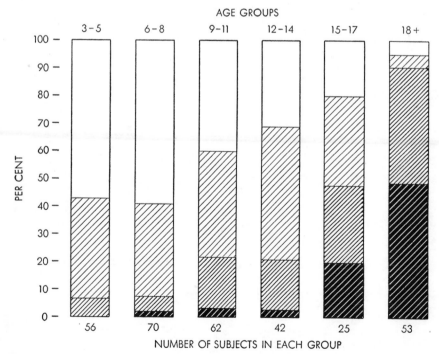

ANTIBODIES against the three types of virus that cause poliomyelitis were determined in 308 individuals from the area of Pittsburgh, Pa. The presence of antibodies against one, two or three types of virus is indicated by the shaded areas.

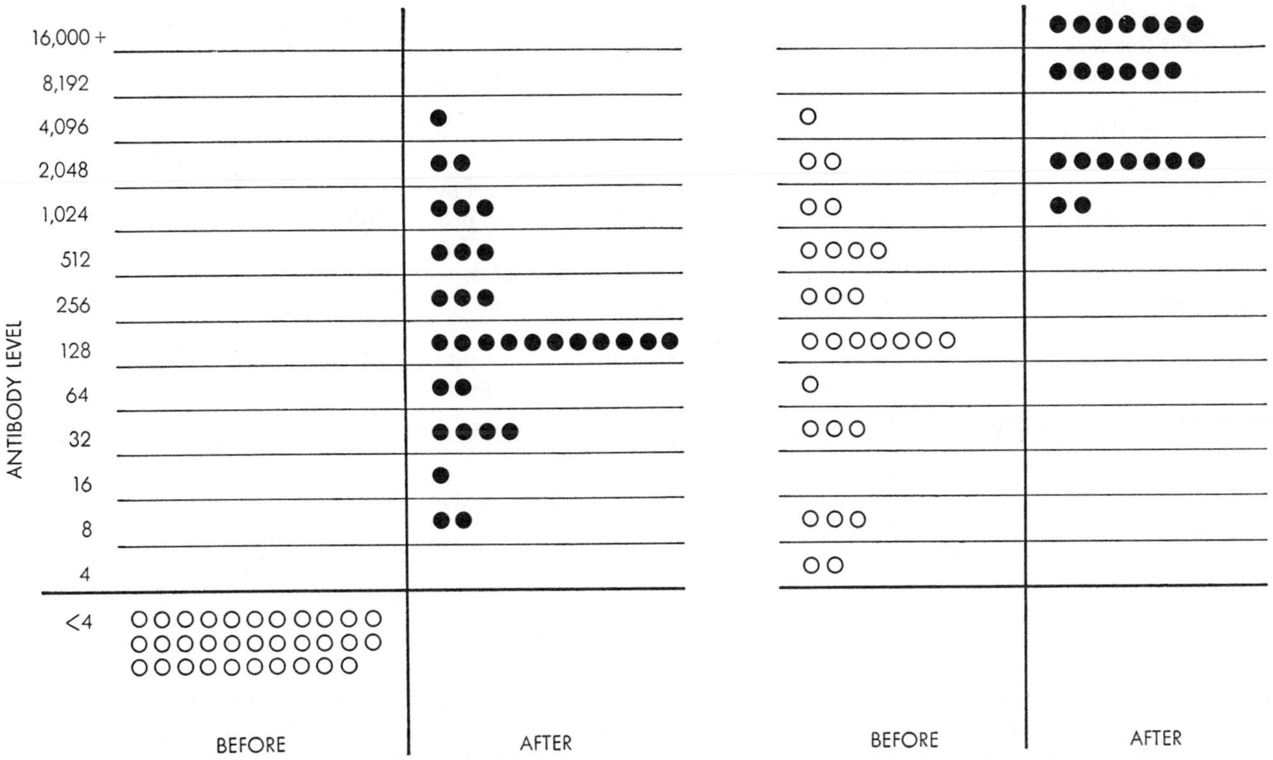

PRIMARY AND BOOSTER EFFECTS of vaccine containing killed poliomyelitis viruses is demonstrated in these two charts. The vaccine contained viruses of all three types. The antibody level is measured in titers. The open circles at the left side of the first chart represent 32 measurements of antibody against any one of the viruses; they indicate that the individuals had less than four units of the antibody measured. The same individuals were then given three doses of the vaccine, the second dose two weeks after the first and the third dose five weeks after the first. Two weeks after the third dose the same antibodies were measured. The primary effect is shown at the right side of the first chart. The open circles at the left side of the second chart represent 28 antibody measurements in another group; they indicate that these individuals had naturally acquired antibodies. The same individuals were then given the same three doses of vaccine. The booster effect is shown at the right side of the second chart.

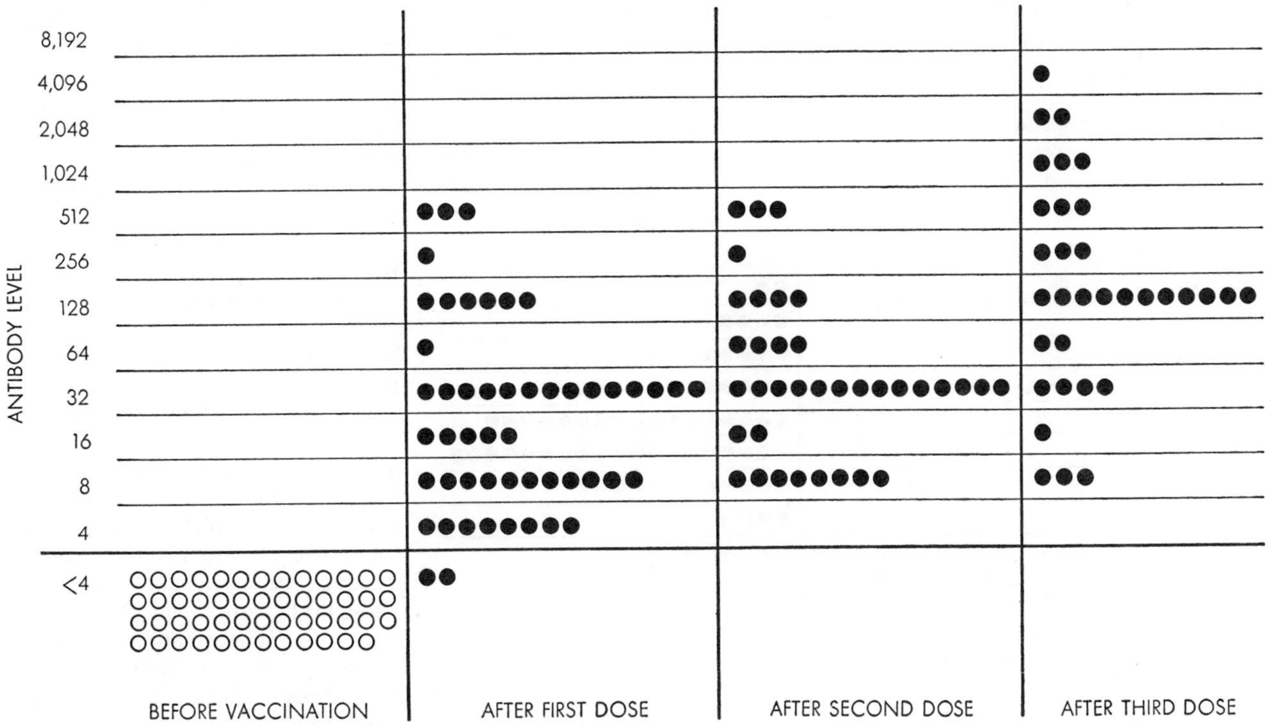

NO BOOSTER EFFECT was observed when doses of vaccine were given at short intervals to individuals with less than four units of antibody. The open circles represent 51 antibody measurements. Here again the second dose was given two weeks after the first and the third dose five weeks after the first. For the full effect the booster dose should be given about seven months after the first.

is how long immunity will last. The vaccine under test has not been in use long enough to give an answer. But we have some clues.

A monkey that has been vaccinated with the killed-virus vaccine at a certain strength will resist a paralyzing dose of poliomyelitis virus injected into its blood. When the vaccine is diluted to one part in four, it still prevents paralysis in every case. Indeed, six out of 10 monkeys suffer no paralysis, as one experiment showed, even when the vaccine is diluted to one part in 256. A vaccine dilution that produces a barely detectable level of antibody in the bloodstream is sufficient to prevent the virus from invading the central nervous system from the blood. The vaccine will prevent paralysis in monkeys even if the virus is introduced into the nervous system, but in that case a somewhat higher level of antibody is required.

Now let us see what happens to the antibody level in human beings when they are vaccinated. As is now well known, there are three poliomyelitis viruses—three different types with more or less independent powers of infection. In a typical U. S. population a majority of the children are not exposed to the virus during their early yeàrs, but as they grow older most of them are attacked by the virus (usually to only a mild, unnoticed degree) and gradually acquire antibodies to one or more of the virus types [see chart on page 222]. Suppose we inject the killed-virus vaccine into two groups, one consisting of persons who have no detectable antibody and the other of persons who have some antibody from an infection at some time in the past. The results of such an experiment are shown in the two upper charts on the preceding page. What

these charts emphasize is that the vaccination has a strong booster effect in the persons who already have some antibody, increasing the amount of antibody against the three virus types to a high level.

We can get the same booster effect by vaccinating previously uninfected persons two or three times at suitably spaced intervals. How long should these intervals be? As the lower chart on the preceding page shows, doses given two and five weeks after the first dose add comparatively little to the antibody level. For the full booster effect, we deduce from studies still not completed, a secondary dose should be given between four and seven months after the primary set of inoculations.

How long will the immunizing effect last? That depends on the capacity of the antigen (the killed poliomyelitis virus) not only to incite antibody formation but also to leave a lasting impression upon the "conditioned" body cells that form the antibody. Some strains of the virus seem to call forth antibody more easily than others. In fact, this accounts for the potency of very small doses of the vaccine. By experimenting with the various strains we have been able to develop vaccines more potent than those with which we started.

We have learned recently that one virus type may have antigenic components like those in another, so that one may call forth antibodies which are also active against the other. For instance, an infection with the type 2 virus seems to reduce the chances that a later infection by type 1 will produce paralysis. This is highly significant, because the type 1 virus appears to be more dangerous than type 2 or 3: among hundreds

of paralyzed poliomyelitis patients examined, infection by type 1 was eight times as frequent as by type 2 or 3.

Now a number of tests show that antibody persists for an appreciable time after vaccination with the killed-virus vaccine. Even after a single dose of the relatively weak preparations used when this vaccine was first made, most of the persons vaccinated had detectable levels of antibody a year after the inoculation [see chart below]. But even more interesting is the fact that when an individual is given a booster injection of the killed vaccine some months after the first, the antibody jumps to a high level— often higher than that after natural infection. This jump occurs even when the second injection is given as long as two years after the first.

Evidently the first exposure to the antigen, whether it is the killed virus or live virus in a natural infection, heightens the reactivity of the body to the antigen. In this hyperreactive state the body responds with rapid formation of antibody to a second invasion, either by live or by killed virus. We do not yet know whether immunity depends on this hyperreactivity or on the actual level of antibody present in the blood. Whichever is the case, the killed vaccine seems to meet both requirements: it produces the hyperreactive state and it maintains antibody in the blood, especially when a booster dose is given some months after the initial vaccination.

Our recent studies suggest that hyperreactivity may be sufficient. Apparently infection with the type 2 virus makes some persons hyperreactive to the type 1 virus, and such individuals seem to be able to resist type 1 paralysis even though there is no measurable antibody against that specific virus in their blood at the time of exposure. This must mean that the new exposure to type 1 causes the sensitized individual to produce type 1 antibody rapidly enough to block the invading virus before it can reach the central nervous system, or perhaps even before it gets into the blood.

This concept of the dynamics of the immunizing process suggests a new outlook toward infectious diseases that behave like poliomyelitis. If the concept is correct, we should test immunity by testing for hyperreactivity. Tests for the degree of hyperreactivity, based on the response to a booster injection, are now being devised. The booster injection would thus serve a double function against poliomyelitis—a test for immunity and a stimulus for the production of more protective antibody.

PERSISTENCE OF ANTIBODIES a year after vaccination is illustrated by this chart. The open circles represent 92 measurements of antibody against any one of the viruses. With a stronger vaccine and a booster dose at the proper interval, the level of antibody sustained after vaccination would be higher. Plus and minus signs indicate traces of antibody.

Rheumatic Fever

by Earl H. Freimer and Maclyn McCarty
December 1965

*It is clear that this baffling disease, which often
damages the heart, stems from streptococcal infection.
No link has yet been found, however, between the
infection and the rheumatic process*

Over the centuries few diseases of childhood have induced a greater feeling of helplessness among physicians or aroused more concern in the families of patients than rheumatic fever. Although the acute symptoms—such as the swollen, tender joints for which the disease was named—were disturbing, it was known that they usually subsided without producing any permanent disability. Rheumatic involvement of the heart, on the other hand, sometimes brought sudden death in a fulminating attack and more often led to chronic heart disease. To this day the menace of rheumatic fever is measured primarily in terms of scarred heart valves that may eventually impair cardiac function.

It is the severity of this end result, which affects several million people in the U.S., that has made rheumatic fever one of the most extensively investigated of mankind's diseases. In the past half-century it has been the focus of a host of clinical investigations and has stimulated fundamental studies in immunology and microbiology. By now it is clear that streptococcal infection may lead to rheumatic fever. Yet no specific link has been found between the infection and its rheumatic sequel. Although streptococcal infections can be cured and the rheumatic symptoms can be allayed, the disease remains mysterious and essentially unconquered.

What is this dread disorder that "licks the joints but bites the heart"? Rheumatic fever is basically an arteritis, an inflammation that involves small blood vessels. The inflammation results in lesions that are widely distributed through the connective tissues of the body. Many organs are affected, but the diverse manifestations appear to be unrelated to one another. Involvement of the joints illustrates the classic description of the inflammatory state: *calor* (heat), *rubor* (redness), *tumor* (swelling) and *dolor* (pain). Sometimes a single joint is affected, but typically the arthritis appears to migrate from joint to joint. One day the right elbow may be involved, the next day the left knee. In young children an early symptom, and often the only one observed, is abdominal pain that is sometimes mistaken for appendicitis. Roughly circular areas of redness may appear on the skin, fade and then reappear from time to time. In severe cases firm, insensitive nodules occur under the skin.

The most striking of all the manifestations of rheumatic fever is Sydenham's chorea, or St. Vitus's dance. This appears late in the course of rheumatic fever, often months after the initiating streptococcal infection; sometimes it is the only sign of rheumatic activity. The irregular and uncontrollable movements of chorea were vividly described by the 17th-century English physician Thomas Sydenham as "a kind of convulsion in which the hand cannot be steady for a moment. It passes from one position to another by a convulsive movement, however much the patient may strive to the contrary. Before he can raise a cup to his lips, he makes as many gesticulations as a mountebank."

In the course of a rheumatic attack various parts of the heart are often affected. The cardiac symptoms are usually vague, but involvement of the pericardium (the outer lining of the heart) or the myocardium (the heart muscle itself) can often be detected by examination with a stethoscope and by X-ray and electrocardiographic studies. In contrast, it is particularly difficult to demonstrate the presence of endocarditis, an inflammation of the endocardium (the inner lining of the heart). And it is endocarditis that is responsible for the scarring and distortion of the valve leaflets that lead to permanent heart disease. Like the submerged portion of an iceberg, the most deadly aspect of the rheumatic process—the extent of involvement of the endocardium—remains undetected until it is disclosed by subsequent valvular dysfunction.

For many centuries rheumatic fever was a totally baffling disorder. Then in the 19th century physicians began to note that acute rheumatism was often preceded by a septic sore throat or by scarlet fever. When, early in this century, streptococci were shown to be the agents responsible for many cases of tonsillitis and for scarlet fever, the way was opened at last for systematic investigations into the cause of rheumatic fever. In recent decades the search has focused to a large extent on the fundamental nature of the bacterium.

Streptococci comprise a biologically diverse collection of microorganisms that have in common a tendency to grow in chains. Some of them lyse, or dissolve, mammalian red blood cells. One group of these hemolytic streptococci, known as Group A, is responsible for most of the streptococcal infections of man. The Group A streptococcus has been studied in great detail, and several independent lines of evidence clearly implicate it in the development of rheumatic fever.

First, the Group A streptococcus is the only bacterium that causes human infections with an epidemiological pattern that parallels the seasonal incidence and geographical distribution of rheumatic fever. Second, this streptococcus can cause repeated infections at intervals throughout childhood, and it is such repetition that probably sets the stage for the first attack of rheumatic fever. Third, rheumatic fever can be prevented by vigorous treatment of streptococcal infections with such antimicrobial agents as penicillin, suggesting that the elimination of the organisms early in the course of the infection interrupts a chain of events that leads to rheumatic fever. Fourth, a specific immune response to streptococcal antigens occurs almost uniformly in patients with acute rheumatic fever; with sufficient antibiotic therapy this response to streptococcal antigens is suppressed.

Although it is clear that streptococcal infections can lead to rheumatic fever, the mechanism by which the streptococci initiate the rheumatic process remains obscure. In an infection a microorganism actively produces the disease state, as the streptococcus produces a sore throat. The symptoms of rheumatic fever, however, do not appear until weeks after the acute infection. By this time hemolytic streptococci are not usually detectable in the affected tissues, and doses of antibiotics large enough to eliminate any that are there do not influence the manifestations or the course of the illness.

The organism must therefore exert its effect through some indirect process rather than by the continued presence of infectious streptococci in the tissues of the host. Many investigators now believe that rheumatic fever represents a state of hypersensitivity resulting from the combination of some streptococcal antigen with host antibody. Hypersensitivity is a special form of the immune reaction, a process by which the body resists the intrusion of foreign substances, or antigens. In the immune reaction specialized cells synthesize antibodies in response to these antigens. The state of hypersensitivity develops in some individuals after one or more exposures to a certain antigen; the reintroduction of the same antigen stimulates increased production of the specific antibody, which reacts with the antigen. When the resulting antigen-antibody complex reaches certain cells, it triggers an acute inflammatory process. Allergies to foreign substances such as pollens or bee venoms are examples of hypersensitivity, and diseases such as hives or asthma are the result of hypersensitive states.

The natural history of rheumatic fever supports the concept that this disease may be the result of a state of hypersensitivity. The interval between the streptococcal infection and the onset of the rheumatic disease is about equal to the time required for an antigenic stimulus to provoke a maximal antibody response. The typical pattern of the rheumatic attack—a latent period during which the patient shows no signs of illness, followed by the sudden development of fever and joint pain—is quite similar to the pattern in acute serum sickness, a disorder in which sensitivity to an antigen is well established. The observed hyperactivity of rheumatic patients in producing antibodies in response to streptococcal antigens also gives support to the hypersensitivity hypothesis. Patients who have rheumatic fever show a greater outpouring of streptococcal antibodies, on the average, than those who have a streptococcal infection without rheumatic fever. Finally, histological examination reveals that rheumatic lesions are very similar to those obtained in studies of experimental hypersensitivity in animals. In rabbits injected with streptococci George E. Murphy of the Cornell University Medical College has found lesions similar to the Aschoff body, which is seen in the heart muscle of people who have had rheumatic fever [see illustration on page 231].

The investigation of rheumatic fever has progressed through several stages. Clinicians described the course of the disease, pathologists studied the lesions, epidemiologists implicated the hemolytic streptococcus and bacteriologists proceeded to study the microorganism. In the past two decades new techniques have been introduced that have made it possible to take the streptococcus apart antigen by antigen. It has been particularly interesting to identify the outer structures of the bacterium and the various substances it releases into its environment during growth.

The streptococcus has a complex surface containing a number of potential antigens [see illustration on this page]. Its outer covering is a capsule composed of a gel, hyaluronic acid. Within this capsule is a tough protective structure, the cell wall. The streptococcal wall can be conceived of as having three layers. The outer layer is made up of a number of different proteins. The middle layer, the major component of the wall by weight, is a carbohydrate; each streptococcal group, such as Group A, has a different carbohydrate. The inner layer of the wall, the one that provides its structural rigidity, is composed of a mucopeptide, repeating units of several amino acids and two amino sugars. Similar mucopeptides form the skeletons of all bacterial cell walls. Inside the cell wall there is a delicate membrane that encloses the cytoplasm of the bacterium.

One of the cell-wall proteins, the M protein, is highly significant. It identifies the various types of Group A streptococci. It also plays a dominant role in determining the virulence of the bacterium by inhibiting phagocytosis, the process in which white blood cells engulf and dispose of foreign particles. The M protein thus aids the streptococcus in its invasion of the host's tissues, where it can multiply. This antiphagocytic effect of M protein can be neutralized by specific antibody that renders the microbe vulnerable to destruction by the white cells. Each type of Group A streptococcus, however, has its own distinct M protein; there are some 50 types, and the body must produce a different antibody to combat each of them. This multiplicity of M proteins, many different types of which may be widely disseminated throughout a human population, explains the repetitive nature of streptococcal infections, since the production of antibodies against one

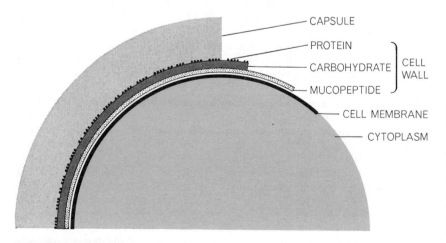

STREPTOCOCCUS, the structure of which is shown schematically, is about a thousandth of a millimeter in diameter exclusive of the outer capsule. The protective cell wall is characteristic of bacteria. The cell membrane is comparable to that of a mammalian cell.

type of streptococcus confers no immunity against a second type.

Another distinctive characteristic of the Group A streptococcus is its ability to synthesize a wide variety of enzymes and toxins. In the never ending struggle between infecting organisms and their hosts, parasites with characteristics that increase their pathogenic capability are favored. Although the precise contribution of the extracellular products to the genesis of streptococcal disease is not clear, they presumably contribute to the survival and propagation of the streptococcus. Indeed, an important part of the host response to a streptococcal infection is the formation of specific antibodies to most of these substances.

There are, first of all, two specific enzymes that lyse the red blood cells. Other enzymes split the coenzyme diphosphopyridine nucleotide (DPN), activate the process that dissolves the blood-clotting agent fibrin, break down hyaluronic acid in the connective tissue of the host, decompose deoxyribonucleic acid (DNA), break down various proteins and hydrolyze glycogen (animal starch). Another identified product of the streptococcus is "erythrogenic toxin," which is responsible for the rash of scarlet fever. John Zabriskie of our laboratory at Rockefeller University has discovered that the ability to produce this toxin depends on a nonlethal infection of the streptococcus by a bacteriophage, or bacterial virus. Apparently a streptococcal infection is capable of generating scarlet fever when the bacteria happen to be carriers of these bacteriophages. (It is because of the persistence of antibodies to erythrogenic toxin that scarlet fever, unlike streptococcal infections in general, usually occurs only once.)

In our laboratory we have been investigating the properties of the streptococcal membrane, the structure that lies inside the cell wall. Unlike most bacterial membranes, it contains lipoproteins in which the lipids, or fatty substances, are essentially identical with those in mammalian tissues. There are variant forms of streptococci, called L forms, that lack a cell wall and in which the membrane is therefore the outer covering. We have prepared similar incomplete forms, called protoplasts, by dissolving the cell wall of the bacteria with enzymes. We find that both L forms and protoplasts are capable of many of the biological functions of the intact bacterial cell. They are also resistant to penicillin, which acts by in-

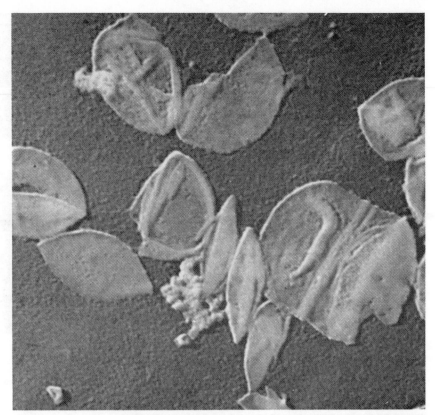

CELL WALLS are enlarged about 12,500 diameters in this electron micrograph made, like the one below, by the authors and Richard M. Krause. Streptococci were disrupted mechanically; their walls were suspended in water, mounted on grids and shadowed with chromium.

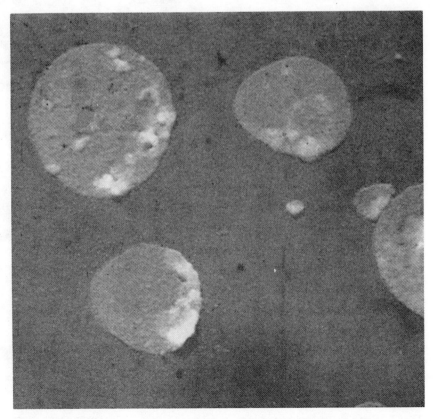

CELL MEMBRANE is much thinner than the cell wall. These membranes were prepared from protoplasts, fragile bacterial forms from which the cell wall had been removed by an enzyme. The protoplasts were disrupted by being placed in water. The membranes were collected by centrifugation, mounted, shadowed and enlarged about 12,500 diameters.

228

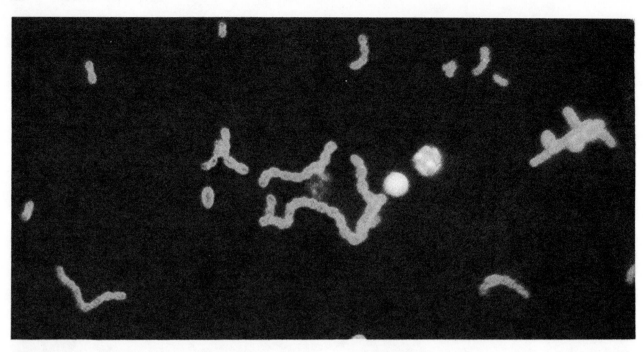

STREPTOCOCCI, the bacteria that cause rheumatic fever, are enlarged 2,500 diameters in a photomicrograph made by one of the authors (Freimer) and John Zabriskie at Rockefeller University.

The bacteria, having combined with antibody tagged with a fluorescent compound, glow under ultraviolet radiation. The antibody is directed against antigens in the streptococcal membrane.

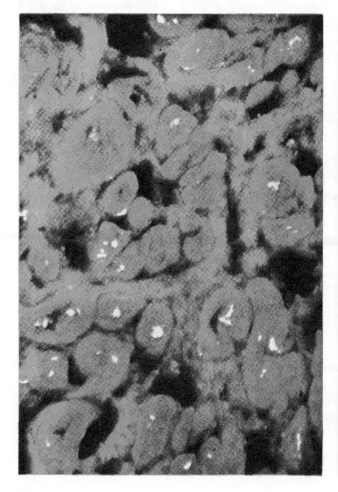

HEART MUSCLE also binds antibody to streptococcal membrane. The fluorescent antibody, applied to a cross section of human cardiac muscle, has combined with antigens in the muscle cells and glows green under ultraviolet. The blue areas are connective tissue.

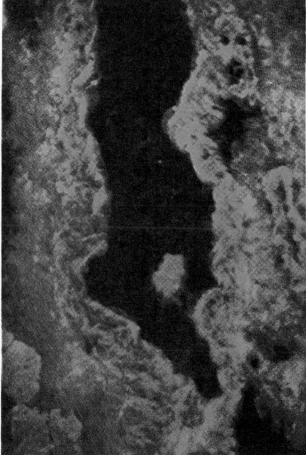

ARTERIAL MUSCLE shows the same immunological relation to streptococcal membrane. Smooth muscle in the wall of a small artery in the heart has bound the fluorescent antibody and glows. Rheumatic fever involves small arteries and may damage the heart.

hibiting the formation of the cell wall. One might postulate that a bacterial variant with a surface of related lipid, rather than of alien cell-wall carbohydrate and protein, might survive unchallenged within the host. The streptococcus would persist as an *L* form, undetectable by the usual bacteriological techniques but with the potential for reversion to an active bacterial form. There is still no firm evidence to support this concept, however.

In 1962 Melvin Kaplan of the Western Reserve School of Medicine reported the existence of an immunological cross-reaction between Group *A* streptococci and cardiac muscle. Following a similar line of investigation, we have found that the membrane of the bacterium appears to contain an antigen that cross-reacts with the membrane of cardiac muscle cells and the muscle layer in small arteries. This may provide a promising clue to the genesis of rheumatic fever; moreover, the discovery of an immunological relation between the membranes of a bacterial cell and a mammalian cell is exciting and may prove to be of broad biological significance.

The experimental procedure begins with the injection of a preparation of streptococcal membranes into rabbits. Over a period of weeks the animals form antibodies to the membranes. Having isolated the globulin (the blood fraction containing the antibodies) from the rabbits' blood, we couple it to a fluorescent substance and layer the fluorescent globulin over the specimen to be tested. If the antibody reacts with an antigen in the specimen, it becomes fixed, and the antigen-antibody complex will fluoresce under ultraviolet radiation. As one might expect, antibody to streptococcal membrane does combine in this manner with streptococci. What is interesting is that this antibody also reacts with muscle from human heart—both from the myocardium and from the wall of small arteries [*see illustration at right*]. It does not react with tissues other than muscle, nor do antibodies to other bacterial species react with the muscle. If instead of rabbit globulin we test globulin from patients with rheumatic fever, we get a similar set of results [*see illustration on page 230*]. It is therefore tempting to form the hypothesis that it is antibody produced to combat the streptococcus that later takes part in a hypersensitivity reaction involving the heart and small blood vessels of the rheumatic fever patient.

There is no dearth of attractive speculations about the possible genesis of rheumatic fever, but none of them is yet

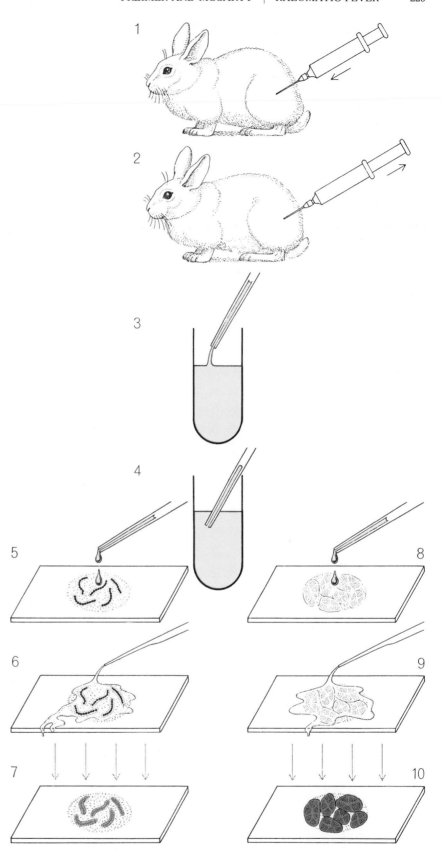

IMMUNOLOGICAL RELATION between the streptococcus and heart muscle is demonstrated by an experiment in which streptococcal membranes are injected into a rabbit (*1*). The globulin fraction, containing antibody formed against the membranes, is isolated from the rabbit's blood (*2*) and coupled to a fluorescent compound (*3*). When the fluorescent antibody is tested on streptococci (*4, 5*), it reacts with antigen in the bacteria, so that in spite of washing (*6*) it remains bound to the bacteria, which glow under ultraviolet radiation (*7*). Tested on heart muscle (*8*), the antibody reacts in the same way (*9, 10*).

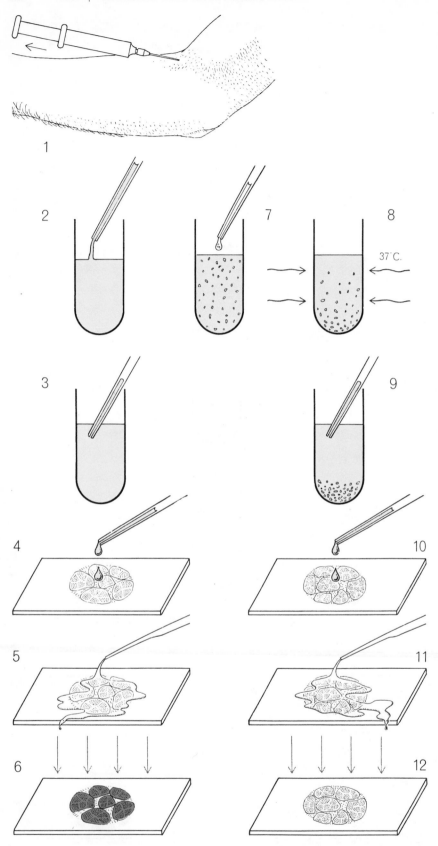

1

2

7   8

37°C.

3   9

4   10

5   11

6   12

HUMAN ANTIBODY from the blood of a rheumatic fever patient (1) is similarly tested. The antibody-containing globulin is isolated, coupled to the fluorescent compound (2) and tested on heart muscle (3, 4). It is bound, and in spite of washing (5) the heart section glows (6). Is the reaction caused specifically by antibody to streptococcal membrane? An indication that it may be comes from the following procedure: Membrane is added to the globulin solution (7) and the suspension is incubated (8). Antibody is bound by the membrane; when the supernatant is tested on a heart section (9, 10, 11), the muscle fails to fluoresce (12).

supported by solid evidence—and "many a beautiful idea has been slain by ugly fact." The rheumatic process is so complex and so diverse that it is difficult to conceive a single scheme that would account for all the observed phenomena. What kind of process can produce localized lesions not only in the joints and the heart but also in the skin all over the body, and by what means does the same process involve the nervous system and express itself in chorea? How can the various rheumatic symptoms continue to appear so long after the inciting infection has disappeared? Why are some people apparently "susceptible" to rheumatic fever and other people not? Rheumatic fever poses many such difficult questions.

Although the genesis of rheumatic fever remains unexplained, enough has been learned about the disease to make it far less of a menace than it was in the past. The identification of the streptococcus as the inciting organism and the development of effective antistreptococcal agents had far-reaching effects. As recently as World War II epidemics of streptococcal sore throat swept through recruit-training camps in the U.S., and roughly 3 percent of those who were infected developed rheumatic fever. The introduction of penicillin and other drugs effective against Group A streptococci essentially eliminated rheumatic fever in military populations and has greatly reduced the risk in the general population. It is clear that the prompt and intensive treatment of a streptococcal infection with penicillin can prevent rheumatic fever.

For those who do develop rheumatic fever the control of streptococcal infection becomes a matter of special significance. The repetitive nature of these infections used to pose a constant threat of recurring rheumatic attacks. Now rheumatic fever patients are first treated intensively with penicillin to eliminate any remaining streptococci and then protected from reinfection by the daily administration of penicillin. The success of this continuous prophylaxis has been dramatic. During the past 15 years very few patients maintained on penicillin have developed another episode of rheumatic fever. The elimination of repetitive attacks, each contributing further damage to the heart valves, should significantly reduce the incidence of serious heart disease in rheumatic individuals.

In view of the deluge of antibiotics with which the U.S. population has been dosed in the past two decades,

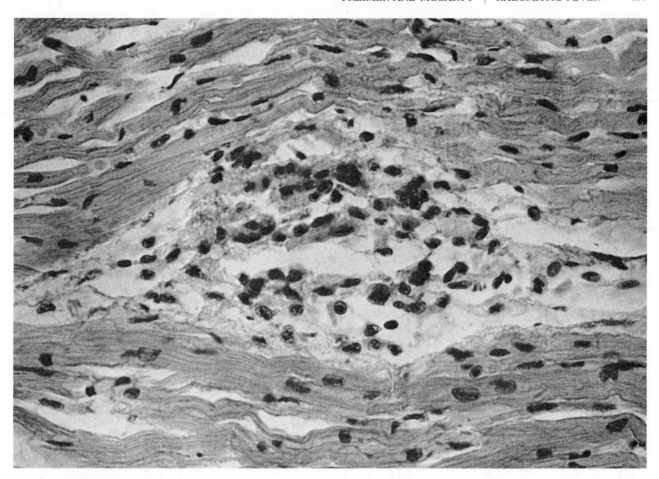

ASCHOFF BODY, the classic lesion of rheumatic fever, is enlarged about 570 diameters in this photomicrograph made by George E. Murphy of the Cornell University Medical College. It is in the striated muscle of the myocardium, the heart muscle itself. Lesions also occur in the endocardium, or inner lining of the heart, in a layer of smooth muscle much like the muscle of a small artery.

one might suppose that streptococcal infection and therefore rheumatic fever should have been all but eradicated by this time. For various reasons, however, both the infection and the disease remain a danger. Three factors are particularly important.

First, many streptococcal infections are so mild that they escape notice, and a "subliminal" infection can incite rheumatic fever in a susceptible individual. Even when the infection is recognized, it is not always treated promptly or vigorously enough.

Second, rheumatic fever is hard to diagnose. Any one of its characteristic manifestations can also be a sign of some other disease. Moreover, the course of the disease is variable. The classic case—in which fever, joint pain, skin lesions and evidence of cardiac inflammation develop some three weeks after a sore throat—is easy enough to recognize, but not every case follows that pattern. Some people become symptom-free in a few days, whereas in others the rheumatic activity may persist for months or even years, or the episodes may come and go in cyclic fashion. In still other individuals who have rheumatic fever no clearcut symptoms ever appear; the disease goes unrecognized until, years later, they are found to have valvular heart disease. Even laboratory tests will not specifically identify rheumatic fever. The blood of a person with the disease shows a high white-cell count and a heightened concentration of fibrinogen, gamma globulin and a substance called C-reactive protein that is not normally present, but all these changes merely indicate the presence of an inflammatory process. A rise in the blood level of antibodies to the Group A streptococcus and its products, on the other hand, only shows that the patient has recently had a streptococcal infection. Even in combination these tests do not prove the presence of rheumatic fever. The physician must therefore season the laboratory data with his evaluation of the broad clinical pattern—history, symptoms and physical signs—and, as we have seen, these are not always clearly defined.

Finally,. rheumatic fever remains a danger because there is no specific therapy for it (as there is against the inciting infection). The only available treatment is the use of aspirin or a steroid hormone such as cortisone to suppress the inflammatory response. This relieves the patient's symptoms but does not eliminate the underlying disease process.

Current therapy, in other words, is largely defensive. The elimination of the disease depends on gaining a clearer understanding of the chain of events whereby an infection with hemolytic streptococci sometimes develops into rheumatic fever. This will require continued investigation not only of the streptococcus but also of the susceptible host. If the role of the bacterium is being stressed in our laboratory and others, that is because the inciting action of streptococcal infections in rheumatic fever is the one key that is currently available to the fundamental nature of the disease. It is this relation to a specific bacterial agent that sets rheumatic fever apart from the other diseases of connective tissue.

25

How the Immune Response to a Virus Can Cause Disease

by Abner Louis Notkins and Hilary Koprowski
January 1973

The body's defense mechanism may not always be beneficial. In many cases the very process that should combat a virus is itself a cause of the damage associated with a viral disease

In biology as in physics it is a truism that the deeper one goes in exploring elementary questions, the more one encounters paradoxical and puzzling phenomena. Such is the case in the investigation of the well-known animal defense mechanism called the immune response, whereby the body fights off infections and other invasions by foreign matter. The classic concept of this mechanism is quite simple: in response to invasion by the foreign substance, or antigen, the body produces specific antibodies that bind to it, thus neutralizing the invader so that it does not harm the invaded organism. Investigators are now learning, however, that this is far from the entire story, that the mechanism of immunity is much more complex than had been supposed.

This is true in particular in virus infections. In the simple case of direct attack by a virus (for example in poliomyelitis) the virus invades a cell and uses the cell's material to replicate, and soon the new crop of viruses bursts the cell and emerges to go on to infect other cells. The timely appearance of antibodies may prevent the spread of infection and the appearance of symptoms. In infections caused by other viruses, however, there is growing evidence that the cells are damaged not directly by the replicating virus but by a specific immune response that produces the symptoms of the disease. The complexities of the immune response to viruses are under exploration in a number of laboratories, including our own at the National Institutes of Health (Notkins) and at the Wistar Institute of Anatomy and Biology (Koprowski). Gradually an account of the immunity mechanism's diverse operations is being pieced together, and

what follows is a review of the emerging picture.

That the immunity system might sometimes be responsible for injurious effects was first suggested more than 60 years ago by Clemens von Pirquet, an Austrian pediatrician who was at one time also a professor at the Johns Hopkins School of Medicine. Von Pirquet noted that in "serum sickness," a disease that can follow injection of foreign blood serum, the patient's blood contained foreign proteins and antibody against them. He speculated that the combination of antibody with foreign proteins (antigen) perhaps produced a toxic substance that gave rise to the symptoms of the sickness: hives, rash, pain in the joints, shortness of breath and, in severe cases, death. He also conjectured that an interaction of antibodies with the viruses of such diseases as smallpox and measles might cause the skin eruptions characteristic of these diseases.

Von Pirquet's speculations that immune response to viruses might cause disease were not followed up at the time, but in the 1950's Wallace P. Rowe, a virus investigator at the National Institutes of Health, came on proof of the hypothesis in an ingenious series of experiments. Rowe was studying the pathology produced by a virus known as lymphocytic choriomeningitis (LCM), which infects rodents and occasionally

man and causes an inflammation of the membranes surrounding the brain (meningitis). He observed that although in infected mice the virus multiplied rapidly in many organs, the animals at first showed no sign of illness. On the sixth day, however, after the mice had begun to show an immune response to the virus, they developed meningitis and died. Was the disease caused by their immunological response to the virus rather than by the virus itself? Reasoning that if he inhibited the immune response, he might be able to prevent the disease, Rowe treated mice with X rays in doses known to suppress the immune response. He then infected both the treated mice and untreated control mice with LCM virus. The irradiated animals did not develop meningitis, although the virus replicated in their tissues just as rapidly as it did in the control mice, which died.

Later a group of investigators at the Johns Hopkins School of Hygiene and Public Health (Donald H. Gilden, Gerald A. Cole, Andrew A. Monjan and Neal Nathanson) took Rowe's experiments a step further. It was known by this time that the immune system responds to foreign substances in at least two ways, one mediated by antibody and the other mediated by a specific group of the cells known as lymphocytes. These "immune lymphocytes" recognize antigens on the surface of foreign cells

IMMUNE COMPLEXES are formed when an antiviral antibody combines with a virus and binds complement. The complexes are detected by a technique in which an antibody to complement is labeled with a fluorescent substance and incubated with tissue; if complexes are present, the antibody binds to them and fluoresces under ultraviolet radiation. The photomicrograph on the opposite page, made by David D. Porter of the University of California Center for Health Sciences, demonstrates the presence of complexes in the kidneys of mink that were infected with Aleutian virus and developed glomerulonephritis.

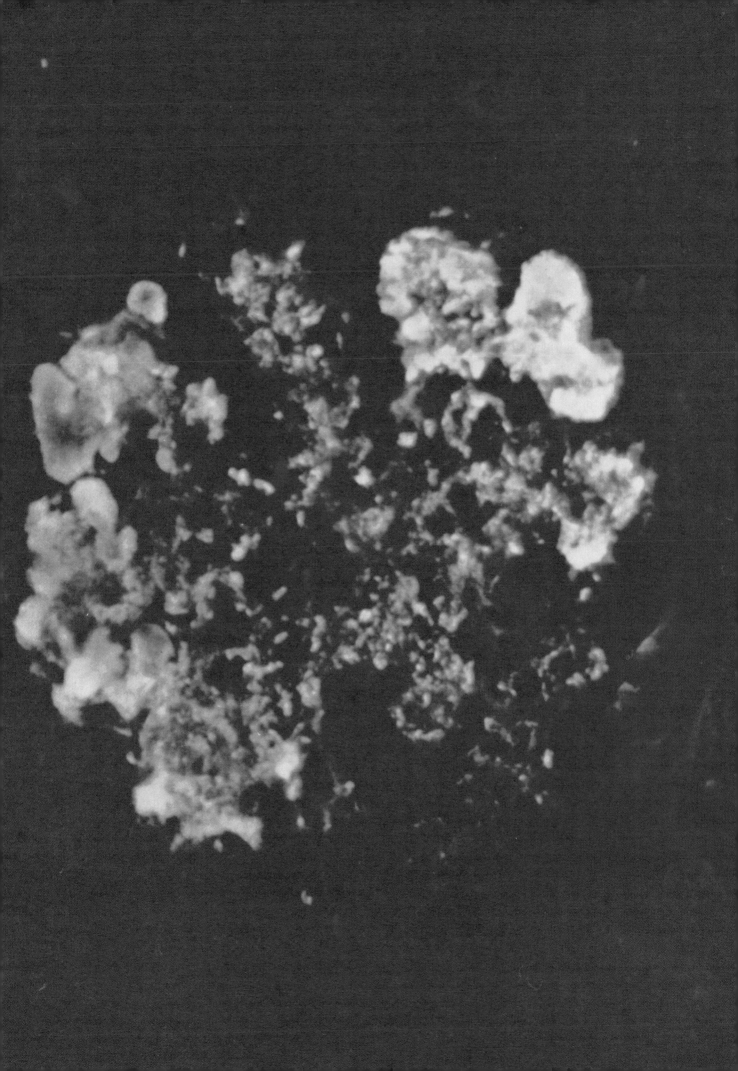

and thereby destroy tissue such as tumors or skin grafts [see "Markers of Biological Individuality," by Ralph A. Reisfeld and Barry D. Kahan, the article beginning on page 202]. Which of these factors was responsible for causing LCM disease in Rowe's experiments: antibodies or lymphocytes? The Johns Hopkins group used drugs to suppress the immunological response in mice, infected them with LCM virus and then divided the animals into three groups. One group received injections of anti-LCM antibody, the second was given anti-LCM lymphocytes and the third normal lymphocytes. The animals receiving the antibody or normal lymphocytes remained well but those given the immune lymphocytes developed the symptoms of LCM disease and died. Evidently in the case of LCM it was the combination of immune lymphocytes and the virus that produced the disease.

Extending their observations, the Johns Hopkins group found that in young rats LCM infection was not fatal but did damage the cerebellum, causing ataxia (inability to coordinate body movements). If the immune response was suppressed at the time of infection, however, the animals remained free of symptoms and cerebellar damage did not occur, even though the virus continued to replicate in the brain. As in the case of mice, development of the rats' disease was thus shown to be immunologically mediated. An interesting suggestion from these experiments is that perhaps other neurological disorders may arise from the immune response to viruses.

It was now time to look into the reasons why lymphocytes destroyed infected cells when the virus itself did not. In order to study this problem Duard L. Walker and his co-workers at the University of Wisconsin Medical School turned from experiments in animals to experiments in tissue culture. It was known that on infecting a cell some viruses induce the formation of viral antigens on the cell's surface. Walker reasoned that if these antigens are recognized by lymphocytes from animals immunized with the same virus, the lymphocytes might attack and destroy cells carrying the label of infection. To test this hypothesis he infected tissue-culture cells with mumps virus, which induced new antigens on the surface of the cells but did not destroy them. When he introduced into the infected cultures lymphocytes taken from animals that had been immunized with that virus, the lymphocytes did indeed destroy the infected cells. On the other hand, lymphocytes from animals that had not been immunized with the mumps virus did not attack the infected cells.

Other investigators soon obtained the same kind of result in tissue-culture experiments with LCM virus and the measles virus. A number of groups are now looking into the possibility that the interaction between immune lymphocytes and viral antigens formed on the surface of infected cells may account for some

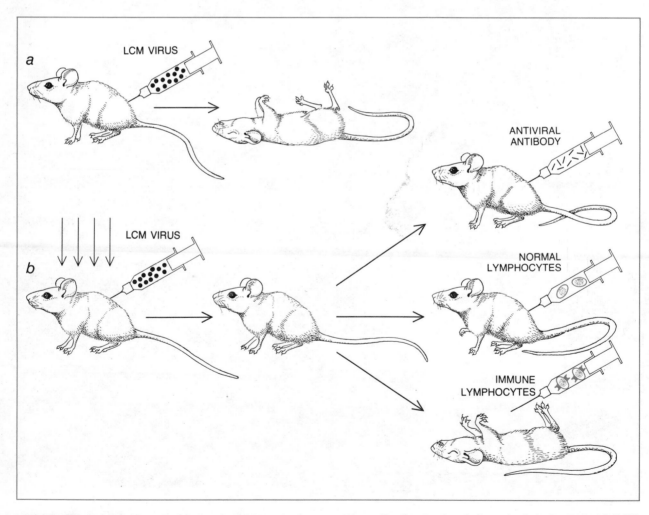

LCM VIRUS kills adult mice (*a*). If the immune response is suppressed by radiation or drugs (*b*), the mouse lives but develops a chronic infection. When immunological competence is restored by injecting lymphocytes from other animals immunized with LCM, test animal dies. Injection of anti-LCM antibody or of normal lymphocytes rather than anti-LCM lymphocytes does not cause death.

of the symptoms associated with viral diseases of man, including hepatitis.

Gary Rosenberg and Paul Farber in Notkins' laboratory at the National Institutes of Health undertook an even more detailed analysis of the behavior of lymphocytes in response to viral antigens. They used herpes simplex virus (HSV), which produces the familiar cold sores in man. They found that when lymphocytes from animals immunized with this virus were incubated in a test tube with HSV antigen, the antigen "turned on" the lymphocytes to replicate their DNA and divide. This reaction began within hours after exposure to the antigen and was quite specific: the anti-HSV lymphocytes were turned on only by the HSV antigen; they did not react at all to antigens of other viruses. In a follow-up study at the Wistar Institute with the rabies virus, Tadeusz J. Wiktor and Koprowski found that lymphocytes from rabbits immunized with that virus could be turned on not only by the complete virus but also by its subunits.

Further research showed that when lymphocytes are stimulated by exposure to viral antigens, they release potent chemical messengers, or mediators, that exhibit a variety of biological properties and are thought to be responsible for some of the inflammatory change and tissue injury associated with many viral infections. One of these mediators is known to attract inflammatory (white) cells and another can keep the inflammatory cells at the site of the infection. A third mediator, lymphotoxin, can destroy uninfected as well as infected cells, and a fourth is the now well-known substance interferon, which can inhibit the replication of viruses. Very likely a number of other mediators will be found to be released by the interaction of viruses with lymphocytes; mediators with at least a dozen different biological properties have been discovered in cultures of lymphocytes that are turned on by nonviral antigens.

If lymphocytes act as agents of tissue destruction and disease, might not antibodies also perform such a role? Mario Fernandas, Wiktor and Ernest Kuwert in Koprowski's laboratory began to explore the antibody phase of the immunity phenomenon. It had been known for some time that the attachment of antibody to antigens on the surface of cells could activate a group of proteins in the serum, known as complement, to break down cells. It was also known that under certain circumstances rabies virus could induce new antigens on the surface of tissue-culture cells without

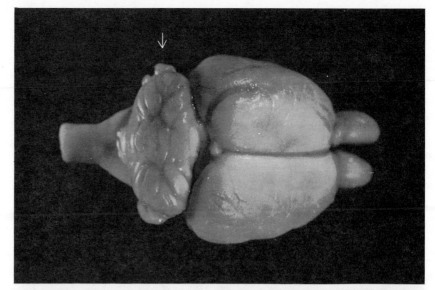

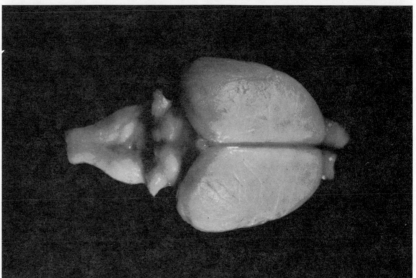

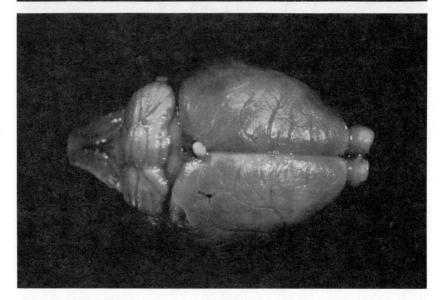

RAT BRAINS show the effects of an immune response to LCM infection demonstrated by Andrew A. Monjan, Gerald A. Cole and Neal Nathanson of the Johns Hopkins School of Hygiene and Public Health. The cerebellum is at the base of the brain (*top*). LCM infection produced severe cerebellar damage (*middle*), impairing the ability to coordinate movements. If the cellular immune response was suppressed, there was no brain damage (*bottom*).

destroying them. The Wistar Institute investigators added antirabies antibody or complement or both to the infected cultures. Neither the antibody nor the complement alone was injurious to the cells, but when they were added together the combination destroyed the rabies-infected cells.

Recent experiments suggest that antibody and complement also may contribute to the breakdown of cells infected with some of the well-known tissue-destroying viruses. Charles Wohlenberg, Arnold Brier and Joel Rosenthal of the National Institutes of Health laboratory showed that viral antigens on the surface

of cells infected with influenza, measles, vaccinia and HSV make the cells vulnerable to destruction by specific antibody and complement long before these cells break down as the direct result of viral replication. It seems highly likely, therefore, that in the body the symptoms and other effects of these diseases are produced by a collaboration between the immunological process and the virus.

How does the interaction of complement with antibody bring about tissue damage and inflammation in the infected animal? Ralph Snyderman of the National Institutes of Health laboratory conducted an experiment that suggested

a likely answer. He found that when complement and antibody to HSV were added to a culture containing cells infected with that virus, a mediator was released from one of the components of complement. This mediator was identified as one that had previously been shown to increase the permeability of blood vessels and to attract white cells. Although white cells are known to be important in the defense against certain infections, they contain potent tissue-destroying enzymes and so they may also act as agents of cell destruction in some viral infections. In fact, several groups of investigators have found that the injection of specific antibody into virus-infected animals has the effect of increasing the number of white cells and the amount of tissue damage in the infected organs. Now it appears that the sometimes fatal shock syndrome associated with dengue fever, a viral disease in Southeast Asia, may be mediated by antibody and complement. Scott B. Halstead of the University of Hawaii Medical School and Philip K. Russell of the Walter Reed Army Institute of Research, who originally proposed the idea, believe mediators released from complement may be one of the factors responsible for the increase in permeability of blood vessels and the consequent shock that marks this disease. Several workers are now attempting to gather proof for this hypothesis.

Up to this point we have discussed primarily mechanisms by which the immune response to viral antigens on the surface of infected cells can cause tissue injury. Von Pirquet's studies in the early 1900's on serum sickness suggested a different mechanism, one involving the combination of antigen and antibody. Again, it was not until the 1950's that firm evidence began to come into view. Frederick G. Germuth, Jr., and his co-workers at the Johns Hopkins Hospital and Frank J. Dixon and his colleagues at the University of Pittsburgh School of Medicine found that they could produce serum sickness in rabbits by injecting combinations, prepared in the test tube, of foreign protein and the antibody to it. They also ascertained that some of these injected complexes, circulating in the rabbits' blood, became trapped in the capillaries of the kidneys and led to inflammation, loss of kidney functions and symptoms characteristic of the human disease known as glomerulonephritis.

In the light of the evidence that the kidney disease was caused by an antigen-antibody complex, it was called "immune complex" disease. Although

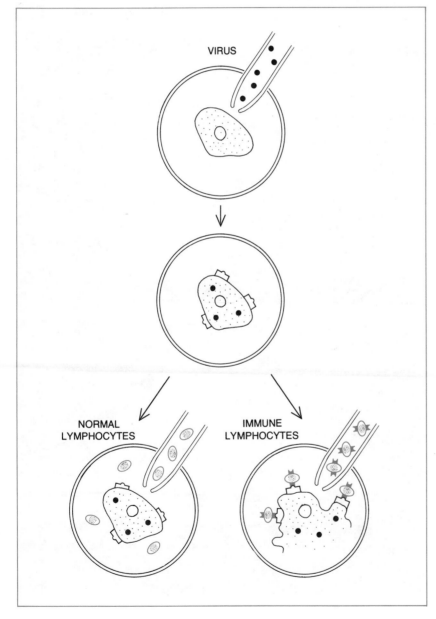

VIRUS-INFECTED CELLS are destroyed by an immune response as shown here. The infecting virus induces the formation of new antigens on the cell surface. Addition of lymphocytes to a culture of infected cells has no effect. Lymphocytes from an animal immunized with the same virus recognize the viral antigen, however, and cell destruction results.

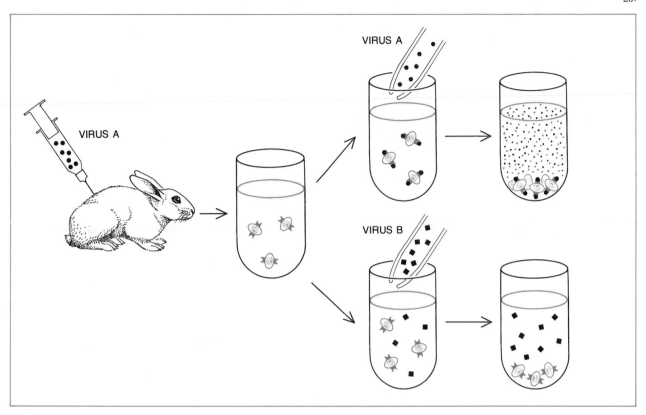

SPECIFICITY of the effect of immune lymphocytes was demonstrated by immunizing rabbits with a virus and then exposing their lymphocytes to the same virus and to another virus. The lymphocytes exposed to the same virus were stimulated to synthesize new DNA and to divide; the others were not. The stimulated lymphocytes produce mediators, some of which destroy normal tissue.

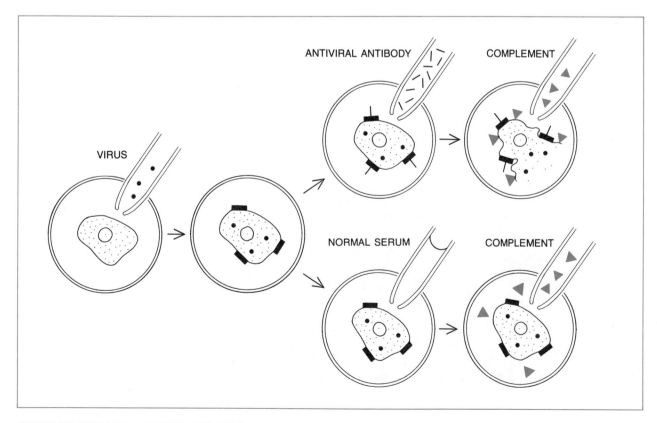

ANTIBODY-MEDIATED IMMUNE RESPONSE is demonstrated in a tissue culture. In the first step antiviral antibody recognizes and binds to virus-induced antigens on the surface of infected cells. Then complement interacts with the newly formed antigen-antibody complex and the cells are destroyed. Neither the antiviral antibody nor the complement alone destroys the infected cells.

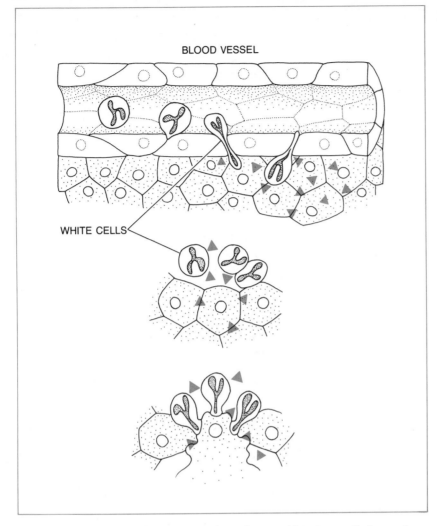

BLOOD VESSEL

WHITE CELLS

SECONDARY EFFECT of the interaction of complement with antigen-antibody complexes is activation of certain components of complement (*color*) that increase the permeability of blood-vessel walls and attract white cells. Inflammation results, and enzymes released from the white cells can injure uninfected tissue, contributing to the symptoms of the infection.

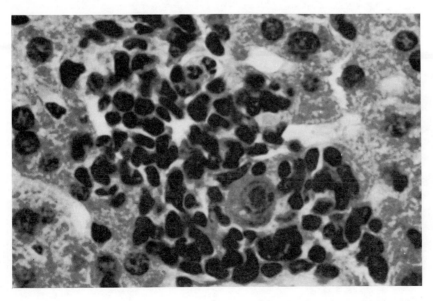

WHITE CELLS (*rounded, dark-staining cells*) are visible in a photograph of mouse-liver tissue made by Donald Henson of the National Institutes of Health. They were attracted to the site of a virus-induced lesion, presumably in the manner diagrammed at the top of the page: the large cell at the center of the clustered cells was infected with cytomegalovirus.

the immune-complex syndrome could readily be produced in animals in the laboratory, the fact that it could also occur in response to viral infections under natural conditions was not demonstrated until a decade later. Virus-antibody complexes were not easy to identify, and the problem became much more manageable when a new technique for doing so was developed.

For a number of years the National Institutes of Health laboratory had been studying an unusual virus called lactic dehydrogenase virus (LDV) because it elevates the level of that enzyme in the blood. Inoculation of mice with the virus produced large amounts of infectious virus in the blood and a chronic infection without any indication of an immune response. It was supposed that the animals were unable to make antibody against the virus, a situation known as immunological tolerance. The laboratory devised a highly sensitive technique for detecting virus-antibody combinations, however, and with this technique [*see top illustration on opposite page*] discovered that the infected mice were indeed making antibody to LDV. The reason it had not been recognized before was that although antibody had combined with the virus, the resulting complex remained infectious and therefore could not be distinguished from the virus itself.

Other investigators proceeded to show that infectious virus-antibody complexes were in fact characteristic of several of the chronic viral infections. What is more, it soon became apparent that some of these chronic infections ended in glomerulonephritis. John E. Hotchin of the New York State Department of Health in Albany had observed several years earlier that infection with LCM virus did not kill newborn mice as it did adults; instead it established a chronic infection that eventually led to glomerulonephritis. How LCM virus produces kidney disease remained unclear until Michael Oldstone and Dixon, who was now working at the Scripps Clinic and Research Foundation in La Jolla, Calif., showed that LCM virus existed in the blood of chronically infected animals as an infectious virus-antibody complex and that the kidneys contained large amounts of LCM antigen, anti-LCM antibody and complement. Moreover, microscopic studies revealed the typical pattern seen when immune complexes are deposited in the kidneys. Similar observations quickly followed with other chronic viral infections, in some of which the inflammatory changes were not confined to kidneys but ap-

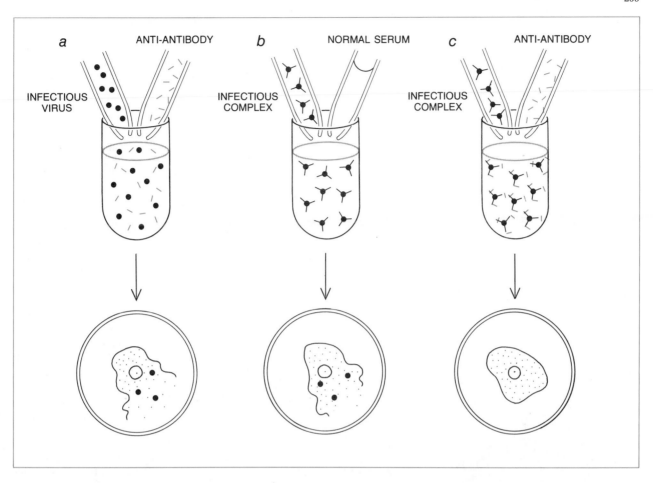

a ANTI-ANTIBODY   b NORMAL SERUM   c ANTI-ANTIBODY

INFECTIOUS VIRUS   INFECTIOUS COMPLEX   INFECTIOUS COMPLEX

INFECTIOUS VIRUS-ANTIBODY COMPLEXES can be detected by a technique utilizing an antibody that recognizes an antiviral antibody as an antigen: an "anti-antibody." When the anti-antibody is incubated with untreated virus, the virus retains its infectivity (a). When virus with antiviral antibody on its surface (in-fectious virus-antibody complex) is treated with normal serum, the complex remains infectious (b). When the infectious complex is treated with the anti-antibody, however, the latter attaches itself to the antibody of the complex, neutralizing the complex (c). Thus the test distinguishes between virus and infectious complex.

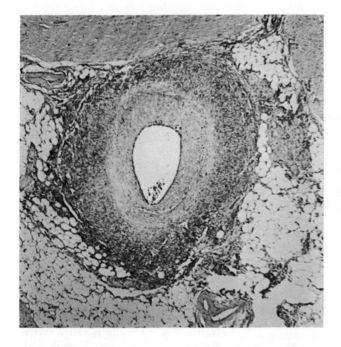

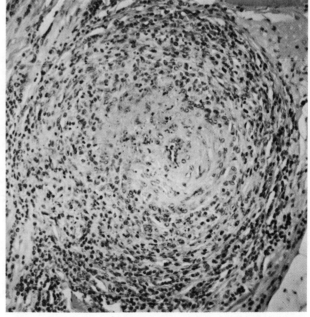

ARTERITIS occurs in some viral immune-complex diseases. Photo-micrographs of the coronary artery of mink infected with Aleutian virus, made by Porter, show mild arteritis (left) and, at higher magnification, severe arteritis with infiltration of white cells (small dark-staining cells) and obstruction of the vessel (right). Dam-aged arteries contained viral antigen, antibody and complement.

INFECTION of mice with leukemia virus depressed their ability to make antibody. Mice, some of which had been infected with virus, were immunized with sheep red blood cells (a). Spleen cells from the mice were spread over layers of sheep red blood cells in laboratory dishes (b) and complement was added (c). Only spleen cells in which antibody to the sheep cells had been induced were able, in the presence of complement, to destroy surrounding sheep cells. Counting the patches of dead sheep cells (white) showed spleens of infected mice contained many fewer antibody-producing cells than spleens of healthy mice.

peared in blood vessels and organs in other parts of the body.

The precise steps involved in the production of immune-complex disease by virus-antibody complexes are still only partly understood. Presumably when the complexes are trapped in the kidneys or on blood-vessel walls, they activate the components of complement; mediators are generated, inflammation results and the tissue-injuring enzymes are released from white cells. There are still many unanswered questions, however. Why does LCM virus produce a severe glomerulonephritis and LDV only a mild one? Why do some animals develop glomerulonephritis when they are exposed to a given virus whereas other animals do not? Are there genetic factors governing susceptibility to the virus or the immunological response to it?

Be that as it may, thousands of people develop glomerulonephritis each year, and so the finding that virus-antibody complexes produce the disease in animals has intensified research interest in such complexes and their possible involvement in human disease. Recently evidence has begun to accumulate that in man the hepatitis virus circulates in the blood as an immune complex and that some of the manifestations of this disease, including the associated high incidence of arthritis, may be due to these immune complexes. If it turns out that the immune response to viruses is actually responsible for glomerulonephritis or other immune-complex diseases in man, then controlling the adverse effects of the immune response may be essential for therapy. In animals many manifestations of these chronic infections, including glomerulonephritis, can be prevented or reduced by drugs that suppress the immune response.

The possibility that viruses and the immune response may also be involved in autoimmune diseases such as rheumatoid arthritis and lupus erythematosus is being investigated in a number of laboratories. An autoimmune disease is one in which the body treats its own tissue as an alien antigen and produces antibodies that attack the tissue. What causes the host suddenly to turn against its own tissues? It has long been suspected that viral infections may be a triggering factor. Several hypotheses about how a virus might bring the immunological system into play against the host's own cells have been suggested. The viral infection may unmask or release a potential antigen that normally is hidden within the cells, out of contact with the immune system. Or a viral antigen may combine with an indigenous protein on the cell's surface and thus form a new "foreign" substance. Another possibility is that a viral infection may activate genes in the cell whose information is ordinarily repressed, thereby causing them to begin producing "new" substances that act as antigens. Wanda Baranska and Wojciech Sawicki at the Wistar Institute found support for this idea in experiments with mouse ova and embryos. They showed that an antigen that was present in the animals' earliest embryonic stage could not be detected in adults, but that when adult cells were transformed into tumor cells by the virus known as SV-40, the embryonic antigen reappeared on the cell surface. Apparently in these transformed mouse cells the genes were again able to redirect formation of the "embryonic antigen."

Still another possibility is that a viral infection may cause the cells of the immune system to behave abnormally and so produce antibodies against some of the host's own tissue. Although proof for this hypothesis is still lacking, there is considerable evidence, particularly from animal studies, that certain viral infections depress the function of the cells of the immune system. Again, it was von Pirquet who first observed that the reactivity to the tuberculin test (an immune response) was depressed in patients infected with measles virus. The effect of viruses on immune function received little attention, however, until 1963, when Robert A. Good and his colleagues at the University of Minnesota College of Medical Sciences showed that mice infected with a leukemia-producing virus were markedly depressed in their ability to make antibody against foreign substances. Other studies, notably by Walter Ceglowski and Herman Friedman at the Albert Einstein Medical Center in Philadelphia, showed that not only was the amount of antibody in the blood reduced but also the number of cells capable of making antibody was curtailed by as much as 99 percent [*see illustration on opposite page*]. Moreover, the immune response was depressed within a few days after infection, long before the animals developed visible signs of leukemia.

It soon became apparent that non-leukemia-producing viruses also could impair immune function. Richard J. Howard and Stephan E. Mergenhagen of the National Institutes of Health laboratory showed this in tests of the reactivity of LDV-infected mice to foreign skin grafts. These animals rejected grafts at a lower rate than uninfected animals. Moreover, there is evidence that the re-

MECHANISMS	PATHOLOGY

1 VIRUS-INDUCED ANTIGENS ON CELL SURFACE:
  a INTERACTION WITH IMMUNE LYMPHOCYTES
  b INTERACTION WITH ANTIVIRAL ANTIBODY AND COMPLEMENT
	DESTRUCTION OF INFECTED CELLS

2 ACTIVATION OF MEDIATORS FROM IMMUNE LYMPHOCYTES OR COMPONENTS OF COMPLEMENT	INFLAMMATION, ALLERGIC REACTIONS, DESTRUCTION OF CELLS
3 FORMATION OF CIRCULATING VIRUS-ANTIBODY COMPLEXES	IMMUNE-COMPLEX DISEASE
4 IMMUNE RESPONSE TO HOST-CELL ANTIGENS ALTERED OR DEREPRESSED BY VIRUS	AUTOIMMUNE REACTIONS
5 INFECTION OF CELLS OF IMMUNE SYSTEM	INHIBITION OR ENHANCEMENT OF IMMUNE FUNCTION

MECHANISMS of the various immune-response disorders that are caused by viral infection and are discussed in the article are summarized, together with the associated pathology.

jection of transplanted tumors also is slowed by viral infection of the immune system. In fact, it seems possible that the virus-induced depression of antibody-mediated and lymphocyte-mediated immunity may be a factor in the initiation and development of tumors and also may account for the chronic nature of certain viral infections.

A curious twist in the already complicated story of immunity and viruses is the finding that lymphocytes, which are the body's major defense against tumors, can actually act as agents for the induction of tumors. It has been known for some time that an unusually high incidence of lymphomas (tumors of the lymphoid glands) occurs in animals or patients undergoing chronic stimulation of these glands as a result of autoimmune disorders or rejection of a graft such as a kidney transplant. It is also known that certain viruses, including the leukemia virus of mice and the mononucleosis virus of man, exist in lymphoid cells in a "latent" state. On the basis of these observations, groups headed by Martin S. Hirsch and Paul H. Black of the Harvard Medical School and Robert S. Schwartz of the Tufts University School of Medicine conducted experiments to see if stimulation of the lymph-

oid elements of the immune system might arouse the latent virus. In order to stimulate the immune system they exposed mice to foreign grafts, and they found that this activated the leukemia virus that had previously been latent in the lymphoid cells. The findings suggest that such activation of leukemia virus from immunologically stimulated lymphocytes may be responsible for the high incidence of lymphomas associated with autoimmune disorders and graft rejection.

All in all, it is now obvious that the interrelations encompassing viruses, immunity and disease are indeed complex. It appears that the immune response to viral infection can have both beneficial and deleterious effects on the host. On the one hand, it may be the chief or only weapon against the infection; on the other hand, it may be responsible for some of the noxious symptoms and even the fatal effects of the disease. Probably the immune response makes some contribution, large or small, to the pathologic picture in most viral infections. Although we must recognize that the immune system is not an unmixed blessing, it is encouraging to know that by learning more about it we may eventually find new approaches to the treatment of viral diseases.

Tetanus

by W. E. van Heyningen
April 1968

*Bacteria that may barely infect a trivial wound
can produce enough toxin to cause the severe and
often fatal symptoms of this disease. Tetanus is
hard to treat, but it could be eradicated
by immunization*

Early in the 19th century the Scottish surgeon Sir Charles Bell made a drawing of a British soldier who had been wounded at the Battle of Corunna, during the Peninsular War in Spain. The soldier was rigid: his back arched, his hands and feet clenched, his jaw set in a terrible grimace—the "sardonic smile" of tetanus, or lockjaw [*see illustration below*]. A victim of tetanus is in a state of spastic paralysis. He is unable to move, although the muscles of his body are contracting with all their strength, because for every muscle pulling in one direction another is pulling as strongly in the opposite direction. Bell's soldier was exerting tremendous energy, pitting himself against himself. He was exhausted but could not possibly rest, and he was suffering intense pain. Soon he would die, because there was no way to save him.

Tetanus is an ancient and ferocious infectious disease that was described by Hippocrates 24 centuries ago. It is a disease of wounding, but not just of serious wounds. Any break in the skin—a superficial scratch or the puncture of a drug addict's needle—is susceptible to the infection. The organism that causes tetanus was identified in 1889; it is the ubiquitous bacillus *Clostridium tetani,* present in soil, dust and clothing. It acts not directly but by producing a nerve toxin that has been isolated and purified and found to be one of the most powerful poisons known. The action of the toxin is now understood in a general way and is being studied at the molecular level. Meanwhile tetanus continues to be one of the world's greatest killers. This need not be, because the disease could be virtually eliminated by an intensive worldwide program of immunization.

The prevalence of tetanus is masked, as B. Bytchenko of the World Health Organization has pointed out, in part by the fact that the disease does not cause epidemics. It strikes individuals rather than large communities or regions, and is therefore less noticed than infectious diseases such as smallpox, cholera, tuberculosis and malaria. Yet it ranks high among the infectious diseases as a cause of death. Tetanus is badly underreported because in many countries it is not a "notifiable" disease. Bytchenko has calculated that if it were reported on the same basis as smallpox, it would be found to account for some 164,000 deaths a year.

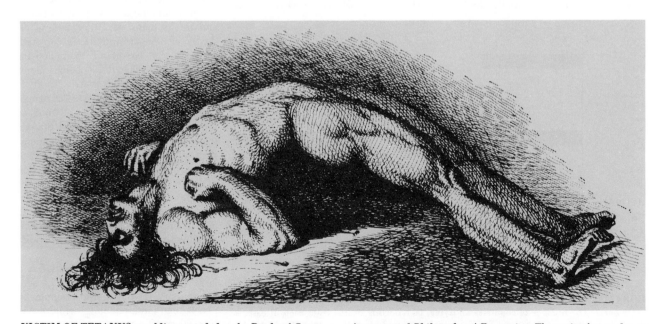

VICTIM OF TETANUS, a soldier wounded at the Battle of Corunna in 1809, is seen in a drawing made by the Scottish surgeon and anatomist Sir Charles Bell and published in 1832 in his book *The Anatomy and Philosophy of Expression.* The patient's muscles are working against one another, leaving him in a state of spastic paralysis; his jaw is set in the "sardonic smile" of tetanus, or lockjaw.

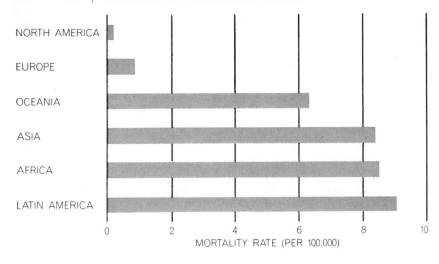

MORTALITY RATES from tetanus vary widely, depending on the stage of development of the region. These rates have been corrected for widespread underreporting of tetanus.

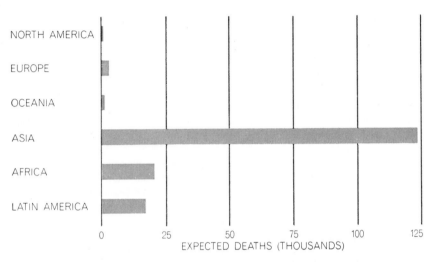

ANNUAL DEATHS, derived from the computed mortality rates, yield the world total of 164,200. Chart data were compiled by B. Bytchenko of the World Health Organization.

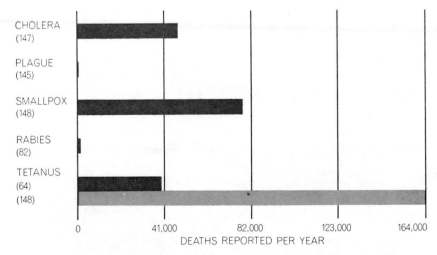

MORTALITY FIGURES for five infectious diseases show smallpox as the leading killer (*gray bars*). The number of countries notifying, or reporting deaths from each disease, is shown in parentheses. If tetanus were as widely reported as smallpox, the World Health Organization estimates, it would account for twice as many deaths as smallpox (*color*).

A remarkably high proportion of the victims of tetanus die of it. The recorded percentage has been as high as 97 percent (based on a study of tetanus cases resulting from July 4 celebrations in the U.S. from 1904 to 1907) and is seldom lower than 40 percent. The very lethality of the disease makes its toll less obvious. As R. Veronesi of the University of São Paulo Faculty of Medicine has remarked, if tetanus did not kill people but rather left them paralyzed, "we would see, every 10 years, more than one million tetanus-crippled individuals in the streets of the world, and confronted with this situation perhaps people and governments would ask immediately for measures to control the problem."

Any tabulation of tetanus mortality rates shows tremendous differences between the developed and the developing regions of the world. The rates tend to increase toward the Equator, and indeed tetanus is listed by the World Health Organization among the 10 leading causes of death in a number of tropical countries. The correlation is not with climatic and soil conditions, of course, but with social and economic conditions; tetanus is closely associated with primitive sanitation. A high proportion of the deaths are caused by "tetanus neonatorum," a disease of newborn babies in the first two or three weeks of life. It results from infection of the umbilicus after the cord has been cut with dirty instruments or under insanitary conditions. (In some countries it is even the practice to apply cow dung to the navel.) Umbilical tetanus accounts for 30 to 80 percent of the deaths from tetanus in tropical countries and for as many as 70 percent of all deaths of newborn infants; in one state in Brazil that has about 15 million inhabitants more than 1,000 babies die of umbilical tetanus every year.

Tetanus appears, however, in people of all ages and as a result of all kinds of injuries. Apart from accidental injuries these include negligent surgical operations, vaccination, circumcision, abortion and ear-piercing as well as the injection of drugs. (In the past 11 years 72 percent of all tetanus cases in New York City occurred in heroin addicts; the fatality rate among these cases was 86 percent compared with 38 percent among nonaddict victims of tetanus.)

Clearly tetanus could be avoided to a large extent by the application of simple sanitary measures, for example by persuading (and enabling) children in tropical countries to wear shoes or sandals and thereby avoid many of the daily small wounds that can lead to infection. The effect of improved sanitation was demonstrated in Japan, where the mortality from tetanus declined steadily from 2.9 deaths per 100,000 inhabitants in 1947 to fewer than .5 in 1964. This last figure was about equal to the rate in France, where preventive immunization had been applied on a nationwide scale since 1940, although immunization had not been widely practiced in Japan. The improvement in Japan can be traced in part to a decreasing death rate from tetanus of the newborn, and that in turn may be correlated with an increase in the proportion of babies delivered in hospitals rather than at home (from 2.4 percent in 1947 to 58 percent in 1961).

The attainment of sanitary conditions in the developing countries is easier said than done, of course, and it will not be possible until their economic condition is greatly improved. Immunization, on the other hand, can prevent tetanus no matter how insanitary the environment or how infested the wound. To understand immunization against tetanus we must first inquire into the nature of the disease and how the infecting bacillus brings it about.

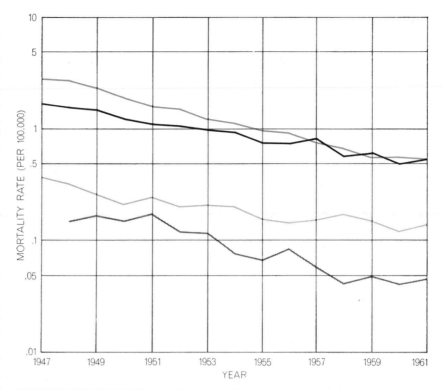

TETANUS DEATH RATE has declined since World War II at roughly the same rate in Japan (*color*), France (*black*), the U.S. (*light color*) and England and Wales (*gray*). Among these countries only Japan was not practicing preventive immunization in those years. The decline there was apparently due to increasingly effective public health and sanitation.

Tetanus is an unusual kind of infection. Not only is the wound that causes it often trivial; there is also no visible pathology that can be detected at postmortem examination. No lesions are produced in the tissues that can be detected even with the electron microscope. The bacillus that infects the wound has hardly any capacity to invade the tissues; it proliferates only to a limited degree, so that the wound hardly appears to be infected. Clearly the mere presence of the infecting organisms cannot account for the violent, widely distributed symptoms of the disease.

This was apparent even in the early days of the germ theory of disease to Arthur Nicolaier of the University of Berlin. He observed that the organisms (which had not yet been identified) that presumably caused tetanus did not seem to be distributed through the body. He also noted that the symptoms of tetanus were similar to those caused by the potent poison strychnine, and in 1885 he suggested that the organism acted by producing a strychnine-like poison. In 1889 the Japanese bacteriologist Shibasaburo Kitasato, working with Emil von Behring in Robert Koch's laboratory in Berlin, isolated *Clostridium tetani*. The following year a Danish investigator, Knud Faber, confirmed Nicolaier's idea. He reproduced tetanus symptoms in ex-

perimental animals by injecting them with filtrates of *C. tetani* cultures from which all the bacilli had been removed. He thus proved that a poison was produced by the germs and was capable of acting independently of them. The first such bacterial toxin, the one produced by the diphtheria bacillus, had been discovered the year before at the Institut Pasteur in Paris by Émile Roux and Alexandre Yersin. In 1896 Émile van Ermengem of the University of Ghent discovered the toxin responsible for the bacterial food poisoning known as botulism. Germ-free filtrates of tetanus bacilli and botulinus bacilli (*Clostridium botulinum*) are extremely toxic: a cubic centimeter may contain enough poison to kill more than a million mice.

When some of these bacterial toxins were isolated and purified during the past 25 years, they turned out to be far more toxic than such poisons as strychnine and arsenic or the snake venoms [*see illustration on page 249*]. An amount of tetanus, botulinus or dysentery toxin weighing no more than the ink in the period at the end of this sentence would be enough to kill 30 grown men; an ounce could kill 30 million tons of living matter; half a pound would be more than enough to destroy the entire human population of the world. (These calcula-

tions are theoretical and somewhat theatrical, since they are based on determinations of the smallest injection that will kill a mouse, and the projection to mass killing of men involves some unrealistic assumptions. Botulinus toxin, for example, has been considered seriously as an agent of warfare, but for a number of reasons—including the fact that such toxins are about a million times less toxic when administered by mouth or through the lungs rather than by injection—its military applications would seem to be limited.)

Why the tetanus and botulinus bacilli should produce these immensely potent toxins is a problem of great philosophical and practical interest. Diphtheria toxin and most other bacterial toxins attack and break down the tissues of the animal infected by the parent organism. In doing so they assist the bacteria in their invasion, because the bacteria grow well in disintegrating tissues. The tetanus and botulinus toxins, however, do not attack animal tissues generally. It does not appear to be of any survival value to the tetanus and botulinus bacilli to produce toxins that not only confine their action to nerve tissue but also, as far as can be seen, cause no damage even in this tissue. Yet on evolutionary grounds it is hardly conceivable that the bacilli should

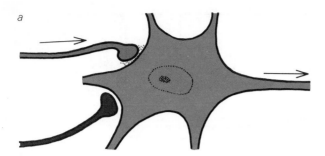

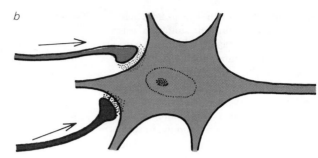

a

b

EXCITATION AND INHIBITION of a motoneuron, a nerve cell controlling a voluntary muscle, are shown schematically. Excitatory (*color*) and inhibitory (*gray*) afferent fibers (*at left in each drawing*) form synapses at the surface of a cell body. Impulses from the

excitatory fiber (*a*) release a chemical transmitter that causes the motoneuron to fire efferent impulses along its axon (*right side of drawing*). Impulses from the inhibitory fiber release a different transmitter (*b*) that opposes excitation, so that no impulse is fired.

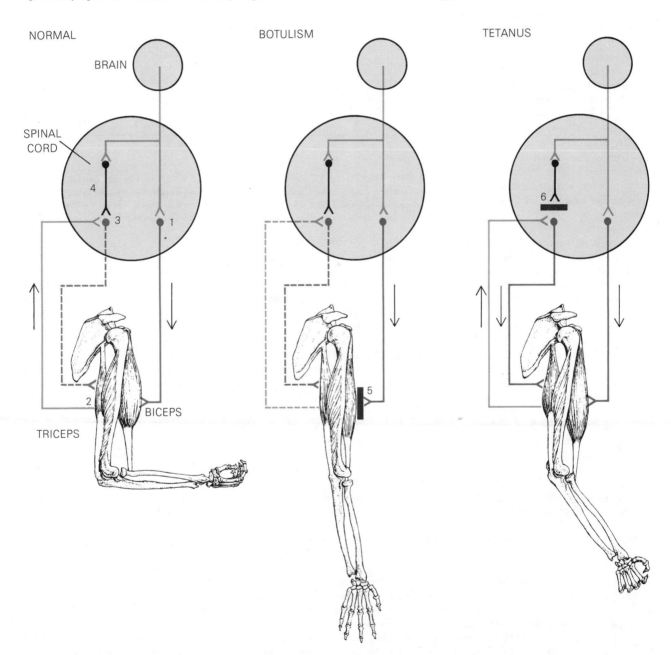

NORMAL   BOTULISM   TETANUS

BRAIN

SPINAL CORD

TRICEPS   BICEPS

NERVOUS CONTROL of muscles that raise and lower the forearm is diagrammed very schematically. In a normal individual (*left*) impulses from the brain can excite a motoneuron (*1*) to cause the biceps to contract, stretching the triceps. A stretch-sensitive receptor (*2*) in the triceps would thereupon cause a triceps motoneuron (*3*)

to fire and oppose the stretching—except that this firing is inhibited by impulses from an inhibitory nerve (*4*). In botulism (*center*) the neuromuscular junction is blocked (*5*), causing flaccid paralysis. In tetanus (*right*) the inhibitory impulses to the triceps motoneuron are blocked (*6*); both muscles contract, causing a spasm.

produce the toxins unless they have some survival value. If we could find out why these toxins are produced, we not only would learn something important about bacterial physiology but also might find clues to the mechanism of the extraordinary action of the toxins on animals.

It is interesting to compare the action of botulinus and tetanus toxins, since they are produced by closely related organisms and since both act on the nervous system and are highly toxic without doing any apparent structural damage. Botulinus toxin prevents muscle activity and thereby causes a flaccid paralysis; tetanus toxin promotes muscle overactivity and thereby causes a spastic paralysis.

Let us consider (in a necessarily oversimplified way) the functions of the voluntary nervous system in raising the forearm. Nerve impulses travel from the brain (or from different sensory regions, such as those in the skin) down a bundle of "afferent" axons, or nerve fibers, to the spinal cord. There the fibers split up and make synapses, or junctions, with motoneurons, the cell bodies of motor-nerve fibers leaving the spinal cord. Each of these "efferent" axons connects with fibers of the biceps muscle of the upper arm. The synapses in the spinal cord are part of the central nervous system; the neuromuscular junctions at the biceps are part of the peripheral nervous system. At each central synapse and at each peripheral junction there is a gap about 200 angstrom units (.00002 millimeter) wide. When an impulse from the brain reaches a central synapse, it causes a chemical substance to be released from the ending, flow across the gap and excite the motoneuron, initiating a new impulse that travels along the efferent fiber to the peripheral neuromuscular junction. There a different chemical transmitter is released from the nerve ending and flows across the gap to the muscle, exciting it and causing it to contract. The excitatory transmitter at the neuromuscular junction is acetylcholine. The transmitters in the central nervous system have not yet been identified.

Now, in the resting state muscle tone is maintained by the constant gentle tension of opposing muscles. For example, the forearm is levered about a fulcrum, the elbow joint, essentially by two sets of muscles: on one side the biceps, whose contraction raises the forearm, and on the other side the triceps, whose contraction pulls the forearm down. When the biceps contracts slightly, the triceps is stretched a little. Stretch-sensitive receptors in the triceps are thereby excited and send impulses up afferent fibers to the spinal cord, where they excite motoneurons that stimulate the triceps in turn to contract and oppose the stretch. The stretch reflex plays a necessary role in maintaining posture and controlling muscle movement, but if every contraction of the biceps were opposed too much by the triceps, there could be no voluntary movement at all because the forearm would be locked in a spastic state. Therefore the afferent impulse that causes the biceps to be excited must at the same time ensure that the triceps will be somewhat relaxed; that is, it must inhibit any stretch-reflex excitation of the triceps. This inhibition is achieved within the spinal cord by the branching of the nerve fiber carrying the impulse from the brain. One branch excites the biceps; the other branch excites a short "interneuron," a nerve cell within the spinal cord that releases not an excitatory but an inhibitory transmitter from its ending. The inhibitory transmitter acts on the triceps motoneuron, opposing the action of the excitatory transmitter released there from the stretch-sensitive afferent nerve. As a result the motoneuron is not excited, the triceps does not contract and the biceps is free to pull the forearm up [see bottom illustration on opposite page].

Botulinus toxin acts at the neuromuscular junctions, as A. S. V. Burgen and his collaborators at Middlesex Hospital in London showed in 1949. It prevents the release of acetylcholine, the excitatory transmitter, from the efferent nerve endings; excitatory impulses are blocked before they can reach the muscles, and the result is a state of flaccid, limp paralysis in which no limbs can be moved.

Tetanus, on the other hand, acts in the spinal cord, apparently by suppressing inhibition. (Strychnine seems to act in the same way, it was suggested by Sir John Eccles and his collaborators in Australia in 1957.) In the absence of inhibition the stretch reflex of the triceps goes unopposed, so that when the biceps contracts, the triceps contracts too. The forearm is locked in a state of spastic paralysis, unable to move in any direction.

Some years ago N. Ambache found, at the Institute of Ophthalmology in London, that an injection of either tetanus or botulinus toxin in the eye of a rabbit paralyzes the muscles that contract the pupil in response to light. It is acetylcholine that excites these involuntary muscles, and so at least in this case tetanus exhibits the same kind of action as botulinus. Tetanus toxin may have other such peripheral effects that are usually masked by its dramatic impact on the central nervous system.

Although the neurophysiology of tetanus toxin's action is reasonably clear, not much is known of what goes on at the molecular level. The first clue to a chemical process that may play an important role came from an observation made in 1898 by August von Wasserman and T. Takaki of the Koch Institute for Infectious Diseases. They found that when the toxin is added to nerve tissue, it is bound, or taken up, by the tissue. This binding is specific: no other bacterial toxin (including botulinus toxin) is bound by nerve tissue and no other tissue of the body binds tetanus toxin. In my laboratory at the University of Oxford we have discovered that the site of this binding is apparently in the synaptic membranes of the nerve endings and that the substance apparently responsible for the chemical fixation of toxin is a ganglioside, a fatty substance found mainly in nerve tissue. There are a number of gangliosides, each somewhat different in chemical structure. They are alike in that each has two portions, one composed of water-repellent fatty acids and sphingosine and the other composed of water-soluble sugars. As a result they are readily water-soluble even though they are fatty, and this ambivalence suggests that they may have an important function in cell membranes. We have found that sialic acid, one of the components of the sugar portion, is essential for the fixation of the tetanus toxin; if the sialic acid is removed, the toxin is no longer bound. It is apparent, however, that only certain sialic acid groups are involved in the fixation of toxin and that their position in the ganglioside molecule greatly affects their binding ability [see illustration on page 248].

Tetanus toxin may be bound to ganglioside in a ratio that is nearly molecule for molecule, but no detectable change takes place in the ganglioside molecule. The part the binding plays in tetanus is not yet established; it may not be an essential stage in the action of the toxin. As I have mentioned, there are hints that tetanus and botulinus toxins may have fundamentally the same mode of action at the molecular level. If that is the case, then (in view of the fact that botulinus toxin is not bound by nerve tissue) it is possible that what the binding of tetanus toxin by ganglioside does is simply to divert this toxin to the central nervous system.

Whatever its basic mode of action,

it is quite clear that the toxin is responsible for all the symptoms of tetanus. These symptoms can be mimicked exactly in experimental animals by the injection of purified toxin (and indeed in humans into whose bodies the toxin has been inadvertently introduced in laboratory accidents). Since the disease is entirely due to the toxin, it is technically rather a simple matter to prevent the disease by immunizing against the toxin. Like other bacterial toxins (and the active principles of snake venoms), tetanus toxin is a protein, and proteins are antigenic: when they are injected, they stimulate the formation of antibodies (antitoxins) that neutralize the toxins and prevent them from acting. The discovery of antitoxins to both diphtheria and tetanus toxins was announced by von Behring and Kitasato in 1890. The antitoxin was present in the blood serum of animals that had been immunized by sublethal doses of attenuated toxin, and its neutralizing activity persisted when the immune serum was transferred into other animals. That is to say, unexposed animals could be made "passively" immune by being injected with the serum of "actively" immune animals.

In 1920 W. T. Glenny of the Wellcome Laboratories in London and G. Ramon of the Institut Pasteur in Paris independently discovered that toxin rendered harmless by treatment with formaldehyde could still remain antigenic, or capable of stimulating antibody formation. This nontoxic antigenic material is called toxoid. Antitoxic serum is made on a large scale by hyperimmunizing horses with repeated large doses of toxoid and then refining their blood serum.

Tetanus antitoxin proved its worth in World War I. During the first months of the war nearly eight British soldiers out of every 1,000 who were wounded died of tetanus—an alarmingly high proportion. By the end of 1914 there was an ample supply of antitoxin for immediate injection of all wounded troops at the front and the death rate from tetanus dropped sharply. In the years between the wars it became the practice, wherever possible in the world, to inject all injured patients routinely with antitoxic serum to prevent the development of tetanus. Antiserum has a serious disadvantage, however; it may give rise to serum sickness, an allergic reaction to the foreign (horse) protein in the serum. The risk of fatal serum sickness is much greater in people who have a history of previous injections of serum, whether against tetanus or some other disease. Indeed, it is now recognized that if reasonable sanitary precautions are taken, the risk of tetanus is less than the risk of fatal serum sickness. Moreover, although passive immunization has some value in preventing tetanus, it has become evident that its therapeutic effect once the disease is established is less than was hoped for. Once the toxin has become attached to the susceptible substance in nerve tissue, antitoxin cannot displace or neutralize it. For these two reasons the administration of tetanus antiserum has now been discontinued in many countries.

Direct, active immunization of human populations with tetanus toxoid is a

STRUCTURE	RELATIVE ABUNDANCE	TOXIN BOUND
I — FATTY ACID / SPHINGOSINE / GLUCOSE / GALACTOSE—SIALIC ACID / GALACTOSAMINE / GALACTOSE	.85	3
II — FATTY ACID / SPHINGOSINE / GLUCOSE / GALACTOSE—SIALIC ACID / GALACTOSAMINE / GALACTOSE—SIALIC ACID	1	3
III — FATTY ACID / SPHINGOSINE / GLUCOSE / GALACTOSE—SIALIC ACID—SIALIC ACID / GALACTOSAMINE / GALACTOSE	.65	20
IV — FATTY ACID / SPHINGOSINE / GLUCOSE / GALACTOSE—SIALIC ACID—SIALIC ACID / GALACTOSAMINE / GALACTOSE—SIALIC ACID	.55	20
TAY-SACHS — FATTY ACID / SPHINGOSINE / GLUCOSE / GALACTOSE / GALACTOSAMINE—SIALIC ACID	.08	0

GANGLIOSIDES are the substances in nerve tissue that bind tetanus toxin. Here general structures are given for the four gangliosides most abundant in nerve tissue and for one that is increased in Tay-Sachs disease. Each has fatty (*gray*) and sugar (*color*) components. The sialic acid groups are specifically responsible for binding toxin. As shown by the number of grams of toxin bound per gram of ganglioside (*right*), only certain sialic acid groups (*dark color*) take part in this process; the others have no effect on the binding.

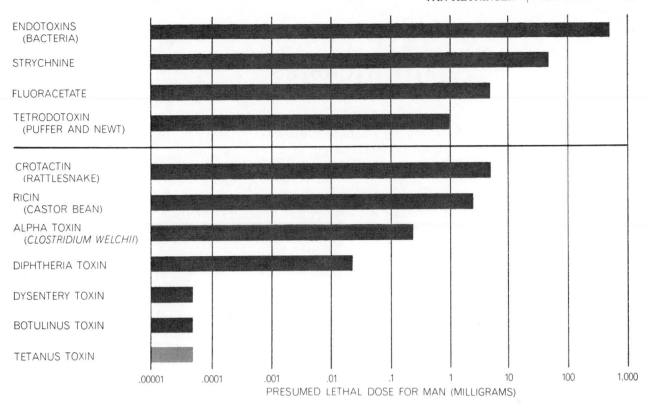

ENDOTOXINS (BACTERIA)

STRYCHNINE

FLUORACETATE

TETRODOTOXIN (PUFFER AND NEWT)

CROTACTIN (RATTLESNAKE)

RICIN (CASTOR BEAN)

ALPHA TOXIN (*CLOSTRIDIUM WELCHII*)

DIPHTHERIA TOXIN

DYSENTERY TOXIN

BOTULINUS TOXIN

TETANUS TOXIN

.00001   .0001   .001   .01   .1   1   10   100   1,000

PRESUMED LETHAL DOSE FOR MAN (MILLIGRAMS)

TOXICITY of the bacterial toxins, including tetanus, is compared with that of other poisons. Crotactin and ricin, like the bacterial exotoxins, are simple proteins. The scale is logarithmic. The dosage figures are theoretical; they assume that the toxin is injected.

much better proposition as a preventive measure. The risk of allergic reaction to the toxoid is negligible. The immunity lasts much longer, since the antibody produced is the subject's own protein, not the protein of a horse. And the immunity is more effective because the antitoxin is present in the body before the toxin produced by infecting bacilli is and can therefore prevent the binding of toxin by nerve tissue.

Deaths from tetanus are now rare in the many countries where active immunization of all children and members of the armed forces against tetanus is routinely practiced. The virtual elimination of tetanus in these countries is one of the great triumphs of combined laboratory research and public health services.

To prevent tetanus in communities (and even whole countries) all that is needed is for every member of the community (or the country's population) to receive two injections of tetanus toxoid spaced six weeks apart. A booster dose after six months and an occasional booster thereafter are considered desirable but are probably not essential. Even the unborn can be protected: J. C. Suri, R. MacLennan and K. W. Newell have demonstrated in India, New Guinea and South America respectively that the active immunization of women (whether they are pregnant or not) virtually elimi-

nates umbilical tetanus in children they bear subsequently. In primitive communities, of course, it is often difficult to make sure that an individual receives two injections some weeks apart. For this reason R. Veronesi in Brazil and C. Merceux in France have been investigating the possibility of active immunization by means of a simultaneous multiple injection of concentrated toxoid over a small area on one occasion. Their preliminary tests indicate that active immunity can be achieved in this way even though antitoxin may not be detectable in the blood.

In contrast to prevention, the treatment of tetanus once contracted is a difficult and expensive procedure. Since 1954 it has been the practice in severe cases to treat the patient with D-tubocurarine, a poison that paralyzes the muscles much as botulinus toxin does. This drastic treatment paralyzes the patient so that even his breathing must be assisted by a respirator, but it does prevent the terrible spasms of tetanus. If the patient can be kept alive long enough, the damage caused by the tetanus toxin is eventually repaired and he is completely restored to health.

Unfortunately this heroic form of treatment has not been as successful as expected. It does prevent death from the

asphyxia that follows the inhalation of vomit during a major spasm or from the chest complications and oxygen depletion that follow recurrent minor inhalations during lesser spasms. Yet the death rate from tetanus remains high, and indeed the prevention of death from spasm appears to have uncovered other sites of action of tetanus toxin that were not known before. There are signs that the toxin may act on the involuntary nervous system, which controls the heart and blood vessels, among other organs. In Alexander Crampton Smith's hospital wards and laboratories at Oxford, evidence is beginning to accumulate that patients with tetanus may die from heart and circulatory abnormalities that are reflected in such symptoms as increased heart rate and blood pressure and constriction of the blood vessels. The possibility that the involuntary system is implicated in death from tetanus suggests new ways to treat tetanus patients, but more research in this area is needed.

Meanwhile it is far simpler to make sure that everybody is actively immune to the disease. At an international conference on tetanus in Switzerland in 1966 the delegates called on organized medical groups and public health authorities to bring about "universal active immunization against tetanus at the earliest practicable date."

27

The Immune Response to Measles

by Sir Macfarlane Burnet
An original article
1976

The signs, symptoms, and subsequent lifelong immunity in measles are all intimately concerned with immune responses to the virus antigens.

Forty years ago measles could be regarded as the classical model of an infectious disease followed by firm immunity. Anyone who had not had the disease was susceptible and every susceptible person infected came down with typical symptoms and was thereafter immune for life. Antibody was known to persist in the circulation for many years and convalescent human serum presumed to contain high-titer antibody was effective in preventing or attenuating measles if administered to children in the first few days after their contact with children or adults in the infectious stage of the disease. It seemed self-evident that immunity to measles was a simple result of the persistence of antibodies and antibody-producing cells in the body.

That simple-minded attitude was permanently destroyed when, soon after agammaglobulinemia was recognized, it became evident to all physicians caring for children with agammaglobulinemia that their patients were susceptible to measles, showed a normal clinical course, and were subsequently firmly immune against a second attack [see "Agammaglobulinemia," by David Gitlin and Charles A. Janeway, page 167]. Antibody was apparently unnecessary for natural cure or for specific immunity. In 1959 J. F. Enders and his colleagues reported another effect of measles on children with an immune defect. Children with acute lymphatic leukemia being treated with corticosteroid drugs were found to be very susceptible to infection with measles virus but showed an entirely different clinical picture. There was no rash and the main pathological feature was a severe giant-cell pneumonia, the cells of which contained large quantities of measles virus. Most of the patients died; some survived with persisting lung lesions and continuing excretion of virus. Subsequently, measles was shown to produce a similar type of giant-cell pneumonia without rash in severe cases of combined immunodeficiency disease involving both B and T cells. Then in 1967 it was discovered that a rare disease of the brain, known for many years as subacute sclerosing panencephalitis (SSPE), could be correlated with intracellular changes in electron micrographs which resembled those already known to occur during measles virus infection, and that a high titer of measles antibody was present in both blood and cerebrospinal fluid of patients with SSPE. With some difficulty measles virus can be isolated from the brain at autopsy. At first it seemed possible that minor differences observed between the behavior of the isolated virus and standard measles strains meant that a special variant of the virus was responsible. Present opinion, however, discounts this suggestion and looks on the factors resulting in this rare condition as being intrinsic to the patient.

The Measles Process in Normal Children

The virus of measles has been well known since around 1960. It is a paramyxovirus, related closely to the viruses of dog distemper and rinderpest and less closely to those of mumps and Newcastle disease. From the epidemiological angle the most important character of the virus is its monotypic quality; a person who has recovered from an attack of measles will resist exposure to any subsequent epidemic. There are three distinguishable antigenic determinants of measles, all present in the virus envelope, but no indication that one is more important than another, and it will be legitimate for our purposes to speak of the measles antigen as a single entity.

In a nonimmune child it is assumed that an active virus particle entering the respiratory tract initiates a symptomless local lesion from which virus passes to local lymph nodes. For the next 10 or 12 days a spreading noncytopathic infection of lymphoid tissue develops without symptoms. The only known pathological change during the incubation period is the development of Warthin's giant cells, which presumably represent the same sort of fusion and syncytium formation seen in measles-infected cell cultures [see the illustration on page 251]. It is not known which cells, B or T, are predominantly (or exclusively) associated with this development; from analogy with Epstein-Barr virus infections, B cells seem likely to be especially involved. What can be said with certainty, however, is that during the incubation period two populations of lymphocytes are building up. One consists of cells within which measles virus is multiplying and disseminating antigen in the cell membranes where, following Parish's rule, which I outlined in an earlier article, it is potent in stimulating T cells to proliferation and less effective with B cells. [See "Tolerance and Unresponsiveness," by Sir Macfarlane Burnet, page 114.] No detectable antibody is present in the blood before the rash, but it seems certain that some proliferation of B cells—the second population of lymphocytes—is going on during the later part of the incubation period, and that these are producing IgM1 receptors. Only in this way can we account for the burst of antibody production that accompanies the appearance of the rash.

With the increase in the two populations, an explosive interaction between them becomes inevitable. [*See the illustration on page 252*]. The nature of the trigger can only be guessed at, but the result is dramatic. Reaction between sensitized T cells and virus-containing "measles cells" takes on a damaging intensity, rupturing the measles cells and liberating virus and soluble measles antigens. The combination of antigen, potentially cooperative T cells, and mitogenic lymphokines now ensures full stimulation of B cells, which proliferate, form plasma cells, and produce large amounts of IgM and IgG antibodies. The focal lesions of the enanthem and exanthem (rash in mucous membranes and skin, respectively) follow the wide dissemination of virus and measles cells in the blood. Virus cells lodge in the capillary beds, and the accumulation there of sensitized T cells and lymphokines liberated locally will account for the character of the rashes. The explosive interaction, producing rash and fever, is apparently sufficient to eliminate the infection in a few days.

The other feature of measles in normal individuals that requires comment is the well-known disappearance of a positive tuberculin reaction and other types of delayed hypersensitivity for a few weeks after measles. This is accompanied by a loss of reactivity of lymphocytes to tuberculin *in vitro*, but it is not clear whether this means elimination of most tuberculin-sensitized cells or a damping down of their reactivity. If the contention is that T-cell reactivity to extrinsic antigens like those of measles virus is passively derived from stimulated B cells, there could be some very interesting possibilities for study of the sequence of immunological change in measles.

Interplay of Immunopathology with Measles

The interpretation of the measles process in normal children allows a more detailed look at the three unusual forms of measles mentioned at the beginning of this article. These are: 1, measles in agammaglobulinemia, showing normal course and recovery without antibody production; 2, measles in leukemic children undergoing corticosteroid therapy, where there is no rash and no immunity;

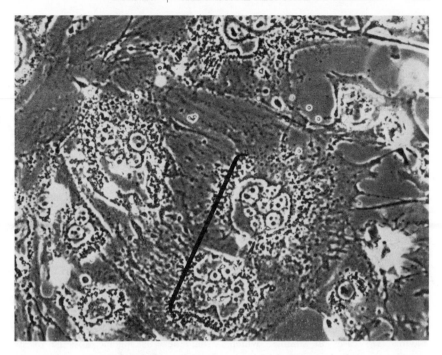

CELLS IN A CULTURE infected with measles virus, showing fusion without other damage. The bracket embraces two groups of previously fused cells that have begun to fuse again to form syncytia, or giant cells (the bracket represents a distance of approximately 32 μm). Such fusion takes place during the measles incubation period. The photo was taken 9 days after infection. It is reproduced from W. Klöne et al, *Archiv für die Gesamte Virusforschung*, **19:**91–106 (1966).

and 3, subacute sclerosing panencephalitis, which is a spreading measles infection in a brain saturated with measles antibody and infiltrated by the plasma cells producing it.

The three conditions considered in sequence may give a clearer picture of the interaction of B and T cells than any other aspect of human immunopathology can.

Agammaglobulinemia appears to be essentially a failure of B cells to give rise to plasma cells, which are the effective producers of circulating antibody. [See "Agammaglobulinemia," by David Gitlin and Charles A. Janeway, on page 167.] Whether there are some forms in which B cells are never produced—these would be equivalent to chickens in which the whole development of the bursa has been inhibited—is uncertain. And since it is obligatory to maintain an artificial level of gammaglobulin in the blood if the child is to survive, it may be impossible to establish the point.

For the most likely situation, one can assume that a B-cell population is genetically incapable of more immunoglobulin formation than is necessary to provide IgM1 receptors and that it responds to stimulation only by producing memory cells. T cells appear to be quite normal and, by hypothesis, capable

of taking up IgM1 to serve as IgT receptors. A main difficulty is in understanding the elimination of virus in the absence of antibody. The simplest way to approach this is to postulate the existence of a large population of specifically cytotoxic T cells whose targets will be cells carrying measles-antigenic determinants in the cell membrane. Like any other myxovirus, an essential part of the construction of the infectious particles (virions) of measles takes place in the cell membrane and antigen is present there before any complete virus has appeared in the cell. In a disrupted cell, synthesized viral components are no longer capable of going on to the final process of self-assembly.

In acute lymphatic leukemia the lymphoid tissue is crowded with malignant cells, presumably greatly reducing the numbers of normal T cells. Corticosteroid therapy reduces the activity and probably the number of those that remain. In the absence of an effective population of specifically cytotoxic T cells, the spread of virus and the formation of syncytial giant cells cannot be cut short. There is no explosive confrontation of the two populations, no rash, no elimination of the virus, and in most patients, no immunity and so, early death.

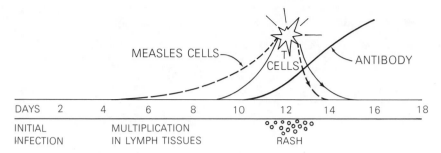

DAYS 2   4   6   8   10   12   14   16   18

INITIAL   MULTIPLICATION
INFECTION   IN LYMPH TISSUES   RASH

THE SEQUENCE OF NORMAL MEASLES, from the day of primary infection until the onset of convalescence. Measles cells, in which virus is present and multiplying, and sensitized T cells increase in numbers till a point of catastrophic interaction is reached, after which both rapidly disappear. Antibodies begin to appear at about the same time.

Subacute sclerosing panencephalitis (SSPE) occurs in a very small proportion of children who have measles, perhaps not many more than one in a million. Two families have been mentioned as having two cases in siblings, which would suggest that a genetic anomaly may be involved. Apart from this, the only clues to its nature must be obtained from what is observed in the patients during life and at autopsy. The immunological features of SSPE are a very high titer of measles antibody in serum and a relatively high titer in cerebrospinal fluid (around one-half to one-tenth of the corresponding serum level). Post mortem, plasma cells are numerous in the brain. In SSPE patients T cells fail to respond against measles antigens. Positive skin tests are given by slightly more than 50 percent of people who have had measles; SSPE patients show no sensitivity, but it should be noted that they also fail to respond to most of the standard skin-test reagents. *In vitro* there is no response of SSPE lymphocytes to measles antigens although *Candida* and tuberculin antigens can be effective. The general conclusion is that there is specific absence or inactivity of T cells toward measles antigens, although other T-cell functions are nearly normal. Probably all that can be said is that in the absence of T-cell activity the progressive infiltration of the brain by virus and by plasma cells goes on unhindered. Details remain to be worked out.

Measles Vaccination

Vaccination against measles is now a fully established and very effective procedure, thanks largely to the pioneering work of J. F. Enders, who in 1958 introduced the first live vaccine virus. His strain has been replaced by other derivatives but the general principle remains the same: an attenuated measles infection is initiated, which in a small proportion of children produces symptoms resembling a very mild attack. The immunity gained by vaccination is not as long-lasting as that resulting from a natural attack, but vaccination appears likely to last effectively for life if there is an occasional opportunity for reinfection by an epidemic virus, which produces a local primary lesion in the respiratory tract. The long incubation period of measles allows an effective secondary immune response to develop in the earliest stages of the spread of the virus in the body, and this is sufficient to abort the clinical manifestations completely at the end of the incubation period.

Killed measles vaccine has not been a success for reasons that may throw some light on B- and T-cell function. Particularly if killed vaccine is followed by administration of live vaccine, a severe bronchiolitis may develop that appears to represent a form of antigen-antibody complex disease. SSPE is perhaps only the limiting example of the rule that a predominant T-cell activity with minor antibody activity is optimal for controlling measles. Reversal of that balance is positively harmful. Administration of killed vaccine presents soluble antigens and provokes a B-cell antibody response, predominantly, which inhibits further T-cell stimulation. The live vaccine will present the virus predominantly on the cell surface, which is optimal for T-cell stimulation, according to Parish, unless this is inhibited by the prior presence of antibody.

IX

AUTOIMMUNITY

28

The Nature of Autoimmune Disease

by Sir Macfarlane Burnet
An original article
1976

The essential features are the presence of an adequate source of autoantigen and of T cells that are abnormally resistant to inactivation by contact with antigen.

An ever-increasing number of conditions of ill health, mostly chronic and of various degrees of severity, are associated with evidence that an antibody has reacted in a damaging way against some body component or that a combined antibody and cell-mediated immune attack has been made on some organ or cell system. Physicians are by no means unanimous about the legitimacy of the term autoimmune disease, or the mechanism by which the abnormal immunological signs arise, and it would be inappropriate to attempt a comprehensive account of autoimmunity in a collection of articles that contains little mention elsewhere of this theme.

However, the strong trend is to regard most of these clinical conditions as manifestations of primary faults—germ cell and somatic cell mutations—in the immune system, and some account of principles in the field of autoimmune disease is necessary to provide a properly rounded picture of the importance of immunology in medicine. Obviously, anything about autoimmune disease must be read in the light of current ideas about mechanisms of immunological tolerance, which exist, according to one commonly held view, to prevent the occurrence of autoimmune conditions. Three sets of conditions only will be discussed, in each case much more from the point of view of what aspects of the normal function of the immune system have been distorted in the illness than in regard to clinical matters. [*See the illustration below.*]

EXAMPLES OF FOUR TYPES OF AUTOIMMUNE DISEASE IN MAN
1. AUTOIMMUNE HEMOLYTIC ANEMIA (WARM, COLD, AND DONATH-LANDSTEINER TYPES); THROMBOCYTOPENIA; THYROTOXICOSIS (GRAVES' DISEASE)
2. HASHIMOTO'S DISEASE; CHRONIC GASTRITIS AND PERNICIOUS ANEMIA; CHRONIC ACTIVE HEPATITIS; ADDISON'S DISEASE
3. RHEUMATOID ARTHRITIS; SYSTEMIC LUPUS ERYTHEMATOSUS; SCLERODERMA
4. GLOMERULONEPHRITIS; AMYLOID DEPOSITION

SOME OF THE COMMONEST FORMS of autoimmune disease in man are shown in this chart. The first three groupings give typical examples of the important groups; some are subsequently discussed under headings having corresponding numbers in the text. Group 1 lists conditions, usually monoclonal, in which damage is done to "target" cells by autoantibody. The second group lists diseases involving specific organs, in which specific T and B cells infiltrate the target tissue. The conditions of Group 3 are still of obscure origin, and suggest a more deepseated abnormality of the immune system than do the other two groups. In the fourth category are two types of pathological changes that may be seen in a variety of autoimmune conditions, especially those of Group 3.

1. Monoclonal Conditions

When it can be shown that a population of cells is acting to produce symptoms in an autoimmune disease and the population is monoclonal in character, we can deduce with some confidence that the condition arises from circumstances that include, at one point, somatic mutation in a single cell. Once this is established, it becomes expedient to consider whether a similar conclusion could be relevant to other autoimmune conditions in which it is not possible to establish the criterion of monoclonality.

Acquired (autoimmune) hemolytic anemia, both "warm" type and "cold" type, cause symptoms by excess destruction (hemolysis) of red cells, which is due in the first instance to a coating of antibody. The antibody coating the patient's own red cells can be released and in a majority of cases this can be shown to be monoclonal, and to have a kappa or lambda light chain, but not both. This can be shown also for another type of hemolytic disease, the so-called Donath-Landsteiner type of "cold hemoglobinuria."

At an earlier stage in the development of immunology one might have said dogmatically that the existence of monoclonal pathogenic antibody indicated that the essential etiological factor was the occurrence of somatic mutation in a B cell or a cell ancestral to a B cell. But answers as simple as that are no longer admissible in modern immunology. Autoimmune disease is an intensely heterogeneous group of conditions occurring in a system whose controlled complexity I have tried to suggest in the phrase "homeostatic and self-monitoring" [see "A Homeostatic and Self-monitoring Immune System," by Sir Macfarlane Burnet, page 158]. No autoimmune disease is simple, and a brief survey of some of the varieties of clinical or hematological conditions that are clearly related to the autoimmune hemolytic anemias may help to give a useful indication of the complexity of the conditions that are concerned in the initiation of any type of autoimmune disease:

1. A positive Coombs test—i.e., a coating of the individual's red cells with specific and usually monoclonal IgG antibody [*see the illustration at the right*]—can occur, without any evidence of hemolytic disease, in (a) a very small proportion of healthy blood donors, and in (b) about 25 percent of patients given long-term treatment for hypertension with the drug α-methyldopa ("Aldomet").

Neither condition produces any symptoms of anemia, making it obvious that, though a coating of autoantibody may be a necessary factor in autoimmune hemolytic anemia (AHA), it is by no means sufficient. Some other abnormal factors must also be present.

2. Careful examination of any typical case of AHA will often show that the autoantibody is specifically directed toward one of the known (blood group) antigens on the patient's red cells. Most often it is directed toward one of the minor Rh antigens *c* or *e* but not infrequently toward what is usually spoken of as a common "core" antigen of the Rh system. An autoantibody against core antigen will react with, and under appropriate circumstances agglutinate, all human red cells except those of the very rare blood type that apparently lacks all Rh antigens and is cited as being of - - -/- - - phenotype.

This emphasizes the important role played by the antigen in stimulating the proliferation of the pathogenic B-cell clone.

3. Autoantibody may have *in vivo* any degree of hemolytic action, including forms in which peripheral cooling of the blood triggers hemolysis. *In vitro* there are autoantibodies that agglutinate red cells only in the cold, others that agglutinate at 37° C, and a small proportion that hemolyze actively at 37° C.

4. Unlike almost all other autoimmune diseases, typical AHA can occur in infants; many recover spontaneously but others may have very severe cases. In at least three such cases physicians

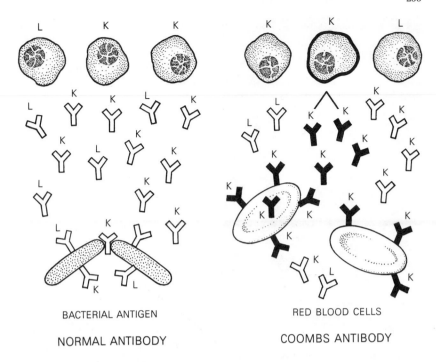

BACTERIAL ANTIGEN

NORMAL ANTIBODY

RED BLOOD CELLS

COOMBS ANTIBODY

THE MONOCLONAL CHARACTER of an autoimmune Coombs antibody is shown at the right in this figure. Individual antibody-producing cells produce antibodies having either kappa (**K**) or lambda (**L**) light chains but never both. Ordinary antibodies are usually derived from numerous clones and will always show a mixture of K and L types. If only one type is regularly found, as is true in most autoimmune hemolytic anemias, one can deduce that all the autoantibody is derived from a single clone, in the last analysis, from a single cell. The drawing is based on one in Macfarlane Burnet, *Cellular Immunology*, Melbourne University Press, 1969.

have credited surgical removal of the thymus with saving life.

No attempt will be made to interpret all these characteristic findings; they are set out to underline the complexity of interactions within the immune system and the many ways by which something can go wrong. Most of the anomalies appear to be genetic and probably all that can be said with certainty is that AHA is a rare condition that depends on the presence in a single precursor cell of anomalous genetic qualities which allow its descendant B-cell clone to proliferate freely, and to liberate autoantibody, if the appropriate red-cell antigen is available. Clearly one must take into account the complications that may arise in the appearance of phenocopy phenomena—possibly induced by a drug or some internal environmental factor—and the likelihood that other genetically-based anomalies must be present if the autoantibody is to induce accelerated hemolysis and anemia. Accepting all this, there is still need for some unique genetic episode in a single cell, i.e., a somatic mutation, to initiate the clonal process that leads to large amounts of

monoclonal antibody. At the physiological level the significant question is to ask what makes the mutant B-cell clone flourish in contrast to the absence of such clones in normal individuals. In broad terms, resistance to processes that normally eliminate cells of autoreactivity must be postulated. In this sense we are dealing with a "forbidden clone" which has survived in virtue of the mutation that initiated it.

Still on the theme of monoclonality, it may be worth noting that a reasonable proportion of myeloma proteins appear to be autoantibodies often directed against an antigen of aggregated immunoglobulin. Since a plasma cell is a derivative of a B cell that has already been stimulated antigenically, the mutation toward unlimited proliferation of the myeloma cells took place after the B cell had differentiated.

2. Thyroid Disease

Functional disease of the thyroid can take three well known forms. One form is Graves' disease or hyperthyroidism, in which the gland is hyperactive and the patient, usually a young woman, is overactive and nervous, with a high

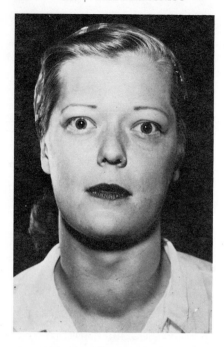

A CASE OF GRAVES' DISEASE in a young woman. Note the enlarged thyroid gland, evidenced by the swelling at the base of the neck, and the protruding eyeballs. The photo is reproduced from P. Beeson and W. McDermott (eds.), *Cecil-Loeb Textbook of Medicine*, W. B. Saunders Company, 1963.

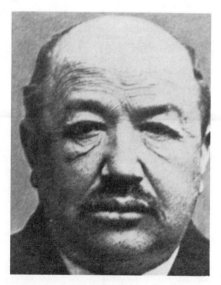

FACIAL APPEARANCE of a myxedema patient in whom thyroid activity is virtually absent. The thickening and dryness of the skin is typical. The photo is reproduced from P. Beeson and W. McDermott (eds.), *Cecil-Loeb Textbook of Medicine*, W. B. Saunders Company, 1963.

basal metabolism, protruding eyeballs, and moderate enlargement of the thyroid. [*See the illustration at the left.*] Another form, Hashimoto's disease, is one of the classical autoimmune diseases, characterized by cellular infiltration by lymphocytes and development of germinal centers in the substance of the gland, reaction of several types of autoantibodies with thyroid antigens, and evidence of suboptimal thyroid function. The third example is myxedema, in which the symptoms are those of complete or nearly complete loss of thyroid function [*see bottom illustration on this page*].

It is not uncommon to see a sequence in which a patient moves from Graves' disease to Hashimoto's disease to myxedema, from hyperactivity through gradual diminution to complete loss of thyroid endocrine function. Detailed immunological study is much more difficult in these diseases than in diseases where red cells of the blood are the target, but enough work has been done to provide an outline of the autoimmune elements. The reality will undoubtedly involve many other factors, but again an outline of the current model will serve to give an idea of how concepts are developing in the field of autoimmunity.

In Graves' disease the recognition of an autoimmune process came from studies by physiologists interested in the control of thyroid activity by pituitary hormones. They found in the blood of some patients with Graves' disease, in addition to thyroid stimulating hormone (TSH) of pituitary origin, a more slowly-acting substance which became known as LATS (long-acting thyroid stimulator). Both were assayed by their effect on the mouse thyroid. Biochemical studies on LATS showed it was a serum protein indistinguishable from IgG and, with reasonable certainty, an antibody directed against the receptors on the mouse thyroid that mediate physiological stimulation by TSH. The fact that many other patients with typical symptoms of the disease showed no LATS in their serum was clarified by the discovery that they had, instead, what became known as a LATS-protector, called this because it protects LATS from neutralization by human thyroid tissue but not by mouse thyroid. Without describing the subsequent investigations, one can summarize the results by saying that all Graves' disease pa-

tients have an unusual autoantibody that reacts with the thyroid through the TSH receptors to produce a chronic long-lasting stimulation. Such antibodies may be of at least two forms. One, in addition to reacting with the human receptor, will also stimulate the corresponding receptors on mouse thyroid cells; this is recognized as LATS. The other form is active against the human thyroid but is inert against mouse thyroid, and it therefore has LATS-protector qualities [*see the top illustration on page 257*]. Between them, the two forms of antibody cover 90 percent of the cases of Graves' disease and virtually establish the classical form of Graves' disease as autoimmune in quality.

Other more conventional antibodies detected by complement fixation or immunofluorescence techniques can be shown to react with the hormone thyroglobulin or with components of the cytoplasm of the thyroid epithelium. These are found in a considerable proportion of patients with Graves' disease, but in an even greater proportion, indeed, in nearly all, of the patients with Hashimoto's disease. The interpretation of these immune responses is complicated by the fact that autoantibodies against thyroid components are often associated with a variety of other antibodies in the same individuals, those against gastric mucosa or adrenal tissue being the most frequently found. The lymphocytes in the thyroid substance, including those in the germinal centers, are B cells, and nothing certain is known of the role of T cells in the natural disease in man. A recent suggestion is that much of the damage produced in the thyroids of patients with Hashimoto's disease may result from the deposition of complexes of autoantibody and thyroid-protein antigen in the thyroid cells. Some researchers are interested too in an antibody-dependent cytotoxic T-cell attack as an explanation. Both suggestions stem from experimental work on animals that do not develop the spontaneous thyroid diseases seen in man. The analogies may be misleading, but there seems to be little doubt in anyone's mind that the slow destruction of thyroid function that eventually results in myxedema is the result of autoimmune processes involving autoantibody, B cells, T cells, and the various potential antigens released from damaged thyroid tissue.

3. Systemic Lupus Erythematosus (SLE)

Most physicians would regard SLE as the autoimmune disease *par excellence.* It is a puzzling disease that may present dozens of different combinations of symptoms. The two features on which diagnosis is based are antibodies against DNA, detected by an indirect procedure known as an LE cell test, and signs of kidney damage; facial rash, pleurisy, joint pains, and fever are the commonest symptoms.

SLE is unique because of the great variety of antibodies against DNA and other nuclear components that may be found in any group of sera from severe cases of the disease. It is in no sense a monoclonal disease and, though no one doubts its autoimmune character, there is no agreement on an interpretation of what immunological errors are basically responsible. In one or two experiments, volunteers have been given transfusions of blood or serum from SLE patients without any ill effect. This, along with the wide variety of antibodies that may be found, makes it unlikely that the primary fault is in antibody-producing cells. What seem to be the most significant clues are the variety of autoantibodies against products of cellular (including nuclear) breakdown and the fact that hematologists seeking antisera against "unusual" red-cell antigens are likely to find them in the sera of SLE patients who have had multiple transfusions. The suggestion is that SLE patients produce antibody against any accessible antigen with abnormal ease.

One reasonable basis for this, in the light of what is known of the qualities of B and T cells, would be to assume the appearance of a clone or clones of T cells that combined high resistance to destruction with active powers of co-operation with antigenically-stimulated B cells. The action of the resistant T cells would be to exert a highly active mitogenic effect on any adjacent specifically-activated B cells. With the exercise of a little ingenuity, such a point of view could be developed to concur with the hypothesis of passive arming of initially-neutral T cells by any initially-stimulated B cells. If a highly resistant T-cell clone came into contact with a clone of a B cell whose receptor-antibody combining site had a high affinity for some surface antigen specific

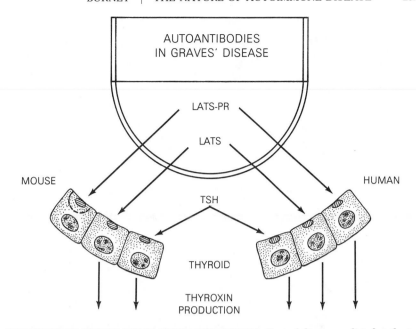

THE THYROID STIMULATING AUTOANTIBODIES in Graves' disease are listed at the top of this diagram. It is highly probable that TSH (thyroid-stimulating hormone) from the pituitary gland and the thyroid autoantibodies LATS (long-acting thyroid stimulator) and LATS-protector (LATS-PR) all act to stimulate the same receptor in human thyroid cells, causing them to secrete thyroxin. LATS is detected by experiments with mice. Only some human beings with Graves' disease produce the LATS autoantibody that stimulates mouse thyroid cells. Other patients with Graves' disease produce autoantibody that stimulates human thyroid cells but combines with the mouse cell receptor without causing stimulation. The blocked receptor "protects" LATS from absorption and inactivation by mouse thyroid.

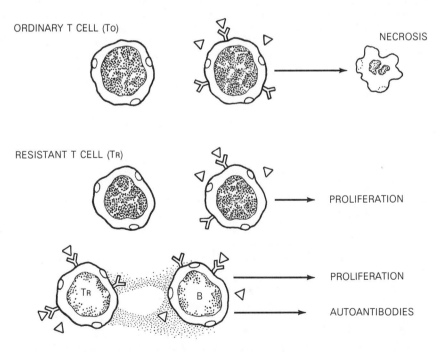

POSSIBLE IMPORTANCE OF A RESISTANT T-CELL CLONE in autoimmune disease can be diagrammed. In this figure the passive origin of the antibody receptors, shown as Y-shaped structures, is assumed. Autoantigen is shown as a triangle. B cells do not liberate autoantibody except when stimulated by antigen in the immediate presence of a reactive T cell.

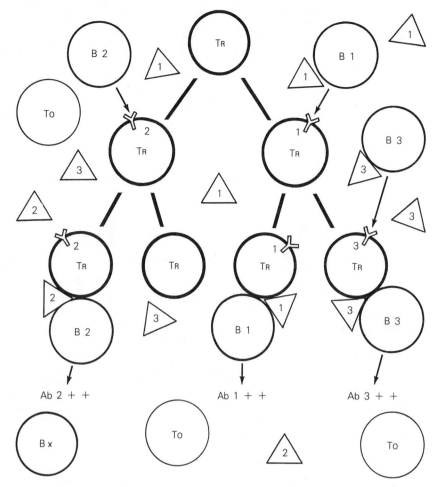

AN APPLICATION OF THE T-RESISTANT CLONE (Tʀ) CONCEPT, diagrammed in the preceding figure, to the conditions in systemic lupus erythematosus (SLE) where numerous antibodies may be produced. The Tʀ clone is shown with heavy circles (ordinary T cells are labeled To); an uninvolved B cell is Bx. Passively obtained IgT receptors are shown as Y shapes. The B cells produce IgM (abbreviated here as Ab 1 + +, etc.), through cooperation with Tʀ cells in response to the presence of an antigen (shown here as triangles). The presence of a foreign antigen (e.g., one resulting from blood transfusion), or any unusual accessibility of autoantigen could give rise to a self-amplifying condition.

Some General Aspects of Autoimmunity

It will be evident even from this brief account of three widely representative forms of autoimmune disease that two rather distinct forms of somatic mutational change seem to be called for. When the pathogenic effect is clearly due to a monoclonal antibody, as in the autoimmune hemolytic anemias, the basic development, by a cell line, of resistance to inactivation upon contact with antigen must be located in a B-cell clone with an intrinsic immune specificity. In the other two examples, where a multiplicity of autoantibodies as well as tissue damage in one or more organs are seen, it is not helpful to think of a whole series of mutant B-cell clones. Two alternative concepts need to be considered. One that has already been suggested for SLE, which may have a wider application too, is the appearance of a mutant clone of T cells that, by hypothesis, carry no actively synthesized IgT receptors but depend on obtaining their receptors passively from initially stimulated B cells [*see the bottom illustration on page 257*]. The mutant, which can be called Tʀ, readily incorporates IgT, as a receptor, into the cell membrane, and in that condition the Tʀ cells can cooperate actively with B cells, which would not be capable of responding with more than limited IgM production without cooperation [*see the illustration at the left*]. Once such a clone came into existence there would be a basic instability in the immune system by which any unusual accessibility of an autoantigen, e.g., by infection or trauma in a specific organ, could give rise to a self-amplifying condition.

The second concept is not necessarily incompatible with the first. It is simply that in a relatively nonspecific fashion any loss of overall efficiency of the immune system will weaken the controls that are needed to prevent the development of an unwanted autoimmune clone or to eliminate it, once it has begun to grow, before it becomes dangerous. This is of necessity a rather vague formulation, called for largely because of the association of autoimmunity with age. In a normal human population the proportion of people with autoantibodies of any of the types normally measured in laboratories of clinical immunology shows an accelerating increase in old age. So does the incidence of high levels of total immunoglobulins and of deposits of amyloid in the senile plaques of the

to lymphocytes, results equivalent to those seen in the blood of SLE patients could develop. The range of autoantibodies found strongly suggests that the accessible autoantigens are present in a tissue undergoing active proliferation and autolysis, as is characteristic of the thymic cortex and the germinal centers in peripheral lymphoid accumulations, such as the spleen, lymph nodes, and tonsils.

This is sheer speculation—no one has reported an autoantibody against lymphocytic-surface antigens in SLE—but it does provide an interpretation of the wide range of autoantibodies that can be found; it is concordant with the general picture of the immune system; and in my opinion it provides rather strong indirect evidence for the passive

origin of Ig receptors on functioning T cells.

The lethal outcome of SLE, when it occurs, is due to failure of kidney function, which is consistently ascribed by pathologists to the accumulation in glomerular basement membranes and elsewhere of antigen-antibody complexes, particularly complexes containing DNA as antigen. An animal model of SLE can be found in the condition that develops in F1 hybrids of New Zealand Black and New Zealand White mice (NZB/NZW). In these hybrids, the antigen-antibody complexes in the kidney also include, as would be expected, complexes of virus antigens with antibodies to any persisting viruses characteristic of the substrain.

brain or elsewhere in the body. All of these are without special symptoms and are within the normal course of senescence. In addition, and hardly to be demarcated sharply from the normal, are the other abnormalities of the immune system that rank as hematological diseases. These diseases are essentially monoclonal, malignant or benign proliferations of T or B cells, and they include the three common blood diseases, chronic lymphatic leukemia, multiple myelomatosis, and Waldenström's macroglobulinemia, as well as a wide range of other lympho-proliferative conditions. It is of interest that many of the monoclonal immunoglobulins found in these conditions have the specificity of an autoantibody. In all of them there is a clear correlation with age. Amyloid disease calls for special mention since modern work on the composition and pathological associations of amyloid points infallibly to its accumulation as a result of confrontations within the immune system such that autoantigens, autoantibodies, and immunocytes, particularly plasma cells, have interacted and been subject to the action of tissue enzymes.

If the picture of the immune system depicted in my article on its homeostatic and self-monitoring qualities [*see page 158*] is approximately correct, the random accumulation of somatic genetic error that is characteristic of the aging process would be expected, in the immune system, to give rise to the same range of effects I have just enumerated. In principle it may be possible to map out the immunological detail of one or two of the particularly well defined patterns of autoimmune disease; but for the autoimmune components of senescence it is not likely that more than a broad general understanding—at most an intellectual model not inconsistent with the facts—will ever be achieved.

EPILOGUE

Finally we can take a brief look at what remains to be done in immunology and venture some tentative forecasts of likely trends for research in the future.

In biology and medicine the infinite complexities of living structures will ensure that there can never be a point in research in any substantial field such as immunology when it can be said that we know all that can be known. This holds particularly for the theoretical and comparative aspects of immunology and, to a considerable extent too, for the clinical and applied sides. It is important, however, to remember that the practical triumphs of the biomedical sciences have been in those fields for which convenient laboratory models were available for study. The application of immunology to infectious disease was successful largely because other mammals respond to the important human pathogens in broadly similar fashion, and it has usually been possible to find a suitable experimental animal as a laboratory model even if, in the case of leprosy, the model is as exotic as the armadillo. The importance of having a valid and convenient laboratory model provides the best lead, if research is to be successful in almost any biological field, in thinking about future prospects in immunological research.

Even when we are concerned as molecular biologists with the finer points of chemical structure and control, the need for a model is still dominant. Antibody structure would still be almost unknown if the significance of the Bence-Jones protein as a monoclonal light chain had not been recognized. No one yet appears to have devised a method by which normal T cells that have not undergone any type of viral transformation or malignant change can be cloned. Success in such efforts is badly needed if knowledge of the nature of the T receptor is to be gained.

Another urgent need for the immediate future is to clarify the process by which transfer factor works. Transfer factor is an agent extractable from human leucocytes that allows the transfer, to a volunteer subject previously nonreactive, of the capacity to respond to any antigen capable of producing a delayed hypersensitivity reaction in the donor of the leucocytes. The response is determinable with a skin test. This is generally accepted as a reproducible phenomenon, but no one has offered any interpretation that can be correlated with other T-cell phenomena. The current suggestions that RNA, double-stranded but of low molecular weight, is responsible seems to make no reasonable contact with current ideas in either immunology or genetics, and if it should be correct, some drastic reshaping of cellular biology will be needed.

In clinical immunology there are major gaps to be filled before we can fully understand or prevent several important human diseases. Most are infectious or parasitic diseases in undeveloped regions of the world, and the only effective way to render them harmless or extinct is by providing capital and technical assistance to bring those countries to a much higher standard of living. Only when this is achieved will the large-scale public health measures needed to control the important parasitic and infectious diseases become possible. Until then, there will be a challenge to alleviate malaria, trypanosomiasis, and other protozoal diseases by immunological means. Trachoma is almost as widespread and presents rather similar problems. Particularly in Africa, schistosomiasis, guinea worm, and other worm infestations are endemic and can cripple the health of whole populations. It is perhaps being unduly optimistic to think of an immunological attack on such conditions, but it may have to be attempted.

Protozoal and metazoan parasites undoubtedly provoke immune responses, but in general these merely hold the infestation in check. The parasite has no difficulty in persisting in the body, but the host suffers little disability. In malaria the surviving adults in hyperendemic areas appear to be completely healthy but are still infected. This is liable to give rise to an intolerable situation: in the course of campaigns to eradicate the disease, a large population of susceptible individuals without malaria are exposed to infection from persons without symptoms who are latently infected. In such circumstances an effective means of immunization would be of enormous value.

Looked at in terms of its evolution, an immune system may be expected to be optimally effective against the infections most commonly experienced by any species during its most recent one to three million years. This creates an interesting picture of the human immune system. The evidence is that for most of the three to five million years that hominids have existed they comprised small bands of nomad hunter-gatherers with relatively few contacts with other groups apart from hostile ones; population density was very low.

During that time the important infectious diseases would have been those enzootic in gregarious vertebrates and spread by mosquitoes or other biting arthropods to any human beings intruding into the enzootic region. Human populations remained too small to generate specifically human infectious diseases; the other main need for defense and immunity then was for protection against the relatively nonspecific bacterial invasions of traumatized areas of the body. With the continued expansion of territorial range and exposure to new pathogens, particularly as populations expanded during the agricultural and urban revolutions, a wide range of more specifically human pathogens emerged, each with its own individual qualities and tricks for survival. Often, no doubt, there were temporary phases when lack of effective defense against some new pathogenic microorganisms caused an excessive mortality. It may well be a general rule that, until a new disease becomes an important factor in limiting survival, it will be countered by standard methods that may be relatively ineffective for some conditions.

In an entirely different field one senses a growing interest at both physiological and clinical levels in the immunological aspects of hormonal and pharmacological control. A number of cell receptors mediating such agents have been identified and one can also look forward to the identification and synthesis of effector groups in both peptide and steroid hormones for use as haptens in synthetic antigens. On the not unreasonable assumption that the therapy of metabolic and degenerative disease will move increasingly in the direction of physiological or near-physiological control of body systems, including the immune system, we can foresee an important future for the immunological approach. With comprehensive knowledge of the control systems such as those postulated for the immune system, it should be possible in principle to bolster inadequate immune function with additional hormone or an equivalent synthetic. Where there is overactivity of hormonal action, or for some reason a damping down of normal function is called for, the use of specific antibody to block either the effector groupings of a hormone or the cell receptors offers a potential approach. There is active work in progress on the possible use of antibody against gonadotrophins as a means of contraception, and no doubt other projects in various fields of clinical endorcinology are also under way.

BIBLIOGRAPHIES

PART ONE **Immunity of the Normal Organism**

I ANTIBODIES AND RECEPTORS

1. The Mechanism of Immunity

AUTO-IMMUNE DISEASE. I: MODERN IMMUNOLOGICAL CONCEPTS F. M. Burnet in *British Medical Journal*, No. 5,153, pages 645–650; October 10, 1959.

AUTO-IMMUNE DISEASE. II: PATHOLOGY OF THE IMMUNE RESPONSE. F. M. Burnet in *British Medical Journal*, No. 5,154, pages 720–725; October 17, 1959.

THE CLONAL SELECTION THEORY OF ACQUIRED IMMUNITY. F. M. Burnet in *The Abraham Flexner Lectures*. Vanderbilt University Press, 1959.

GENES AND ANTIBODIES. Joshua Lederberg in *Science*, Vol. 129, No. 3,364, pages 1,649–1,653; June 19, 1959.

IMMUNOLOGICAL SPECIFICITY. David W. Talmage in *Science*, Vol. 129, No. 3,364, pages 1,643–1,648; June 19, 1959.

THEORIES OF IMMUNITY. F. M. Burnet in *Perspectives in Biology and Medicine*, Vol. III, No. 4, pages 447–458; Summer, 1960.

THE UNIQUENESS OF THE INDIVIDUAL. P. B. Medawar. Basic Books, Inc., 1957.

2. How Cells Make Antibodies

ELABORATION OF ANTIBODIES BY SINGLE CELLS. G. J. V. Nossal and O. Mäkelä in *Annual Review of Microbiology*, Vol. 16, pages 53–74; 1962.

SINGLE CELL STUDIES ON 19S ANTIBODY PRÓDUCTION. G. J. V. Nossal, A. Szenberg, G. L. Ada and Caroline M. Austin in *The Journal of Experimental Medicine*, Vol. 119, No. 3, pages 485–502; March, 1964.

STRUCTURE AND SPECIFICITY OF GUINEA PIG 7S ANTIBODIES. G. M. Edelman, B. Benacerraf and Z. Ovary in *The Journal of Experimental Medicine*, Vol. 118, No. 2, pages 229–244; August, 1963.

3. The Structure of Antibodies

IMMUNOGLOBULINS. Julian B. Fleischman in *Annual Review of Biochemistry*, Vol. 35, Part II, pages 835–872; edited by Paul D. Boyer. Annual Reviews, Inc., 1966.

IMMUNOGLOBULINS. E. S. Lennox and M. Cohn in *Annual Review of Biochemistry*, Vol. 36, Part I, pages 365–406; edited by Paul D. Boyer. Annual Reviews, Inc., 1967.

THE STRUCTURE OF IMMUNOGLOBULINS. R. R. Porter in *Essays in Biochemistry: Vol. 3*, edited by P. N. Campbell and G. D. Greville. Academic Press, 1967.

4. The Structure and Function of Antibodies

ANTIBODIES. Cold Spring Harbor Symposia on Quantitative Biology, Vol. 32. Cold Spring Harbor Laboratory of Quantitative Biology, 1967.

THE ANTIBODY PROBLEM. Gerald M. Edelman and W. Einar Gall in *Annual Review of Biochemistry*, Vol. 38; edited by Esmond E. Snell. Annual Reviews, Inc., 1969.

THE COVALENT STRUCTURE OF AN ENTIRE γG IMMUNOGLOBULIN MOLECULE. Gerald M. Edelman, Bruce A. Cunningham, W. Einar Gall, Paul D. Gottlieb, Urs Rutishauser and Myron J. Waxdal in *Proceedings of the National Academy of Sciences*, Vol. 63, No. 1, pages 78–85; May 15, 1969.

GAMMA GLOBULINS—STRUCTURE AND CONTROL OF BIOSYNTHESIS. Nobel Symposium 3. Edited by Johan Killander. Interscience Publishers, 1968.

5. The Immune System

ANTIGEN DESIGN AND IMMUNE RESPONSE. Michael Sela in *The Harvey Lectures 1971–1972*, Series 67. Academic Press, 1973.

ANTIGEN SENSITIVE CELLS: THEIR SOURCE AND DIFFERENTIATION. J. F. A. P. Miller, G. F. Mitchell, A. J. S. Davies, Henry N. Claman, Edward A. Chaperon and R. B. Taylor in *Transplantation Reviews*, Vol. 1, edited by Goran Möller. Williams & Wilkins Co., 1969.

THE CLONAL SELECTION THEORY OF ACQUIRED IMMUNITY. F. M. Burnet. Cambridge University Press, 1959.

INDIVIDUAL ANTIGENIC SPECIFICITY OF IMMUNOGLOBULINS. John E. Hopper and Alfred Nisonoff in *Advances in Immunology*, Vol. 13, pages 57–99; 1971.

THE PROBLEM OF MOLECULAR RECOGNITION BY A SELECTIVE SYSTEM. Gerald M. Edelman in *Studies in the Philosophy of Biology: Reduction and Related Problems*, edited by F. Ayala and T. Dobzhansky. University of California Press, 1974.

THE REGULATORY INFLUENCE OF ACTIVATED T CELLS ON B CELL RESPONSES TO ANTIGEN. David H. Katz and Baruj Benacerraf in *Advances in Immunology*, Vol. 15, pages 1–94; 1972.

THE TAKE-HOME LESSON–1971. Melvin Cohn in *Annals of the New York Academy of Sciences*, Vol. 190, pages 529–584; December 31, 1971.

6. The Development of the Immune System

THE FUNCTIONS OF THE THYMUS SYSTEM AND THE BURSA SYSTEM IN THE CHICKEN. Max D. Cooper, Raymond D. A. Peterson, Mary Ann South and Robert A. Good in *Journal of Experimental Medicine*, Vol. 123, No. 1, pages 75–102; January, 1966.

THE IMMUNE SYSTEM: A MODEL FOR DIFFERENTIATION IN HIGHER ORGANISMS. L. Hood and J. Prahl in *Advances in Immunology*, Vol. 14, page 291; 1971.

MODIFICATION OF B LYMPHOCYTE DIFFERENTIATION BY ANTI-IMMUNOGLOBULINS. A. R. Lawton and M. D. Cooper in *Contemporary Topics in Immunobiology*, Vol. 3, edited by Max D. Cooper and Noel L. Warner. Plenum Press, 1974.

T AND B LYMPHOCYTES IN HUMANS. Edited by G. Möller. *Transplantation Reviews*, Vol. 16; 1973.

T AND B LYMPHOCYTES: ORIGINS, PROPERTIES AND ROLES IN IMMUNE RESPONSES. M. F. Greaves, J. J. T. Owen and M. C. Raff. American Elsevier, 1974.

II CELL-MEDIATED IMMUNITY

7. Delayed Hypersensitivity

CELLULAR AND HUMORAL ASPECTS OF THE HYPERSENSITIVE STATES. Edited by Henry Sherwood Lawrence. (Paul B. Hoeber Book) Harper & Brothers, 1959.

THE DELAYED TYPE OF ALLERGIC INFLAMMATORY RESPONSE. H. Sherwood Lawrence in *The American Journal of Medicine*, Vol. 20, No. 3, pages 428–447; March, 1956.

EXPERIMENTAL ALLERGIC ENCEPHALOMYELITIS AND THE "AUTO-ALLERGIC" DISEASES. B. H. Waksman in *International Archives of Allergy*, Vol. 14, Supplement; 1959.

REACTIONS OF GRAFTS AGAINST THEIR HOSTS. R. E. Billingham in *Science*, Vol. 130, No. 3,381, pages 947–953; October 16, 1959.

8. The Thymus Gland

THE IMMUNOLOGICAL SIGNIFICANCE OF THE THYMUS. J. F. A. P. Miller, A. H. E. Marshall and R. G. White in *Advances in Immunology*, Vol. 2, edited by W. H. Taliaferro and J. H. Humphrey. Academic Press, Inc., 1962.

THE IMMUNOLOGICAL SIGNIFICANCE OF THE THYMUS: AN EXTENSION OF THE CLONAL SELECTION THEORY

OF IMMUNITY. F. M. Burnet in *Australasian Annals of Medicine*, Vol. 11, No. 2, pages 79–91; May, 1962.

THE INTEGRITY OF THE BODY. F. M. Burnet. Harvard University Press, 1962.

9. The Thymus Hormone

CELLULAR GENETICS OF IMMUNE RESPONSES. G. J. V. Nossal in *Advances in Immunology*, Vol. 2, edited by W. H. Taliaferro and J. H. Humphrey. Academic Press, Inc., 1962.

EVIDENCE FOR FUNCTION OF THYMIC TISSUE IN DIFFUSION CHAMBERS IMPLANTED IN NEONATALLY THYMECTOMIZED MICE: PRELIMINARY REPORT. R. H. Levey, N. Trainin and L. W. Law in *Journal of the National Cancer Institute*, Vol. 31, No. 2, pages 199–217; August, 1963.

THE IMMUNOLOGICAL SIGNIFICANCE OF THE THYMUS. J. F. A. P. Miller, A. H. E. Marshall and R. G. White in *Advances in Immunology*, Vol. 2, edited by W. H. Taliaferro and J. H. Humphrey. Academic Press, Inc., 1962.

INITIATION OF IMMUNE RESPONSES BY SMALL LYMPHO-CITES. J. L. Gowans, D. D. McGregor, Diana M. Cowen, and C. E. Ford in *Nature*, Vol. 196, No. 4855, pages 651–655; November 17, 1962.

10. The Human Lymphocyte as an Experimental Animal

IMMUNOGLOBULIN PRODUCTION: METHOD FOR QUANTI-TATIVELY DETECTING VARIANT MYELOMA CELLS. Philip Coffino, Reuven Laskov and Matthew D. Scharff in *Science*, Vol. 167, No. 3915, pages 186–188; January 9, 1970.

IMMUNOGLOBULIN PRODUCTION BY HUMAN LYMPHO-CYTOID LINES AND CLONES: ABSENCE OF GENIC EXCLUSION. Arthur D. Bloom, Kyoo W. Choi and Barbara J. Lamb in *Science*, Vol. 172, No. 3981, pages 382–383; April 23, 1971.

SYNTHESIS OF PLASMA MEMBRANE-ASSOCIATED AND SECRETORY IMMUNOGLOBULIN IN DIPLOID LYMPHO-CYTES. Richard A. Lerner, Patricia J. McConahey, Inga Jansen and Frank J. Dixon in *Journal of Experimental Medicine*, Vol. 135, No. 1, pages 136–149; January, 1972.

III IMMUNE TOLERANCE

11. Tolerance and Unresponsiveness

"ACTIVELY ACQUIRED TOLERANCE" OF FOREIGN CELLS. R. E. Billingham, L. Brent, and P. B. Medawar in *Nature*, Vol. 172, No. 4,379, pages 603–606; October 3, 1953.

IMMUNOLOGICAL TOLERANCE: MECHANISMS AND POTEN-TIAL THERAPEUTIC APPLICATIONS. Brook Lodge Symposium, April-May, 1974. Edited by D. H. Katz and B. Benacerraf. Academic Press., Inc., 1974.

"INTRINSIC" IMMUNOLOGICAL TOLERANCE IN ALLO-PHENIC MICE. B. Mintz and W. K. Silvers in *Science*, Vol. 158, No. 3,807, pages 1,484–1,487; December 15, 1967.

THE RELATIONSHIP BETWEEN HUMORAL AND CELL-MEDIATED IMMUNITY. C. R. Parish in *Transplantation Reviews*, Vol. 13, pages 35–66; 1972.

SPECIFIC INHIBITION OF ANTIBODY PRODUCTION. II. PARALYSIS INDUCED IN ADULT MICE BY SMALL QUANTITIES OF PROTEIN ANTIGEN. D. W. Dresser in *Immunology*, Vol. 5, No. 3, pages 378–388; 1962.

IV NONSPECIFIC ASPECTS OF IMMUNITY

12. The Lymphatic System

THE LYMPHATIC SYSTEM WITH PARTICULAR REFERENCE TO THE KIDNEY. H. S. Mayerson in *Surgery, Gynecology & Obstetrics*, Vol. 116, No. 3, pages 259–272; March, 1963.

LYMPHATICS AND LYMPH CIRCULATION. István Rusznyák, Mihály Földi and György Szabó. Pergamon Press Ltd., 1960.

LYMPHATICS, LYMPH AND LYMPHOID TISSUE. Joseph Mendel Yoffey and Frederick Colin Courtice. Harvard University Press, 1956.

OBSERVATIONS AND REFLECTIONS ON THE LYMPHATIC SYSTEM. H. S. Mayerson in *Transactions & Studies of the College of Physicians of Philadelphia*, Fourth Series, Vol. 28, No. 3, pages 109–127; January, 1961.

13. The Lysosome

LYSOSOMES. Alex B. Novikoff in *The Cell, Vol. II: Biochemistry, Physiology and Morphology*. Edited by Jean Brachet and A. E. Mirsky. Academic Press, Inc., 1961.

LYSOSOMES: A NEW GROUP OF CYTOPLASMIC PARTICLES. C. de Duve in *Subcellular Particles*. Edited by Teru Hayashi. The Ronald Press Company, 1959.

14. The Complement System

DEVELOPMENT OF THE ONE-HIT THEORY OF IMMUNE HEMOLYSIS. Manfred M. Mayer in *Immunochemical Approaches to Problems in Microbiology: A Symposium Held at the Institute of Microbiology, Rutgers University, September 6–8, 1960*, edited by M. Heidelberger and Otto G. Prescia. Rutgers University Press, 1961.

MECHANISM OF CYTOLYSIS BY COMPLEMENT. Manfred M. Mayer in *Proceedings of the National Academy of Sciences of the U.S.A.*, Vol. 69, No. 10, pages 2,954–2,958; October, 1972.

THE MOLECULAR BASIS OF THE BIOLOGICAL ACTIVITIES OF COMPLEMENT. Hans J. Müller-Eberhard in *The Harvey Lectures 1970–1971*, Series 66. Academic Press, Inc., 1972.

V A SUMMARY VIEW OF PART I

15. A Homeostatic and Self-monitoring System

THE IMMUNE SYSTEM—A WEB OF V DOMAINS. N. K. Jerne in *The Harvey Lectures* (March 20, 1975), Series 70. Academic Press, Inc., in press.

PART TWO Immunity in Relation to Medicine

VI MANIFESTATIONS OF IMMUNE DEFICIENCY

16. Agammaglobulinemia

AGAMMAGLOBULINEMIA. Ogden C. Bruton in *Pediatrics*, Vol. 9, No. 6, pages 722–728; June, 1952.

17. Immunodeficiency: Investigations since 1957

DRUG-INDUCED IMMUNOLOGICAL TOLERANCE. R. S. Schwartz and W. Dameshek in *Nature*, Vol. 183, No. 4,676, pages 1,682–1,683; June 13, 1959.

IMMUNE SURVEILLANCE. Brook Lodge Symposium, May 11–13, 1970. Edited by R. T. Smith and M. Landy. Academic Press, Inc., 1970.

IMMUNOLOGIC DEFICIENCY DISEASES IN MAN. Sanibel Island Conference, February 1967. Edited by D. Bergsma and R. A. Good. Birth Defects—Original Article Series, Vol. 4, No. 1, National Foundation (March of Dimes), New York, 1968.

RISK OF CANCER IN RENAL-TRANSPLANT RECIPIENTS. R. Hoover and J. F. Fraumeni in *The Lancet*, Vol. 2, No. 7820, pages 55–57; July 14, 1973.

VII TRANSPLANTATION

18. Skin Transplants

ENZYME, ANTIGEN AND VIRUS: A STUDY OF MACRO-MOLECULAR PATTERN IN ACTION. F. Macfarlane Burnet. Cambridge University Press, 1957.

QUANTITATIVE STUDIES ON TISSUE TRANSPLANTATION IMMUNITY. III: ACTIVELY ACQUIRED TOLERANCE. R. E. Billingham, L. Brent and P. B. Medawar in *Philosophical Transactions of the Royal Society of London*, Series B, Vol. 239, No. 666, pages 357–414; March 15, 1956.

THE UNIQUENESS OF THE INDIVIDUAL. P. B. Medawar. Basic Books, Inc., 1957.

19. The Transplantation of the Kidney

EXPERIENCES WITH RENAL HOMOTRANSPLANTATION IN THE HUMAN: REPORT OF NINE CASES. David M. Hume, John P. Merrill, Benjamin F. Miller and George W. Thorn in *The Journal of Clinical Investigation*, Vol. 34, No. 2, pages 327–382; February, 1955.

KIDNEY TRANSPLANTATION BETWEEN SEVEN PAIRS OF IDENTICAL TWINS. Joseph E. Murray, John P. Merrill, J. Hartwell Harrison in *Annals of Surgery*, Vol. 148, No. 3, pages 343–359; September, 1958.

SUCCESSFUL HOMOTRANSPLANTATION OF THE HUMAN KIDNEY BETWEEN IDENTICAL TWINS. John P. Merrill, Joseph E. Murray, J. Hartwell Harrison and Warren R. Guild in *The Journal of the American Medical Association*, Vol. 160, No. 4, pages 277–282; January 28, 1956.

20. Skin Transplants and the Hamster

HOMOGRAFT SENSITIVITY: AN EXPRESSION OF THE IMMUNOLOGICAL ORIGINS AND CONSEQUENCES OF INDIVIDUALITY. H. Sherwood Laurence in *Physiological Reviews*, Vol. 39, No. 4, pages 811–859; October, 1959.

STUDIES ON THE HISTOCOMPATIBILITY GENES OF THE SYRIAN HAMSTER. R. E. Billingham, G. H. Sawchuck and W. K. Silvers in *Proceedings of the Na-*

tional Academy of Sciences of the U.S.A., Vol. 46, No. 8, pages 1079–1090; August, 1960.

TRANSPLANTATION OF TISSUES AND CELLS. Edited by R. E. Billingham and Willys K. Silvers. The Wistar Institute Press, 1961.

21. Markers of Biological Individuality

THE IMMUNOLOGY OF TRANSPLANTATION. P. B. Medawar in *The Harvey Lectures 1956–1957*, Series 52. Academic Press, Inc., 1958.

MARKERS OF BIOLOGICAL INDIVIDUALITY: THE TRANSPLANTATION ANTIGENS IMMUNOLOGY. Edited by Barry D. Kahan and Ralph A. Reisfeld. Academic Press, Inc., 1972.

TRANSPLANTATION ANTIGENS. Barry D. Kahan and Ralph A. Reisfeld in *Science*, Vol. 164, No. 3879, pages 514–521; May 2, 1969.

TRANSPLANTATION ANTIGENS. R. A. Reisfeld and B. D. Kahan in *Advances in Immunology*, Vol. 12, pages 117–200; 1970.

TRANSPLANTATION OF TISSUES AND CELLS. Edited by R. E. Billingham and Willys K. Silvers. The Wistar Institute Press, 1961.

THE UNIQUENESS OF THE INDIVIDUAL. P. B. Medawar. Basic Books, Inc., 1957.

22. The Prevention of "Rhesus" Babies

PREVENTION OF RHESUS ISO-IMMUNISATION. C. A. Clarke in *The Lancet*, Vol. 2 for 1968, No. 7558, pages 1–7; July 6, 1968.

PREVENTION OF RH-HAEMOLYTIC DISEASE. C. A. Clarke in *British Medical Journal*, Vol. 4, No. 5570, pages 7–12; October 7, 1967.

THE PREVENTION OF RH HAEMOLYTIC DISEASE. R. B. McConnell in *Annual Review of Medicine*, Vol. 17, pages 291–306; 1966.

PROPHYLAXIS OF RHESUS ISO-IMMUNIZATION. C. A. Clarke in *British Medical Bulletin*, Vol. 24, No. 1, pages 3–9; January, 1968.

SUCCESSFUL PREVENTION OF EXPERIMENTAL RH SENSITIZATION IN MAN WITH AN ANTI-RH GAMMA$_2$-GLOBULIN ANTIBODY PREPARATION: A PRELIMINARY REPORT. Vincent J. Freda, John G. Gorman and William Pollack in *Transfusion*, Vol. 4, No. 1, pages 26–32; January–February, 1964.

TRANSFUSION, Vol. 8, No. 3. May–June, 1968.

VIII IMMUNITY AND INFECTIOUS DISEASE

23. Vaccines for Poliomyelitis

STUDIES IN HUMAN SUBJECTS ON ACTIVE IMMUNIZATION AGAINST POLIOMYELITIS. Jonas E. Salk and others in *The Journal of the American Medical Association*, Vol. 151, No. 13, pages 1081–1098; March 28, 1953; and *American Journal of Public Health*, Vol. 44, No. 8, pages 994–1009; August, 1954.

24. Rheumatic Fever

THE HEMOLYTIC STREPTOCOCCI. Maclyn McCarty in *Bacterial and Mycotic Infection of Man*, edited by René J. Dubos and James G. Hirsch. J. B. Lippincott Co., 1965.

RHEUMATIC FEVER. Maclyn McCarty in *Cecil-Loeb Textbook of Medicine*, edited by Paul B. Beeson and Walsh McDermott. W. B. Saunders Company, 1963.

RHEUMATIC FEVER: DIAGNOSIS, MANAGEMENT AND PREVENTION. Milton Markowitz and Ann G. Kuttner. W. B. Saunders Co., 1965.

THE STREPTOCOCCUS, RHEUMATIC FEVER AND GLOMERULONEPHRITIS. Edited by Jonathan W. Uhr. The Williams & Wilkins Co., 1964.

25. How the Immune Response to a Virus Can Cause Disease

DESTRUCTION OF VIRUS-INFECTED CELLS BY IMMUNOLOGICAL MECHANISMS. David D. Porter in *Annual Review of Microbiology*, Vol. 25, pages 283–290; 1971.

EFFECTS OF VIRUS INFECTIONS ON THE FUNCTION OF THE IMMUNE SYSTEM. Abner Louis Notkins, Stephan E. Mergenhagen and Richard J. Howard in *Annual Review of Microbiology*, Vol. 24, pages 525–538; 1970.

IMMUNE COMPLEX DISEASE IN CHRONIC VIRAL INFECTIONS. Michael B. A. Oldstone and Frank J. Dixon in *The Journal of Experimental Medicine*, Vol. 134, No. 3, Part 2, pages 32S–40S; September, 1971.

IMMUNOPATHOGENESIS OF ACUTE CENTRAL NERVOUS SYSTEM DISEASE PRODUCED BY LYMPHOCYTIC CHORIOMENINGITIS VIRUS. Donald H. Gilden, Gerald A. Cole, Andrew A. Monjan and Neal Nathanson in *The Journal of Experimental Medicine*, Vol. 135, No. 4, pages 860–869; April, 1972.

INFECTIOUS VIRUS-ANTIBODY COMPLEXES: INTERACTION WITH ANTI-IMMUNOGLOBULINS, COMPLEMENT, AND RHEUMATOID FACTOR. Abner Louis Notkins in

The Journal of Experimental Medicine, Vol. 134, No. 3, Part 2, pages 41S–51S; September, 1971.

Das Leben und Wirken des Wiener Klinikers Clemens Freiherrn v. Pirquet. Dissertation. E. Hoff. Verlag G. H. Nolte, 1937.

26. Tetanus

The Fixation of Tetanus Toxin by Ganglioside. W. E. van Heyningen and Pauline Allan Miller in *The Journal of General Microbiology*, Vol. 24, No. 1, pages 107–119; January, 1961.

The Neurotoxins of Clostridium botulinum and Clostridium tetani. G. Payling Wright in *Pharmacological Reviews*, Vol. 7, No. 4, pages 413–465; December, 1955.

Principles of Tetanus. Proceedings of the International Conference on Tetanus, Bern, July 15–19, 1966. Edited by Leo Eckmann. Hans Huber Publishers, 1967.

Tentative Identification of the Tetanus Toxin Receptor in Nervous Tissue. W. E. van Heyningen in *The Journal of General Microbiology*, Vol. 20, No. 2, pages 310–320; April, 1959.

27. The Immune Response to Measles

Conference on Measles Virus and Subacute Sclerosing Panencephalitis. Edited by J. L. Sever and W. Zeman, in *Neurology*, Vol. 18, No. 1, Part 2, pages 1–192; January, 1968.

Isolation of Measles Virus at Autopsy in Cases of Giant-cell Pneumonia without Rash. J. F. Enders, K. McCarthy, A. Mitus, and W. J. Cheatham in *New England Journal of Medicine*, Vol. 261, No. 18, pages 875–881; October 29, 1959.

Measles as an Index of Immunological Function. F. M. Burnet in *The Lancet*, Vol. 2, pages 610–613; September 14, 1968.

IX AUTOIMMUNITY

28. The Nature of Autoimmune Disease

Clinical Aspects of Immunology. Edited by P. G. H. Gell and R. R. A. Coombs. Blackwell Scientific Publications, Ltd., 1968.

The Immunology and Pathology of NZB Mice. J. B. Howie and B. J. Helyer in *Advances in Immunology*, Vol. 9, pages 215–266. Edited by F. J. Dixon and H. G. Kunkel, Academic Press, Inc., 1968.

Present Concepts in the Aetiology of Thyrotoxicosis. D. D. Adams in *Quarterly Journal of Surgical Sciences*, Vol. 7, No. 4, pages 179–187; December, 1971.

Structural Aspects of Human Erythrocyte Autoantibodies. I. L Chain Types and Electrophoretic Dispersion. J. P. Leddy and R. F. Bakemeier in *Journal of Experimental Medicine*, Vol. 121, pages 1–17; January, 1965.

Systemic Lupus Erythematosus. National Institutes of Health Conference. *Annals of Internal Medicine*, Vol. 82, No. 3, pages 391–404; March, 1975.

INDEX

Del Villano, Bert, 112
Dempster, W. J., 183, 187
Dengue fever, 236
Deoxyribonucleic acid (DNA).
  antibody, 23, 27, 28, 30, 47, 68,
    70, 71
  antibody against, 257
  antigen and, 186, 235
  antigen-antibody complex and, 258
  cell function and, 103
  enzyme action and, 227
  immune response and, 107, 109
  immunosuppressive drug and, 174
  polymerase, error-prone, 8
  RNA and, 110
  thymus and, 88, 90, 94, 95
  transplantation markers and, 208
Desensitization, antigen, 83
Diabetic, 15–16
Di George, Angelo M., 61
Di George's syndrome, 61, 172–174
Diphtheria, 154, 155, 245, 248
Disease
  immune complex, 232–241
  immune system and, 12, 20, 21, 55,
    100, 103, 109, 110, 112, 116
Dixon, Frank J., 116, 201, 236, 238
Donath-Landsteiner hemoglobinuria,
  254
Donnan effect, 149
Donohoe, W. T. A., 216
Donor
  anti-Rh, 215–218
  host, 202, 204–205, 209–210
  transplant and, 187, 190, 192
Dourmashkin, Robert R., 150, 153
Dresser, David W., 53, 116
Dreyer, William J., 69
Drinker, Cecil K., 124, 126
Drug, immunosuppressive, 174–175,
  250, 251
Dumont, Allan E., 133
Dutton, Richard W., 55
Duve, Christian de, 121

Eccles, Sir John, 247
Edelman, Gerald M., 29, 36, 52
Edema, 124
Edidin, Michael A., 206
Edman, P., 46
Eeckhout, Yves, 140
Egg albumin allergy, 83, 85
Ehrlich, Paul, 4, 12, 105, 114
Eichwald, E. J., 185
Eigen-behavior, immune system, 56
Elephantiasis, 132
Embryo
  antigen, 241
  cell mutability of, 15, 18–19
  immune system, 6, 61–63
Enders, John, 252
Endocarditis, 225
Enzyme, 8, 9, 32, 33, 34, 207
  circulation of, 131
  clonal selection theory and, 21
  function, 227
  linked, 120, 143–155
  lysosome, 134–142
  properdin system, 148–150, 154, 155

protein chains and, 37, 38
synthesis, 107
See also Complement system
Ephrussi, Boris, 103
Epitope, 49, 52–53, 55, 56–57, 76
  See also Antigenic determinant
Epstein-Barr virus, 76, 176, 250
Ermengem, Emile van, 245
Error-prone DNA polymerase, 8
Erythrogenic toxin, scarlet fever
  and, 227
Escherichia coli, 47, 121–122
Evolution
  antibody binding site, 45, 46
  lymphatic system, 123, 126

Faber, Knud, 245
Fabricius ab Aquapendente,
  Hieronymus, 60
Fagraeus, Astrid, 22
Fahey, John L., 106
Farber, Paul, 235
Feedback mechanism, antibody, 67
Feldman, Joseph, 105
Fell, Honor B., 142
Fernandas, Mario, 235
Ferrone, Soldano, 206, 209
Fertilization, lysosome enzyme
  and, 140
Fetus, Rh factor and, 212–218
Fibrinogen, 130
  See also Plasma, protein
Filtration mechanism, 126–130
Finn, Ronald, 215
Flagella, 22, 117
Florey, Sir Howard, 131
Fluid exchange, circulatory systems,
  127–128
Ford, E. C., 61
Frank, Michael, 155
Freda, Vincent J., 216
Friedman, Herman, 241
Fudenberg, H. Hugh, 69
Furth, Jacob, 61

Gally, Joseph A., 36, 42
Gamma globulin, 12, 26, 29, 36, 145
  agammaglobulinemia, 168–171
  anti-Rh, 216
Garrod, Sir Archibald, 202
Gell, Philipp G. H., 52
Gene
  antibodies and, 8, 29, 30
  coding by, 38
  cross-over, 213
  expression of, 202–204
  histocompatibility antigen, 196–198
  immunoglobulin and, 64–66, 67, 69
  mutation, 44–45, 46–47
Gene pool, 70, 202, 209
Genetic code
  antibody and, 46, 54, 56, 66, 67, 69
Genetic recombination, 38, 44–45, 47,
  54, 70
Genetics
  anomalies of, 255
  antibody and, 6, 8, 15, 18, 21, 35
  complement protein deficiency,
    154–155

histocompatibility antigen, 195–196
immune system and, 70, 71, 158–159
immunodeficiency and, 170, 171,
  172–176
immunological tolerance and,
  114–115
lymphatic system and, 108, 132
mimicry, 212–213
Rh factor, 212–218
Genetic variability, 202, 211
Genome, viral, 110, 112
Germuth, Frederick G., Jr., 236
Gilden, Donald H., 232
Glenny, W. T., 248
Glick, Bruce, 6, 60
Globulin, 127–130. See also Plasma,
  protein
Glomerulonephritis, 236–237, 238, 240
Goldberg, Burton D., 149, 154
Gomori, George, 139
Good, Robert A., 60, 61, 69, 171, 241
Gorer, P. A., 180
Gorman, John G., 216
Gottlieb, Paul D., 47
Gowans, James L., 52, 65, 101,
  161, 205
Graft
  blood-group and, 182–183, 187, 190
  host cells and, 6, 16–17, 76, 77, 79,
    205–206, 209–210
  kidney, 187–193
  rejection, 81, 85, 187, 190, 203,
    204–205
  restored immunity, 61, 71
  thymus cells, 172, 173
  tolerance, 179
  virus and, 241
  See also Autograft; Homograft; Skin
    graft; Transplantation
Graft-versus-host, 6, 16–17, 76, 77, 79,
  205–206, 209–210
Granner, Daryl, 107
Graves' disease, 255–256, 257
Green, Howard, 107, 149
Green, N. Michael, 31, 34, 53, 54
Gross, Erhard, 42–43
Grubb, Rune, 46

Halsted, Scott B., 236
Hamster, homograft and, 194–201
Hapten. See Antigen
Harris, Henry, 107
Harrison, J. Hartwell, 190
Hashimoto's disease, 256
Heart, rheumatic fever and, 225, 228,
  229, 231
Hellström, Ingegerd, 115
Hellström, Karl E., 115
Hemolytic anemia, 92, 95
Hepatitis virus, 240
Herpes simplex virus (HSV), 175,
  235–236
Hers, H. G., 142
Herzenberg, Leonard A., 56
Heterograft, 194, 196, 199
High blood-pressure. See Hypertension
Hildemann, William H., 195
Hill, Robert L., 42, 46
Hilschmann, Norbert G. D., 42, 46